Memory Impairment and Occupation

Memory Impairment and Occupation

A Guide to Evaluation and Treatment

Jonathon O'Brien, SROT, PhD

Lecturer, Department of Occupational Therapy
University of Liverpool
Liverpool, UK

WILEY Blackwell

This edition first published 2024

© 2024 John Wiley & Sons Ltd

The right of Jonathon O'Brien to be identified as the author of this work has been asserted in accordance with law.

Registered Offices

John Wiley & Sons, Inc., 111 River Street, Hoboken, NJ 07030, USA

John Wiley & Sons Ltd, The Atrium, Southern Gate, Chichester, West Sussex, PO19 8SQ, UK

For details of our global editorial offices, customer services, and more information about Wiley products visit us at www.wiley.com.

Wiley also publishes its books in a variety of electronic formats and by print-on-demand. Some content that appears in standard print versions of this book may not be available in other formats.

Limit of Liability/Disclaimer of Warranty

The contents of this work are intended to further general scientific research, understanding, and discussion only and are not intended and should not be relied upon as recommending or promoting scientific method, diagnosis, or treatment by physicians for any particular patient. In view of ongoing research, equipment modifications, changes in governmental regulations, and the constant flow of information relating to the use of medicines, equipment, and devices, the reader is urged to review and evaluate the information provided in the package insert or instructions for each medicine, equipment, or device for, among other things, any changes in the instructions or indication of usage and for added warnings and precautions. While the publisher and authors have used their best efforts in preparing this work, they make no representations or warranties with respect to the accuracy or completeness of the contents of this work and specifically disclaim all warranties, including without limitation any implied warranties of merchantability or fitness for a particular purpose. No warranty may be created or extended by sales representatives, written sales materials or promotional statements for this work. This work is sold with the understanding that the publisher is not engaged in rendering professional services. The advice and strategies contained herein may not be suitable for your situation. You should consult with a specialist where appropriate. The fact that an organization, website, or product is referred to in this work as a citation and/or potential source of further information does not mean that the publisher and authors endorse the information or services the organization, website, or product may provide or recommendations it may make. Further, readers should be aware that websites listed in this work may have changed or disappeared between when this work was written and when it is read. Neither the publisher nor authors shall be liable for any loss of profit or any other commercial damages, including but not limited to special, incidental, consequential, or other damages.

Library of Congress Cataloging-in-Publication Data applied for

Paperback ISBN: 9781119708865

Cover Design: Wiley

Cover Images: © Stefano Madrigali/Getty Images; Yuji Sakai/Getty Images

Set in 11.5/13.5pt STIXTwoText by Straive, Pondicherry, India

Printed and bound by CPI Group (UK) Ltd, Croydon, CR0 4YY

C9781119708865_191223

Contents

Preface

When I think about my reasons for writing this book, a number of memories seem to pop up spontaneously. Some are professional, some personal.

First, a young man who had a traumatic brain injury as a result of tripping up on a night out. He worked in an office. I took him to the treatment room and showed him the old computer we had there. When I asked him if he knew what it was, he indicated he did not. When I asked him if he could use it, he began typing his name without a problem. I now recognise that this was probably a case of visual agnosia accompanied by intact procedural memory.

Second, a man with global aphasia following a stroke. His mental capacity to make a decision about returning home, as he and his family wished, was being questioned by the multidisciplinary team. I went on annual leave and, for some reason, a medical doctor sent him for assessment to a private neuropsychologist. On my return from leave, I was accosted by his daughters demanding to know why their dad was being sent to a 'nursing home'. Why indeed?

It seems that he had been tested with a battery of language-based standardised assessments. Being aphasic, he had scored very poorly, and this was taken as evidence of profound cognitive impairment. However, I had been conducting repeated kitchen assessments with this man. I had evidence, therefore, that he was making fewer errors each day when preparing a complex hot meal. Using this evidence, I was able to make the case that he could indeed perform activities of daily living, with a bit of support. Eventually, with the supervision of his daughters, he was able to return to his own home after all.

This taught me the importance, and, in this case, superiority, of the occupational therapist's task-based approach to assessment and treatment. However, the therapist needs the theoretical background so that they can recognise and label what they are observing. One aim of this book is to provide that background.

Now for the personal memories. I was able to interview my grandmother about her life prior to her death in 1998. One of her most startling memories was of the unemployment riots in our home town, Birkenhead, in 1932. Her recall was precise and emotive. However, her subsequent memories were vague. Major events, such as the Second World War and the foundation of the National Health Service, were brushed over in a few words.

Why the contrast? I am not sure I can explain this exactly, but I now have words to describe it. The memories of the riots were episodic memories, while those vaguer statements belong to semantic memory.

Another personal note. While studying occupational therapy, also in 1998, a friend, who was later the best man at my wedding, almost surreptitiously passed me a copy of *The Making of Memory: From Molecules to Mind* by Steven Rose. I was gripped by Professor Rose's descriptions of the memory feats of the ancients, long-term potentiation and, of course, neural plasticity. In my memory I read the entire book in one sitting, although, as we will see, episodic memory is vulnerable.

The Making of Memory inspired my subsequent occupational therapy career. I have since had a chance to thank Professor Rose. His somewhat old-world academic courtesy and encouragement when he learned I was writing my own book on memory have stayed with me.

This book was started in January 2020, three months before Britain was locked down. My autobiographical memories of the time involve novel concepts such as 'home schooling' and 'online learning'. Also, on a roasting hot day in the depths of the first lockdown, our second child was born.

The media at that time were full of stories of people reassessing their lives and doing new things. I felt irritated back then, when simply keeping on top of work and family life seemed like the most we could do. Looking back, though, I suppose this book is what *I* did. The reader will judge how successful I have been.

Dedicated to Catalina, Emma and Daniel.

Acknowledgements

I would like to thank Dr Bethan Collins for first suggesting that my ideas could be turned into a book. Also, thank you to the anonymous reviewers of the original book proposal: their suggestions were very useful. My editors at Wiley-Blackwell, Anne Hunt and Christabel Daniel Raj, gave encouragement throughout; they also knew when to, tactfully, apply some pressure so that deadlines were met. Especial thanks to Dr Sally Osborn, whose superbly efficient copyediting and personal engagement with the content have contributed greatly to the final text. Associate Professor Melissa Nott and Dr Mark Morgan-Brown provided generous feedback on my descriptions of their respective research programmes, which I hope I have represented accurately. Colleagues at the University of Liverpool have been consistent in their support. In particular, Mrs Vikki Barnes-Brown and Dean of School of Health Sciences Professor Denise Prescott arranged for me to take some valuable study leave towards the end of the writing process. Finally, thank you to the patients, families, occupational therapists and occupational therapy students who have provided inspiration and ideas over the years.

1 Concepts of Memory

The chapter opens by defining learning and memory. Their neurophysiological basis is explained. A strong emphasis is placed on the role played by modification of the synapse, the point of communication between neurons. It is shown how this process of modification underpins neural plasticity and may facilitate learning and memory.

There is a brief overview of the history of memory theory. It is shown, in particular, that the work of some early theorists in this field, such as James and Bartlett, fits well with some occupational therapy concepts. There is also a discussion of the 'cognitive revolution' that took place in psychology in the United States in the 1950s. Some practical applications of the 'information processing' turn that this involved are explained.

The chapter also contains a detailed description of the case of Henry Molaison. This is justified by the far-reaching implications of these findings for learning and memory theory. Following from this, space is devoted to a detailed discussion of the 'hippocampal memory system'.

Some leading theorists have developed models of memory. The chapter includes a detailed discussion of Tulving's hierarchal model of procedural, semantic and episodic memory. In addition, there is consideration of the 'multicomponent working memory' model, which is particularly associated with the work of Baddeley. Also, there is discussion of the concept of prospective memory and reflection on the work of Luria and Vygotsky on the socio-historical origins of cognitive processes.

Defining Learning and Memory

The learning process allows the acquisition of novel information (Gazzaniga et al. 1998, 2009). Memory is the persistence of this learned content in a condition in which it can be retrieved in the future (Gazzaniga et al. 1998, 2009; Schacter and Wagner 2013). This linkage means that scientific accounts have often discussed learning and memory in combination (Tulving and Madigan 1970; Gazzaniga et al. 2009).

Memory's role in occupation has been explored by occupational therapy theorists including Hagedorn (2000, p. 31), who defined it as a 'skill component' of performance, and Radomski (2002, p. 198), for whom it was a 'primary

Memory Impairment and Occupation: A Guide to Evaluation and Treatment, First Edition.
Jonathon O'Brien.
© 2024 John Wiley & Sons Ltd. Published 2024 by John Wiley & Sons Ltd.

cognitive capacity' underpinning 'higher level thinking abilities'. Kielhofner (2008, p. 18), meanwhile, described memory as an aspect of cognition that could support 'performance capacity'. For all these authors memory, then, is fundamental to effective occupational performance.

For Kandel et al. (2000), learning and memory are the supreme processes through which the environment influences our behaviour. So, learning and memory formation imply a *change* in the organism at some level and this requires both stable body structures and the capacity to modify these in response to experience (Kielhofner 1995; Rose 1992). The persistent stability of the organism is called 'specificity'; the ability to change, 'plasticity' (Rose 1992, p. 137).

These themes of change and stability have also been discussed by occupational therapy theorists. Kielhofner (1995, p. 10), for example, drew on 'general, dynamical and open systems theories' in his examination of human occupation. A system is made up of components that function in concert for a specified purpose: an 'open system' constantly changes and organises itself as it interacts with its environment, while 'dynamical systems' describe the process by which a novel order emerges following an epoch of flux (Kielhofner 1995, p. 9). In the following section, these themes are explored in relation to learning and memory from within a 'physiological frame of reference' (Hagedorn 1992).

Neurophysiological Mechanisms of Learning and Memory

In order to understand the 'organic substrate' (Trombly 2002, p. 7) that allows the changes brought about through learning to take place while maintaining the continuity of the organism, it is first important to grasp that communication within the nervous system requires the transfer of information between neurons (Bear et al. 2016). Neurons are nerve cells that possess electrical excitability and underpin functions such as learning and memory (Tortora and Derrickson 2011). Communication between neurons occurs at sites called synapses, where a presynaptic neuron signals to a postsynaptic neuron; typically, the 'presynaptic element' is the terminal ending of an axon, while the postsynaptic component is a dendrite on the postsynaptic neuron (Bear et al. 2016). This communication is discussed in more detail later in the chapter.

In most synapses, the presynaptic and postsynaptic neuronal membranes are separated by a microscopic gap, the synaptic cleft (Bear et al. 2016). The presynaptic axon terminal houses 100–200 microscopic spheres named 'synaptic vesicles' that contain chemicals called neurotransmitters, the medium of communication between the neurons (Bear et al. 2016; Siegelbaum and Kandel 2013). Vesicles release their neurotransmitter into the synaptic cleft in response to an electrical signal called an action potential, or nerve impulse, travelling to the axon terminal of the presynaptic neuron (Bear et al. 2016; Siegelbaum and Kandel 2013; Tortora and Derrickson 2011). The neurotransmitters bind to receptor sites on the postsynaptic neuron; these sites are normally closed, but they open when particular neurotransmitters cleave to them

(Bear et al. 2016). The synaptic cleft, then, is the region of communication between the pre- and postsynaptic neurons.

The receptor sites are located on channels in the postsynaptic cell membrane. When neurotransmitters bind to these sites, the channels open. The channels are specialised to permit only certain ions to enter or exit the cell (Bear et al. 2016; Tortora and Derrickson 2011). Ions are atoms or molecules with an electrical charge, conventionally labelled as either 'positive' or 'negative', meaning that they can cause a force of attraction or repulsion when close to another ion. The movement of these ions creates a current across the cell membrane, with implications that are explained later.

The ions that cross the postsynaptic membrane enter from the extracellular fluid and cause changes in the *voltage* of the membrane of the postsynaptic neuron (Bear et al. 2016; Tortora and Derrickson 2011). Voltage is a measure of the difference in electrical energy between two locations, in this case between the outer membrane and inner membrane of the neuron. The difference is created as a result of the varying amounts of negatively and positively charged ions on either side of the membrane. This difference results in a *membrane potential*, typically of -70 mV, a value indicating that the inner membrane of the neuron is negatively charged when compared with the outer membrane (Gazzaniga et al. 2009). As already stated, the neuron is electrically excitable, meaning that the membrane potential can change as a result of a stimulus, so this value is named the *resting* membrane potential (Martini 2018). The resting membrane potential, then, can change as result of ions entering the neuron.

Sodium ions have a positive charge, so if sodium ion channels open and these ions enter the postsynaptic cell, they cause an increase of positive charge in the region around the cell's inner membrane (Tortora and Derrickson 2011). This leads to a reduction in the negativity of the membrane potential, a phenomenon labelled *depolarization* (Siegelbaum and Kandel 2013; Bear et al. 2016). If potassium ion channels open, leading to an outflow of these positively charged ions, this leads to a rise in negative charge at the inner cell membrane, resulting in an increase in the negativity of the membrane potential, a phenomenon labelled *hyperpolarisation* (Tortora and Derrickson 2011). The opening of chloride channels will lead to an inflow of these negatively charged ions, also leading to hyperpolarisation (Tortora and Derrickson 2011).

These variations in the membrane potential make it more or less likely that an action potential, also called a nerve impulse, will be generated. The action potential is an electrical signal that conducts along the axon of the neuron without losing strength, a process called propagation (Tortora and Derrickson 2011). As already shown, once the action potential reaches the axon terminal it causes neurotransmitter to be released into the synaptic cleft, so that interneuronal communication can occur. If hyperpolarisation occurs in the postsynaptic neuron, this results in an *inhibitory postsynaptic potential*, meaning that an action potential will not be generated (Siegelbaum and Kandel 2013; Bear et al. 2016). However, when *depolarisation* occurs in the postsynaptic neuron, there will be an *excitatory postsynaptic potential* (Siegelbaum and Kandel 2013; Bear et al. 2016). If the excitatory postsynaptic potential results in a change in the membrane potential to a threshold value of -55 mV, then an action potential will be generated (Tortora and Derrickson 2011).

Long-Term Potentiation

Since the nineteenth century, researchers have suggested that the process of learning and formation of memories is underpinned by modification of the synapse (Rose 1992; DeFelipe 2006). This concept was given a clear formulation by Hebb (1949), who proposed that, if a presynaptic neuron repeatedly partook in activating a postsynaptic cell, then its ability to activate that cell would increase; he commented that 'this changed facilitation . . . constitutes learning' (Hebb 1949, p. 65). Hebb's (1949) postulate, therefore, was that learning involved the strengthening of the connection between synapses, and this required simultaneous activity at the pre- and postsynaptic neurons (Lamprecht and LeDoux 2004).

Neurophysiological evidence that provided support for Hebb's postulate was first described in detail by Bliss and Lømo (1973; Bliss and Collingridge 1993). These researchers had noticed that electrical stimulation in one part of the rabbit hippocampus (a brain region that is known to be involved in learning and memory and that will be discussed further later in the chapter) led to an increase in electrical activity in neurons in another hippocampal region that had not been directly stimulated (Bliss and Lømo 1973). The depolarisation of these latter cells lasted for up to 10 hours, a phenomenon they labelled 'long lasting potentiation' (Bliss and Lømo 1973, p. 339).

The phenomenon described by Bliss and Lømo (1973) is now called 'long-term potentiation' (LTP). LTP has been reproduced in many laboratory studies and has been found to be a feature of synaptic excitation throughout the cerebral cortex (Malenka 2003). LTP has been identified in the neocortex, the amygdala, the cerebellum and the neostriatal region of the basal nuclei (Bauer et al. 2007).

It is known that LTP occurs when neurotransmitter released from a presynaptic neuron activates a specific receptor on the postsynaptic neuron called the AMPA receptor, causing inflow of sodium ions and depolarisation at the postsynaptic membrane (Lamprecht and LeDoux 2004). Another receptor in the postsynaptic membrane, the NMDA receptor, is then opened up as a result of the depolarisation, leading to an inflow of positively charged calcium and sodium ions, an event that is believed to facilitate plasticity, in Hebb's sense of increased effectiveness of activation between the pre- and postsynaptic neurons (Eichenbaum 2012; Lamprecht and LeDoux 2004).

The finding that synaptic plasticity requires both presynaptic release of neurotransmitter *and* depolarisation of the postsynaptic membrane has been seen as a confirmation of Hebb's postulate (Bliss and Collingridge 1993; Lamprecht and LeDoux 2004). Furthermore, plasticity has been noted at the level of the structure of the synapse following LTP, as spines, extensions of the dendrites that function to increase the available surface area for inputs from presynaptic cells, have been found to increase in number and also change their shape during LTP (Lamprecht and LeDoux 2004). This suggests a strengthening of the synapse, as predicted by Hebb. Baddeley (2015a) suggests that LTP may facilitate consolidation of the memory trace following initial encoding.

LTP is only observed following electrical stimulation of presynaptic cells in laboratory conditions; however, similar changes have been noticed in animals' brains following learning, and researchers have found that blocking the NMDA receptor leads to impaired spatial learning in rats (Eichenbaum 2012; Lamprecht and LeDoux 2004). Overall, LTP is felt by many researchers to be a 'universal plasticity mechanism' that provides a model of the neural events that occur following learning and memory formation and that aligns with Hebb's postulate (Eichenbaum 2012, p. 62).

Occupation and Neural Plasticity

For occupational therapists it is crucial to grasp that plasticity is influenced by experience, so what we *do* shapes brain structure. Development is distinguished by 'sensitive periods', in which plasticity is more likely to occur, and 'critical periods', in which deprivation of occupational opportunities impedes neural plasticity with potentially irreversible results (Sanes and Jessell 2013, p. 1260). Evidence for this comes from a study by Eluvathingal et al. (2006), who conducted magnetic resonance imaging (MRI) scans of seven children, with an average age of 9.7 years, who had been raised from birth in Romanian orphanages during the Ceausescu period, where they had been socially and emotionally deprived (Gluck et al. 2008), and who had subsequently been adopted by families in the United States. The control group consisted of seven 'normal' children, with an age of 10.7 years (Eluvathingal et al. 2006). The images were processed using diffusion tensor imaging (DTI), which allows visualisation of white matter tracts in the brain (Eluvathingal et al. 2006). It was found that the left uncinate fasciculus, a tract connecting the anterior temporal and frontal lobes of the brain, had significantly lower fractional anisotropy values for the adopted children, indicating structural deficiencies in the tract. The authors comment that abnormalities in this structure have also been noted in people with schizophrenia, where they have been linked to impaired verbal, episodic and declarative memory (Eluvathingal et al. 2006). This is evidence of how occupational deprivation may affect brain development.

Striking evidence for the way in which occupation influences neural plasticity was also provided by Maguire et al. (2000). These authors scanned the brains of 16 licensed London cab drivers. This occupational group has specific skills: in order to gain their licence, drivers must learn the location of 25 000 streets, training that takes two years (Maguire et al. 2000, 2006). Maguire et al. (2000) compared the scans with those from a control group of non-taxi drivers and found that the taxi drivers had a significantly larger mass of grey matter, the segment of the brain consisting of neuron cell bodies (Tortora and Derrickson 2011), in the posterior hippocampus on both sides (Maguire et al. 2000). In addition, they found that the number of years driving a taxi was positively correlated with the volume of grey matter in the right posterior hippocampus (Maguire et al. 2000). Subsequent research compared taxi drivers with a group of London bus drivers who drove fixed routes that did not require the navigational skills of cab drivers (Maguire et al. 2006). In this study, the authors found a greater volume of grey matter in the right and left mid-posterior regions of the hippocampus in the taxi drivers (Maguire et al. 2006). They interpreted their results as evidence supporting experience-dependent plasticity (Maguire et al. 2000, 2006). These findings suggest that productivity occupations can shape brain structure.

Historical Theories of Memory

Associationism and Occupation

Aristotle, writing in the fourth century BCE, argued that learning and memory occur as a result of the 'association' of items (Gluck et al. 2008, p. 4). For example, if trying to remember the word 'Autumn', one 'might pass swiftly in thought from one point to another, e.g. from milk to white, from white to mist, and thence to moist, from which one remembers Autumn (the season of mists)' (Aristotle and McKeon, 1941, p. 614). He also believed that we may recollect things more quickly if we think about them 'frequently' or by thinking about things that are similar to those items we are trying to remember (Aristotle and McKeon, 1941, p. 614). This 'associationist' perspective has continued to be influential in memory theory (Tulving and Madigan 1970; Gluck et al. 2008, p. 10).

One person who developed associationism was William James (1890). First, he argued that an item could only be recognised as a memory once it was associated with other items from our past, otherwise it would appear as a kind of dream isolated from any context (James 1890). Second, this association of items with each other constituted the 'elementary law of habit in the nerve-centres' (James 1890, p. 1522). Thus, he stressed that both retaining and retrieving memories depended on the modification of neural pathways shaped by habit and that memory was the conscious aspect of this process; this novel proposal was not adopted by mainstream psychology until many years later (Gluck et al. 2008). Third, retention and retrieval benefited from increasing the number and elaborateness of the associates of the item, with each association giving the person an extra 'hook' to locate the item when trawling the memory (James 1890, p. 1536). Fourth, he argued that memory was strongest for those items linked to our preferred occupations; an athlete, for example, may retain vast knowledge of information linked to their sport, while retaining little of anything extraneous. This occupation-linked memory formed a 'concept-system' that associated otherwise isolated pieces of information together (James 1890, p. 1537).

In the nineteenth century the application of experimental methods to memory research was pioneered by Ebbinghaus, who used lists of nonsense words to test learning, retention and forgetting (Gluck et al. 2008; Schacter 2008). Meanwhile, Semon developed the notion of the 'engram', the fleeting or more long-lasting changes in the brain stemming from experience (Schacter 2008).

Schema Theory

Bartlett, working in Britain in the early twentieth century, referred to the earlier work of Head, who had suggested that conscious awareness of a change in posture was, unconsciously, related to earlier postures (Bartlett 1995). This amalgamation of previous postures, against which the incoming sensation of postural change is evaluated prior to consciousness awareness,

Bartlett (1995, p. 199) labelled a 'schema'. Bartlett (1995, p. 200) objected to the idea of the cortex as a 'storehouse' of impressions of the past, arguing that schemata were constantly active and developing. Applied to remembering in general, Bartlett argued that this meant that memory does not simply reproduce the past, but involves 'construction' on a schema (1995, p. 205). Construction may involve condensing and elaborating items from the past, or even inventing and adding material (Bartlett 1995). This ongoing reconstruction of schemata allows a complex organism to adapt to an ever-changing environment and, in Bartlett's (1995) view, is both the origin of and explanation for consciousness. The elements of the schema that are foregrounded depend less on *when* the experience occurred and more on the 'interests and ideals' that shape the 'attitude' of the person, so that schemata are organised according to 'vocation', or divisions of 'human knowledge', for example (Bartlett 1995, pp. 210, 211, 213). So, in this view, memory traces are not stored passively, but change as our own inclinations change, and are linked to our occupations.

Bartlett (1995) based his arguments on the results of a range of experimental work. In one study, people were shown images of faces of men in military caps. This was done during the First World War and, suggested Bartlett (1995), the memories of the images were influenced by his participants' attitudes. For example, a picture of a 'regular army type' was remembered after a delay as having a moustache, which was not actually in the image; Bartlett (1995, p. 54) suggested that the memory was actually shaped by imported details from cartoons of 'Tommy Atkins', the stereotypical British soldier, which were then popular. In addition, the image of a captain was remembered subsequently as being more angular and serious than was actually the case, and one person, on being shown the original picture once more, initially believed that the experimenter had made a switch (Bartlett 1995). These were examples of what Bartlett (1995, p. 44) called 'effort after meaning', where the person attempts to connect a stimulus with something else, in this case military stereotypes, and which he believed underpinned all human cognition.

In another experiment, participants were asked to read a folk story from North America, 'The War of the Ghosts'; they were then asked to recall the story after 15 minutes, 20 hours and sometimes after several years (Bartlett 1995). With time, Bartlett (1995) noted that the retelling became more concise, the language more modern, and more magical aspects of the tale were missed out. He also noted that when some men remembered the story they tended to foreground details concerning the anxiety of family members of absent warriors; he points out, once more, that these men were tested at the time of the war and their remembering may therefore have been influenced by their own attitudes concerning actual or immanent military service (Bartlett 1995). Bartlett (1995, p. 52) insisted on the adaptive nature of constructive remembering, commenting that in everyday life 'meticulous accuracy of detail' in memory was of little importance. If this view is correct, then it perhaps calls into question the real-world applicability of the standardised cognitive screening tests often used by occupational therapists. Overall, Bartlett's experimental work provides evidence of the ways in which occupation, and awareness of occupational roles, may contribute to the construction of memory.

Information Processing Approaches

Prior to the 1950s, psychology in the United States was dominated by 'behaviourism', an approach premised on the idea that only externally observable behaviours could be meaningfully studied (Miller 2003). In this view, the mental processes underpinning memory, for example, could not be measured, and only learning, which could be observed and controlled, was appropriate for research (Miller 2003). It is important to state that different approaches prevailed in other parts of the world, for instance Bartlett's (1995) research in Britain, described earlier, and Luria's work focusing on the neural process underpinning the mind in the Soviet Union (Luria 1966; Miller 2003). However, Tulving (1983) argues that the decline in memory research throughout much of the twentieth century, despite the early work of Ebbinghaus, Semon and James, resulted from the dominance of the behaviourist approach.

The situation changed in 1956, largely as a result of presentations from researchers in computer science, linguistics and experimental psychology at an interdisciplinary symposium at the Massachusetts Institute of Technology (Miller 2003). In particular, the presentation by Noam Chomsky on language is considered to have had a major impact (Miller 2003; Gazzaniga et al. 2009). The symposium contributed to the analysis of learning and memory as mental *information processing*, an approach that eventually fed into the emergence of cognitive science in the 1970s (Miller 2003). Miller (2003) has described cognitive science as an interdisciplinary field linking neuroscience, linguistics, anthropology, computer science, psychology and philosophy. One result of this 'cognitive revolution' seems to have been an increase in research on memory, as Melton (1963) noted a large increase in published experimental work from 1958 onwards.

A parallel development was the use of analogies from computer science. Melton (1963, pp. 7, 12), whose earlier experimental work had been sponsored by the US Army Electronics Command, for example, argued that memory theory should be seen as a subfield of learning theory that focused on 'storage and retrieval of memory traces' and he also used the term 'encoding'. These concepts have become part of the toolkit of cognitive neuroscientists, with the key stages of the information processing model of learning and memory being *encoding*, as the sensory stimuli are converted to neural representations; *storage*, as the representations are permanently cached for later extraction; and *retrieval*, when they are retrieved for use (Gazzaniga et al. 2009). Encoding is divided sometimes into two further steps: *acquisition*, where sensory inputs are temporarily stored and analysed; and *consolidation*, where these representations are fortified with time (Gazzaniga et al. 2009). Tulving (1983) argues that the application of these 'two principles' of encoding and retrieval led to a renaissance in memory research following the era of behaviourism.

One of the key contributions in this new area came in an article by Miller (1956) that explored constraints on learning and memory in relation to information processing. In this account, a communication system requires a connection between input and output. The degree of correlation between input and output is an index of the degree to which the output is related to the input and how much output is down to random variation, or 'noise', in the system (Miller 1956, p. 82). In experiments where a person was asked to make judgements on different stimuli, the individual was conceived of as an 'information channel' (Miller 1956). A unit of information was defined as the amount of information needed to halve the degree of uncertainty in a situation where there are two equally possible alternatives, meaning that the chances of accuracy are 50 : 50 (Miller 1956; Schmidt and Lee 2005). The unit of information was expressed as a binary digit or 'bit' (Miller 1956, p. 82; Schmidt and Lee 2005). One bit allows us to choose between two alternatives, two bits between four, three bits between eight and so on, meaning that each doubling of the number of choices requires one extra bit of information (Miller 1956). The upper boundary of the amount of information a person can process when asked to make judgements about stimuli, the point at which confusion starts to occur, is called 'channel capacity' (Miller 1956, p. 82).

Miller (1956) surveyed the results of a number of studies of discrimination over a range of modalities, including loudness levels, degree of curvature of visually presented lines and salt content of water when tasted, and estimated that the mean channel capacity was about 2.6 bits, meaning that the upper limit for categorisation was about 6.5 items. He suggested that these limits may be a function of the human nervous system or of learning processes (Miller 1956).

Miller's (1956) concepts have application to the work of occupational therapists, when recommending strategies for people with memory impairments. In a personal care task, for instance, the occupational therapist might recommend a carer to reduce the number of choices the person with dementia needs to make by laying out their clothes for them in advance, thus cutting the number of bits of information needed to complete the task. A simplified representation of this is shown in Table 1.1.

Table 1.1 gives examples of instructions that could be used in a dressing task. In line with Miller's (1956) theory, one bit is needed to choose between two alternatives and two bits are needed to choose between four alternatives. By decreasing the number of alternatives, the occupational therapist can reduce the amount of information, or bits, needed to carry out the task. Alternatively, the therapist could increase the number of bits needed by increasing the number of alternatives. This approach would allow the therapist to grade the task for a person with memory impairment, according to their capacity.

Another of Miller's concepts that has relevance for occupational therapists originated from his work on the 'span of immediate memory' (Miller 1956, p. 92). He argued that this was limited by the number of 'chunks of information' to be memorised, which seemed to be unaffected by the quantity of bits in each chunk. Miller (1956, p. 93) maintained that this independence resulted from

Table 1.1 Instructions in a personal care task in relation to bits of information required to respond correctly.

Statement	Number of bits required
'Put your shirt on'	0
'Put on your red shirt or your blue shirt'	1
'Put on your red shirt or your blue shirt or your white tee-shirt or your red tee-shirt'	2

'recoding', whereby the initial code, which had a large amount of information organised into a lot of chunks, was recoded so that there was a smaller number of chunks but more bits in each chunk. He argued that the easiest way to do this would be to recode the original inputs by labelling them with a name and remembering the name in place of the inputs (Miller 1956).

Miller (1956) suggested that humans were recoding information into chunks almost constantly in daily life and that this process underpinned the majority of mnemonic techniques and could actually be equivalent to memorisation itself. Melton (1963, p. 11) was later to describe Miller's concept of the chunk as 'the unit of measurement of human information-processing capacities'. Miller also suggested that verbal recoding was a reflection of the individual's life history, in that it depended on their particular inclinations and was actually the 'life-blood' of thought (Miller 1956, p. 95). In this sense, then, recoding is, in part, a function of our occupational history. In addition, occupational therapists can apply 'chunking' when adapting activities for people with memory impairment, for example by grouping the tasks required in preparation of a complex hot meal under the labels of 'preparation', 'cooking', 'serving' and 'safety'. This is illustrated in Table 1.2. In addition, the concept of chunking will be encountered in more detail again in Chapter 5.

Despite the use of analogies from computing, the information processing approach to learning and memory was *not* based on a model of the person as a non-conscious device. This has also been stressed by other authors. Occupational scientists, for example, have insisted that the human person responds to an environment that challenges them at various levels, including the 'symbolic-spiritual', via occupational engagement (Yerxa 2000, p. 197).

Table 1.2 Chunking the tasks required to make hot tea and beans on toast.

Chunk	Tasks
Preparation	Put bread in toaster
	Open can of beans
	Fill kettle with water
	Plug in toaster
	Put tea bags in teapot
	Take pan and plate out of cupboard
Cooking	Place beans in pan and switch on hob
	Pull lever down on toaster
	Switch kettle on to boil water
	Pour boiled water into teapot
Serving	Place toast on plate
	Pour beans onto toast
	Pour tea into cup and add milk
Safety	Do not put hand near lit hob
	Do not put fingers in toaster
	Turn off hob
	Unplug toaster

Luria (1973, p. 284), a pioneer of neuropsychology, also stressed that encoding was an *active* process whereby the person chooses the 'system' that would complete it, while recall of information was a 'complex and active' process involving selection of relevant items according to 'the purpose of the task' in hand. Similarly, as shown later, early work in the cognitive science tradition also provided evidence for the active nature of memory.

Levels of Memory Processing

Craik and Lockhart (1972) produced a critical view of contemporary memory research. They took issue with the contemporary 'multistore models', based on computer analogies, of memory that portrayed items as passing through a sensory (SS), short-term (STS) and long-term store (LTS) (Craik and Lockhart 1972, p. 671). SS was a transient store, which operated independently of whether the person was paying attention to the stimulus or not; STS required attention to the stimulus, had a limited capacity and stored information in a manner specific to the sensory modality of the stimulus, so that the storage format mirrored that of the input; and LTS was thought to have an unlimited storage capacity and items were stored related to meaning, in a 'semantic' format (Craik and Lockhart 1972, p. 672).

Craik and Lockhart (1972, p. 671) argued that some of the assumptions of these 'multistore models' could be questioned. STS, for example, had been shown to store semantic as well as modality-specific items. In addition, estimates of the rate of decay of items in STS varied widely, with research showing that a visual stimulus could persist for anywhere between 1 and 25 seconds. They also cited evidence that people could recognise non-verbal but relatively non-semantic items, such as faces and voices, over long periods, calling into question the nature of long-term storage. All this suggested that the demarcations of the multistore models could be questioned.

Craik and Lockhart (1972) proposed that research on encoding and retrieval should focus on the *level* of processing. Their concept was that a perceived stimulus moves through stages of processing, from basic sensory and physical features to association with prior learning, and recognition of patterns and semantics. In this view, greater depth of processing implies more cognitive and semantic analysis. Coding may also be 'elaborated', meaning that an item may be linked to images or other associations based on the person's experience (Craik and Lockhart 1972). Also, these authors redefined the 'memory trace' as resulting from perceptual analysis, while its longevity is a function of the depth of processing, such that deeper processing leads to longer retention (Craik and Lockhart 1972, p. 675). Furthermore, a cue to retrieve an item would be more effective if it matched the initial coding, meaning that the original 'learning context' could be restored (Craik and Lockhart 1972, p. 678). Craik and Lockhart's (1972) views point to a role for personal experience in shaping the encoding process, and align with the suggestions of occupational scientists that memory may act as a 'buffer' between genes and culture on one side, and behaviour on the other, and also that a person's interests and history of 'engagement in occupation' shape the development of their nervous system (Wilcock 2006; Yerxa 2000, p. 197).

A widely discussed early study focusing on encoding and retrieval was carried out by Craik and Tulving (1975). These authors suggested that their work was part of a 'new look in memory research', in that it focused on the 'mental operations' conducted on the stimulus by the person, rather than the properties of the stimulus; this focus resulted from a belief that differences in retention reflected different encoding strategies (Craik and Tulving 1975). They suggested that, just as perception can progress from basic awareness of sensation to high-level semantic processing, so material to be memorised could be analysed at different levels and retention was a function of the level of elaboration of the analysis. This meant that material processed only at the sensory level would be less well retained than material analysed with greater attention and elaborated with associations and images (Craik and Tulving 1975).

Craik and Tulving (1975) ran experiments in which participants were questioned about a word presented for encoding. Questions were asked about words at three different levels: structural (e.g. is it written in upper case?); phonemic (e.g. does it rhyme with 'crate'?); and semantic (e.g. is it an animal name? Would it fit in this sentence?). They were then shown the word for 200 milliseconds and asked to answer yes or no to the question. Following this, their retention of the words was tested, without warning, in conditions of 'free recall', where the person simply listed recalled words in any order; 'cued recall', where a fragment of the initial 'word event' was provided as a cue; or 'recognition', in which the initial words were viewed alongside 'distractors' that were not part of the original presentation (Craik and Tulving 1975, p. 272).

The results showed that semantic decisions took slightly longer than structural decisions (Craik and Tulving 1975). Taking processing time as an index of depth, Craik and Tulving (1975) argued that the longer processing time was a function of the depth of processing. Crucially, the words presented with semantic questions were recalled better than those presented with structural or phonemic questions, and the authors concluded that this manipulation of the level of processing had affected the strength of retention (Craik and Tulving 1975).

Craik and Tulving (1975) argued for the concept of 'spread', rather than depth, as a key determinant of retention. This suggests that the stimulus can be elaborated by structural, phonemic or semantic coding (Craik and Tulving 1975). Preservation of memory, then, depends on the quality of encoding, so that a basic analysis of semantics is more effective than a complex analysis of structure (Craik and Tulving 1975). 'Memory performance', in this view, is a function of how elaborate the encoding is and the 'memory trace' is, in fact, the history of the observer's cognitive analyses of the stimulus (Craik and Tulving 1975, p. 290).

Another important finding was that retention was improved when the coding question or context was congruous with the target word, so that the two form a single unit, and the authors suggested that this explained the higher retention of words that required a positive response in their experiments (Craik and Tulving 1975). In addition, Craik and Tulving (1975) argued that congruity meant that retrieval of only a part of the presented stimulus allowed more rapid access to the entire memory. Furthermore, they suggested that this 'unitising' of stimulus and context may involve coding the item in relation to the person's world knowledge, their 'semantic memory', meaning that when they encounter a cue they can draw on these structures and construct the primary coding once more (Craik and Tulving 1975, p. 291). This idea seems congruous with Bartlett's concept of 'effort after meaning' (1995, p. 44), described earlier.

For occupational therapists in clinical practice, these ideas can be applied when considering how instructions are presented to a service user, or a team member in training. For example, asking a patient with memory impairment to explain each of the steps involved in a kitchen activity prior to practice, rather than the therapist simply listing the different tasks, may facilitate deeper and more elaborate processing, aiding recall. For occupational therapists involved in education or training, encouraging the student or supervisee to work through problems on their own may have a similar impact. (The author has successfully applied these principles to the teaching of anatomy and physiology to year one undergraduate occupational therapy students.) Overall, the message is that more active engagement with the information facilitates better encoding and retrieval.

The Case of Henry Molaison

As well as the experimental work already discussed, important insights into learning and memory have come from clinical case studies. One historically significant case is discussed here, while another will be discussed in Chapter 3.

In 1953, a 27-year-old man, Henry Molaison from Hartford, Connecticut, in the United States, underwent brain surgery. His case, known as that of 'H.M.' until his death in 2008, was to become one of the most widely cited in the field of neuroscience, and was to open the contemporary era of memory investigation by providing the first evidence that memory could be separated from other perceptual and cognitive brain functions and also localised to specific brain regions (Corkin 2002, 2013; Squire 2009).

At the age of either 7 (Corkin 2002; Eichenbaum 2002, 2012; Squire 2009) or 9 years old (Scoville and Milner 1957; the confusion may result from inconsistencies in medical records and family accounts: Corkin 2013), Molaison had struck his head and lost consciousness after being knocked over by a bicycle, and a few years later he started experiencing mild epileptic seizures. Whether these resulted from the fall or from inherited genetic factors is not clear, but certainly by early adulthood the seizures had become frequent and severe, marked by 'urinary incontinence, tongue biting and loss of consciousness' leaving him 'unable to work' (Scoville and Milner 1957 p. 11; Eichenbaum 2002).

Although doctors could not identify a regional source of the epileptic discharges, evidence suggested that the medial temporal lobes were, often, the origin of such activity (Corkin 2013). Accordingly, a neurosurgeon, William Beecher Scoville, proposed bilateral removal of a brain region called the hippocampus, which is located in the floor of the medial temporal lobe (Scoville and Milner 1957). Molaison gave consent, and 5 cm of the medial temporal lobes, including the anterior hippocampi, anterior parahippocampal gyri encompassing the entorhinal, perirhinal and anterior parahippocampal cortices, and the amygdalae, were removed (Corkin 1968, 2013; Squire 2009). (Scoville (1968) stated that 8 cm of the lobe had been removed; however, subsequent neuroimaging showed that this was incorrect.) The amygdala, as part of the limbic system, is discussed in detail in Box 1.4 later in the chapter.

Following the operation, although the epileptic seizures subsided, he began to display marked memory impairments: he could no longer find his way around the ward, could not remember having eaten lunch half an hour earlier or people he had just met, and only seemed vaguely aware of having had surgery (Scoville and Milner 1957). He had developed comprehensive anterograde amnesia that persisted when researchers used different types of tests, with varied stimuli, from words to faces and public and personal episodes, and in every sensory domain (Corkin 2002).

The profundity of this amnesia is shown by Milner et al. (1968), who describe Molaison visiting his mother, who was his main carer, while she was in hospital, three times in one week. When tested, he had no memory of this, despite one visit having happened that morning. He did express a sense of unease that there may have been a problem with one of his parents, but by the next day he seemed to have forgotten this altogether and did not evidence any emotion in connection with the worry he had mentioned (Milner et al. 1968). Corkin (2013) commented that, in this situation, Molaison had forgotten the fact that his mother was in hospital, but seemed to retain the emotional salience, leading to his sense that something was wrong. In later life, he showed only vague awareness that his father had died. His mother eventually developed dementia and moved to a care setting and, in 1977, a researcher noted that Molaison carried a note in his wallet stating 'Dad's gone . . . Mum's in nursing home' (Corkin 2013, p. 205), to remind him of these important personal events.

Molaison likened his state to that of just waking from a dream (Milner et al. 1968). Milner et al. (1968) commented that it was as if he were approaching awareness of his circumstances but was unable to completely understand them, as he had no memory of what had happened previously. This temporal disorientation is illustrated by an exchange with a researcher in 1992: asked what he had done that morning, or what he had had for lunch, he could not answer; asked what he would do the next day, he replied 'whatever's beneficial' (Corkin 2013, p. xiii). The reader will be reminded of William James's (1890) speculation, explained earlier, about the dreamlike state that would result if one were unable to associate items with other memory traces.

Molaison's amnesia was predominantly anterograde; that is, it was for events occurring *after* his lobectomy. He did have some degree of retrograde amnesia for one to two years prior to surgery, but his memory for events prior to this was mainly intact (Milner et al. 1968). Once, for example, when directing researchers to his home, he guided them to the house he had lived in *before* the operation (Milner et al. 1968). He also knew his date of birth, but could not state his age, and remembered events from his first years in school and a job he had had in his 20s (Milner et al. 1968).

Molaison maintained good language abilities: he could work with complex sentences and was able to understand and make jokes (Corkin 2013; Milner et al. 1968). The intersection of vocabulary knowledge and amnesia was shown dramatically in an experiment involving 'word stem completion priming', where he was given a list of words to study, then shown a list of word stems that include both studied and non-studied words. Priming, a form of 'implicit' or 'non-declarative memory' in which learning takes place without conscious recollection, would be evidenced if he were able to complete the word stems of the studied words more rapidly (Gazzaniga et al. 2009, p. 338; Postle and Corkin 1998). Molaison was presented with a list of study words that had been introduced in US dictionaries only *after* 1965, several years subsequent to his surgery, such as 'jacuzzi' (Corkin 2002). He was then presented with a list of word stems to complete, but showed no evidence of a priming effect for the studied words (Postle and Corkin 1998).

The authors suggested that this was evidence that priming of word stem completion in people with amnesia, a form of *implicit* memory, must rely on 'modification' of a memory representation of the word from before the onset of amnesia, during the study stage of the test. Molaison's lack of memories for words introduced following his surgery meant that the priming effect was absent because there were no memories to modify (Postle and Corkin 1998, p. 433). In a following trial, Molaison was tested for priming using a study list of words appearing in the dictionary *prior to* his operation in 1953. Here, the word stem priming effect was present and was similar to that of non-amnesic control participants (Postle and Corkin 1998).

Despite this marked anterograde amnesia, some domains of memory appeared, remarkably, unimpaired. In one experiment, conducted when he was 40, he was required to maintain a stylus on a target on a rotating disc; in another he had to maintain a stylus bimanually on two tracks on a rotating drum, using both left and right hands together (Corkin 1968). Molaison was able to learn the tasks and showed significantly improved performance when tested over several days (Corkin 1968). At the age of 60, he learned to trace a star when the only visual guide was the view of his hand and the pattern being copied in a mirror (Gabrieli et al. 1993). He was able to achieve this, and the researchers found that he had retained this skill when tested one year later; this was despite him having hardly any recall of having learned the skill and failing to recognise the task even on the first day of practice (Gabrieli et al. 1993). In later life Molaison developed osteoporosis, suffered fractures and had a hip replacement. Despite having no memory of being in hospital or of having osteoporosis, he was still able to learn to use a walking frame (Corkin 2013). These discoveries showed that learning and maintenance of visual-motor abilities do not depend on the medial temporal lobes, which had been removed by the surgery (Corkin 2002).

The key findings from Molaison's case were, first, that the medial temporal lobe – that is, the hippocampus and surrounding regions, discussed in detail in Box 1.1 – is essential for converting immediate items into long-term memory (Squire 2009; Milner et al. 1968). Second, the fact that Molaison had good capacity for retaining information over a short period, for example when remembering digits or in conversation, until he stopped attending to the task, confirmed the distinction between immediate memory and long-term memory (Squire 2009). Squire (2009) points out that an associated finding was that immediate memory is not, primarily, based on the length of time that items can be retained, but on the storage capacity of the system and the ability of the person to attend to the information. The third finding was that memory is not unitary but made up of different systems, in this case 'declarative' memory, of which we are consciously aware, and 'procedural' memory, such as the visual-motor skills Molaison learned, of which we may not be aware

(Eichenbaum 2012; Squire 2009, p. 8). Fourth, because he was found to have intact memories from up to two years prior to surgery, it suggested that the medial temporal lobe region was not the site where such long-term information was stored (Squire 2009).

BOX 1.1   THE STRUCTURE AND FUNCTION OF THE HIPPOCAMPUS

The 'hippocampal memory system' is located within the medial temporal lobe of the cerebrum (Eichenbaum 2012, p. 236). It consists of the hippocampus, which is made up of the dentate gyrus, the subiculum and the horn of Ammon. The latter section is subdivided into four regions, CA1, CA2, CA3 and CA4 (CA stands for 'cornu ammonis', or 'horn of Ammon') (Eichenbaum 2012; Gazzaniga et al. 2009). It should be noted that there is some variation in the terminology that authors use, and the hippocampus is also described as consisting only of CA1–CA4, while the hippocampus, dentate and subiculum together are referred to as the 'hippocampal formation' (Amaral and Strick 2013, p. 349).

The parahippocampal region comprises the perirhinal cortex, the parahippocampal cortex and the entorhinal cortex (Bear et al. 2016; Eichenbaum 2012). The hippocampus and these linked cortical regions make up the floor of the lateral ventricle's temporal horn and are located within the ventromedial aspect of the temporal lobe (Gazzaniga et al. 2009; Amaral and Strick 2013).

The location of the hippocampus in the cerebrum is shown in Figure 1.1.

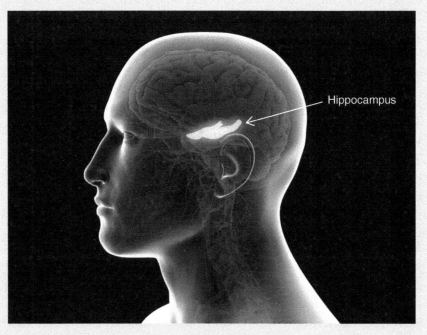

Figure 1.1 Location of the hippocampus in sagittal view of the brain.
Source: SciePro/Adobe Stock.

The parahippocampal region is involved with 'bidirectional' communication with neocortical areas and with the hippocampus (Eichenbaum 2012, p. 237). The various areas of the parahippocampal region receive information that has been highly processed by the different neocortical areas, ultimately by the cerebral association areas of the parietal, temporal and frontal lobes, meaning that only high-level representations based on 'visual, auditory, and somatic' information, rather than basic sensory inputs, are received (Kandel et al. 2000, p. 1231; Bear et al. 2016). These are transmitted to the hippocampus for further processing and then returned to the parahippocampal region, from where they are relayed back to the same neocortical regions they first came from (Eichenbaum 2012). The key function of these medial temporal lobe regions is to modify, reorganise and improve storage of information represented in the neocortex (Eichenbaum 2012).

The hippocampus is connected to subcortical brain regions, including the thalamus and hypothalamus, via a white matter bundle called the fornix, and to the neocortical areas by way of the parahippocampal region, mainly via the entorhinal cortex (Eichenbaum 2012). The entorhinal cortex projects to the dentate gyrus via an axon bundle called the perforant path (Kandel et al. 2000, p. 1231; Bear et al. 2016). The dentate gyrus then projects axons called mossy fibres to CA3, which in turn projects one branch of axons to the fornix and another branch, called the Schaffer collateral, to CA1 (Bear et al. 2016). The parahippocampal cortex and fornix are shown in Figure 1.3 later in the chapter.

The hippocampal 'return circuit' involves projections to subcortical regions via the fornix, and also projections from CA1 and the subiculum back to the parahippocampal region, particularly the entorhinal cortex. From there, projections from the entorhinal and perirhinal cortices relay the information back to the neocortical regions from which the signals first came (Eichenbaum 2012, p. 241). The principal theme here is that signalling from the neocortex affects the parahippocampal region and the hippocampus and the processing of the signals that takes place in these areas in turn influences the neocortex (Eichenbaum 2012).

As shown in the case of Henry Molaison, damage in the hippocampus impairs the ability to convert short-term memories in order to form new long-term memories (Amaral and Strick 2013). In addition, damage to CA1 is a feature of Alzheimer's disease, a key feature of which is memory impairment (Padurariu et al. 2012).

Taxonomies of Memory

Researchers have developed models of the human memory system, many of which are based on the work carried out with patients such as Henry Molaison (Corkin 2013; Eichenbaum 2012). Insights from these models can inform occupational therapists' practice with individuals with memory impairment. They are discussed in the following section.

Tulving's Hierarchy of Procedural, Semantic and Episodic Memory

Tulving (1985a, p. 386) conceived of memory as a 'complex' that could be subdivided into three 'memory systems' consisting of brain mechanisms and their associated cognitive skills and behaviours. The systems were organised hierarchically: 'higher' systems depended on a 'lower' system or systems, but also possessed specific capacities that the lower system did not (Tulving 1985a). Tulving (1985b) listed the systems, in order from lower to higher, as procedural, semantic and episodic memory. In Tulving's scheme, procedural memory underpins semantic, and semantic underpins episodic, so one can have procedural memory without semantic and episodic, and semantic without episodic, but not the other way round (Tulving 1985b). These memory systems are discussed in more detail next.

Procedural memory involves gaining, retaining and using skills of perception, movement and cognition (Tulving 1985a). It underpins the learning of appropriate responses to stimuli, which may be arranged in complex patterns and require chained responses (Tulving 1985a).

Acquiring procedural memory necessitates an observable behavioural response (Tulving 1985a). It does not require any memory of the context in which knowledge was acquired, but prescribes a pattern for action when the stimulus is encountered again (Tulving 1985a). This means that procedural memory can only be expressed through the performance of the learned response (Tulving 1985b).

Tulving (1985b, p. 3) also argued that procedural memory is accompanied by 'anoetic' consciousness, which does not require knowledge of anything beyond the stimulus. An example might be the skill of riding a bicycle. Here, the performance of the skill does not require us to remember the event of learning it, and does not necessitate any additional information about the world in order to perform it. In addition, procedural memory may support the motor and process skills identified by Kielhofner (1995), such as postural alignment, calibration of the necessary force or speed, or organisation of the tools and space needed to complete a task or activity.

Semantic memory encompasses information about the world that can be represented internally using symbols (Tulving 1985a). The information units of semantic memory may be 'facts', 'ideas', 'concepts', 'rules', 'propositions', 'schemata' and so on (Tulving 1983, p. 38). Although no specific behavioural response is required during semantic memory performance, the memory could potentially be expressed in a variety of ways, not necessarily aligned to the manner and circumstances in which it was acquired (Tulving 1985a).

Semantic memory is associated with 'noetic' or 'knowing' consciousness, which facilitates mental operations on items and events that are no longer present in the outside world (Tulving 1985b, p. 3). To return to the example of riding a bicycle, knowledge of the meaning of road signs, traffic lights and the different types of cycles would be part of semantic memory. We could, for instance, understand the messages of signs while on the road, which are conveyed visually, but we could also explain their meanings using words or drawing to another person in a room with no view of the signs. Semantic memory is also needed to complete daily living tasks, for example by providing the knowledge needed to recognise items such as a kettle or cooker.

Episodic memory, first proposed by Tulving in 1972, entails the recollection of events we have experienced ourselves (Tulving 1985b, 2002). This starts with a person 'witnessing or experiencing' an 'event or episode' and finishes when they subsequently remember it (Tulving 1983, p. 11). The episodic memory mode allows us to mentally travel back in time; its correlate is 'autonoetic' or 'self-knowing' consciousness, which imbues the act of remembering with the feeling that we did truly experience the event (Tulving 1985b, p. 1). Autonoetic consciousness gives the person an awareness of their identity and location in time as someone with a past and a future (Tulving 1985a).

Drawing on cycling once more, we may have a clear episodic memory of the first time that we rode a bike without stabilisers; this could involve memories of the person helping us, the location it occurred and our feelings as it happened. Autonoetic consciousness also involves 'subjective time', the capacity to be aware of our past, while also imagining ourselves in the future (Tulving 1985b; Hassabis and Maguire 2007). Thus, episodic memory and autonoetic consciousness allow an organism to act more decisively in the present and plan more efficiently for the future.

Occupational therapy authors have also highlighted the 'temporality' of the experience of human occupation (Kielhofner 1995, p. 3). Kielhofner (1995), for example, presented a rudimentary definition of human occupations as activities with cultural meaning that develop through time, imbuing human experience with the sense of past and future. Other occupational therapy theorists have used the concept of 'becoming' to show how humans change in time as they aspire to achievements that require engagement in occupation (Hitch et al. 2014). Law et al. (1996) also stressed the temporal nature of occupations as grouped actions undertaken repeatedly as part of a role, potentially throughout life, in order to meet inherent personal needs. Arguably, then, episodic memory and autonoetic consciousness would be involved in providing the sense of personal continuity that would allow occupations defined in these ways to be undertaken.

Episodic memory also has an affective element, which semantic memory does not; the mood of the person during the remembered experience is part of the trace of the memory and is also important when retrieving the memory (Tulving 1983). An interesting application of these concepts is in 'Gibbs' Reflective Cycle', a tool used by some occupational therapy practitioners to support reflective practice. Here, the therapist is asked to think about a specific episode, usually a critical incident from clinical experience, remember their feelings as it happened, and think about what they would do if the same situation occurred again, an example of 'memory for the future' (Tulving 1985b; Hargreaves and Page 2013). This is an instance of drawing on episodic memory in order to support effective reflection.

Another clinical case, that of 'K.C.', provided evidence that episodic memory could also be considered a separate domain (Rosenbaum et al. 2005). At the age of 30, K.C. was involved in a motorbike accident that left him with head injuries (Rosenbaum et al. 2005). MRI scans revealed extensive bilateral damage in the hippocampal formation and the parahippocampal gyrus, and damage to other regions thought to be involved with memory, including the left amygdala and left mamillary bodies (Rosenbaum et al. 2005).

K.C. did not show evidence of general cognitive impairment and was able to learn new procedures such as basic computer programming (Rosenbaum et al. 2005). His memory for semantic items learnt prior to the injury was intact (Tulving 2002). He was also able to learn new semantic information, for example he could remember novel definitions of everyday words that the researchers taught him, although he had no recollection of the learning event (Rosenbaum et al. 2005; Tulving 2002). However, K.C. was unable to recall any episodes from his life (Tulving 2002). For example, he could not remember being told of the death of his brother, to whom he was very close, nor a fall that led to surgery and using crutches for six months, nor being forced to evacuate his house following a local chemical spill (Rosenbaum et al. 2005; Tulving 2002).

K.C. also had an impaired sense of himself as a person in time and could not make statements about his future: when asked to think about what he might do the following day, he described his mind as 'blank' (Tulving 1985b, 2002). This is comparable to Henry Molaison, who commented on one occasion that 'every day is alone in itself, whatever enjoyment I've had, and whatever sorrow I've had' (Milner et al. 1968, p. 217). Following Tulving (1985b, p. 5), it could be argued that K.C. and Molaison were incapable of the 'mental time travel' that is a function of episodic memory and did not possess 'autonoetic consciousness'.

Schacter et al. (2007) stress that 'episodic thought' can encompass the future as well as the past, referring to evidence that people with amnesia have been found to have reduced ability to imagine novel events in detail (Schacter et al. 2007). Older people have also shown impaired capacity for episodic reminiscence and for generating episodic content when imagining future happenings (Schacter et al. 2007). Schacter et al. (2007) therefore argue that imagining future events depends on the recombination of past memories, and put forward a 'constructive episodic simulation hypothesis' suggesting that imagination of future happenings is dependent on the recombination of previous memories (Schacter et al. 2007, p. 659).

It may be the case that Molaison and K.C. had a diminished sense of personhood, which, as Farah (2010, p. 296) has argued, may include 'self-awareness' and 'cognition about the future'. Occupational therapy theorists such as Wilcock (2006, p. 153) have also foregrounded the drive to order experience over time as a feature of personal 'becoming'. Kielhofner (1995, p. 30), meanwhile, explained how reflection on past experience supports the 'self-knowledge' that allows a person to project themselves into the future and make choices to engage in specific occupations. It appears that neither K.C. nor Henry Molaison was able to do this, suggesting that episodic memory may be a key component of personhood and 'occupational choice' (Kielhofner 1995, p. 30).

The Relationship Between Episodic and Semantic Memory

The registering of information in episodic memory is directly based on experience, while in the semantic system registration is symbolic, for example using language (Tulving 1983). The encoding stage of episodic memory consists of converting information about the episode, including knowledge of when and where it occurred, into a 'trace' or 'engram' (Tulving 1983, p. 11).

We may retrieve knowledge of the past from episodic or semantic memory systems, or a combination of both. The experience is different in both cases: for (Tulving 1985b), episodic retrieval is autonoetic 'remembering', while semantic retrieval is noetic 'knowing'. The experience of recollection is, then, governed by the degree of episodic and semantic information involved in retrieval and a 'trade-off' exists whereby access to poorly remembered episodes can be supported by semantic cues, and impaired semantic cues are strengthened by episodic remembering, a process described as 'synergistic ecphory' (Tulving 1985b, p. 7). 'Ecphory' is a term coined by Semon and indicates 'the process of activating or retrieving a memory' (Schacter 2008, p. 57). An example can be drawn from the case of Henry Molaison: when asked to retrieve episodes relating to celebrating Christmas, he responded with semantic information about the difference between festivities in the south, where his father was born, and the north, where Molaison was brought up (Corkin 2002).

Vulnerability of Episodic Memory

Tulving (1985b, 2002) suggests that episodic memory and autonoetic consciousness are uniquely human. In addition, he argues that they are not present in children under the age of four, but develop later. Furthermore, episodic information is more subject to change, modification and loss, and is therefore selectively vulnerable in amnesia (Tulving 1983). This may be because of the complexity of the information, being based on many combinations of elements, its looser organisation and its basis in a single event (Tulving 1983).

Tulving (1985b) described a patient, N.N., with a closed head injury who could not recall any incidents from his past. His procedural and semantic memory were intact but his episodic was markedly impaired. He had, for example, abstract knowledge of concepts related to time, but no personal sense of time (Tulving 1985b). When asked to describe what he would do tomorrow, or what he did yesterday, he described only blankness (Tulving 1985b). Tulving calls this lack of subjective time awareness 'chronoagnosia', stating that N.N. was living in a 'permanent present' (Tulving 1985b, p. 4). He had anoetic and noetic consciousness but not autonoetic consciousness (Tulving 1985b). N.N. was incapable of 'mental time travel' and the lack of awareness of his past also meant he could not project into the future (Tulving 1985b). It may be recalled that Henry Molaison showed a similar inability to describe past events or to predict what he might do the following day.

Hassabis and Maguire (2007, p. 299) develop these themes, and suggest that 'self-projection' into the future requires a shunt in perception from one's immediate situation to a different, imagined alternative, while maintaining the focus on oneself. They suggest that episodic recollection, future self-projection, navigation and imagination of fictional scenarios all share 'scene construction' as a shared process (Hassabis and Maguire 2007, p. 299). This is characterised by retrieval of information from brain areas specialised for specific sensory modalities and assembly of this into a coherent spatial scene that can be manipulated and also allows visualisation (Hassabis and Maguire 2007, p. 299).

Hassabis and Maguire (2007, p. 300) hold a 'constructivist' view of episodic memory, meaning that recollection involves reconstruction of scenes, not perfect recall. They argue that episodic memory, memory for previously remembered fictitious events and creation of new fictions activate the hippo-campus and other regions, including the posterior parietal cortex and ventromedial prefrontal cortex, and show that patients with bilateral damage to the hippocampus have reduced ability to imagine novel fictitious happenings (Hassabis and Maguire 2007). Furthermore, while non-mnemonic cognitive functions might also depend selectively on processes such as autonoetic consciousness, those linked to the sense of self and scene construction, episodic memory is posited to draw on all these. This complexity may explain why it is peculiarly vulnerable, compared with other memory processes, if the brain is damaged and also why it only emerges at around 4 years old (Hassabis and Maguire 2007).

Episodic Memory and Human Occupation

The concepts of episodic memory and autonoetic consciousness fit well with the notion of 'temporality' as applied to human occupation (Hitch et al. 2014, p. 239). This, in turn, can be associated with Wilcock's (2006, p. 148) concept of 'becoming', referring to the unending process of change, negative as well as positive, that occurs throughout the human lifespan. In addition, it may the case that 'becoming' is a process supported by a wider network of family and community (Hitch et al. 2014). For example, episodic memory impairment is a prominent feature of Alzheimer's type dementia (ATD) and also retrograde amnesia following traumatic brain injury (TBI) (Chatzikostopoulos et al. 2022; Kopelman 2002). It may the case that occupational therapists can encourage family members or carers of people with these conditions to support retrieval of episodic memories with items such as photographs, aromas, music or food. These ideas are revisited in Chapter 7, in relation to interventions such as cognitive stimulation therapy.

Working Memory

Working memory is the capacity for temporarily remembering information and actively processing it at the same time, in order to accomplish an immediate goal (Baddeley 2015b; Corkin 2013). It is conceived of as a 'mental workspace' where action, perception and long-term memory interact (Baddeley 2003; Corkin 2013, p. 65). Occupational therapists' concern with the environment-bound performance of goal-directed, purposeful tasks and activities means that working memory concepts are especially relevant to their practice (Law et al. 1996; Kielhofner 1995). Several accounts of working memory have evolved and some of these are explored next.

The Atkinson and Shiffrin Model of Working Memory

The term 'working memory' was first used by Miller et al. (1960, p. 65) to describe a rapid access storage site for plans that were under formation, trans-formation or execution, and also for 'intentions', the yet-to-be completed aspects of any interrupted plans. Atkinson and Shiffrin (1968) developed these ideas and proposed a three-part structure for memory consisting of a 'sensory register', where information is held very briefly in the sensory modality in which it was encountered, prior to dissolution; and short-term and long-term stores.

It is perhaps important to stress that, up to this time, it was widely believed that memory was not divisible into short- and long-term components, and Atkinson and Shiffrin's (1968) paper, which drew on analogies from computing and cited Milner's work with Henry Molaison and other hippocampal patients as evidence, played an important role in establishing this division.

In Atkinson and Shiffrin's model, the short-term store constitutes working memory and it accepts items copied from both the sensory register and the long-term store. These are then worked with so as to guide ongoing actions. Items in the short-term store had a life of around 30 seconds, but this could be extended by 'control processes' that the person deploys voluntarily (Atkinson and Shiffrin 1968, p. 14). Such processes could include a range of mechanisms. Rehearsal of the information, for example, could strengthen coding and storage and act as a temporary 'buffer', such as when we repeat a telephone number to ourselves while dialling in order to remember it (Atkinson and Shiffrin 1968, p. 111). The authors also mention chunking of information, which was discussed earlier in this chapter. In addition, they describe the use of mnemonic devices, such as forming visual images of items to aid recall (Atkinson and Shiffrin 1968). Hopefully, it is clear that, in both Miller et al. (1960) and Atkinson and Shiffrin's (1968) accounts, working memory is a temporary site in which information drawn from different sources is worked with dynamically, and that, in occupational therapy terms, it supports occupational performance.

Atkinson and Shiffrin's (1968) account of memory was questioned from different perspectives. First, Craik and Lockhart (1972) challenged their model of sequential structured memory stores. As already discussed, these authors questioned the evidence for discrete memory storage sites and suggested that Atkinson and Shiffrin's (1968) emphasis on 'control processes' indicated that the multistore approach was not sufficient, in itself, to explain the mechanisms involved (Craik and Lockhart 1972, p. 673). Craik and Lockhart (1972, p. 671) argued instead that research should focus on the 'levels of processing' involved in remembering.

Shallice and Warrington (1970) also questioned the assumptions of Atkinson and Shiffrin's (1968) model, based on neuropsychological evidence from studies with a neurological patient, K.F. K.F. had severely impaired short-term memory, which was evidenced by reduced ability to remember lists of words (Shallice and Warrington 1970). However, in one test it was found that K.F.'s impaired performance was consistent with a pattern normally observed when performing *long-term* memory tasks, suggesting that he was relying on long-term memory processes (Shallice and Warrington 1970). In addition, earlier work had shown that K.F.'s long-term memory performance appeared to be unaffected (Shallice and Warrington 1970).

These results indicated that the Atkinson and Shiffrin (1968) model, in which information was copied sequentially from the short-term store to the long-term store, was problematic, as K.F. performed normally on tasks requiring long-term memory while having severely impaired short-term capacity. Shallice and Warrington (1970) proposed instead a model for processing auditory–verbal information in which the inputs to the short-term store arrived in parallel, rather than serially. In this model, the short-term store processed information about the *sound* of words, or phonemics, while the long-term store simultaneously processed semantic information, related to the *meaning* of words (Shallice and Warrington 1970).

The Multicomponent Model of Working Memory

Stemming from these criticisms of Atkinson and Shiffrin's (1968) model, Baddeley and Hitch focused on the role of short-term memory as a putative working memory system (Baddeley 2015b; Baddeley and Hitch 2017). The participants in their early research were asked to perform digit span tasks, involving memorising strings of digits, at the same time as other tasks considered to be underpinned by working memory (Baddeley 2007; Baddeley and Hitch 2017). They found that digit spans of three items had very little impact on the other tasks, while spans of six digits were associated with marked performance impairment, for example with greater time needed to complete verbal reasoning activities (Baddeley and Hitch 2017). They proposed, therefore, that working memory might consist of a 'phonemic buffer' that stored and rehearsed 'speechlike' items, such as digits, relatively autonomously, and a more flexible 'central executive' that only became involved once the capacity of this buffer was breached, in this case when the number of digits in the string increased (Baddeley and Hitch 2017, pp. 68, 69). They also cited evidence showing that visuo-motor tasks disrupted the capacity to recall visually presented items, but had no effect on recall of the items presented phonemically, suggesting that there was a separate storage area for visual information (Baddeley and Hitch 2017). The researchers argued that their proposed model could account for Shallice and Warrington's (1970) findings about K.F. It could be that his phonemic buffer was impaired, while his central executive remained functional, allowing him to complete the task successfully (Baddeley and Hitch 2017).

The working memory scheme outlined by Baddeley and Hitch (2017) was developed and became known as the 'multicomponent model' (Baddeley 2007, p. 7). This model 'assumes that a range of subsystems may be brought to bear upon the performance of any task' (Baddeley 2007, p. 78). The original model comprised three components: the 'phonological loop', the 'visuospatial sketchpad' and the 'central executive' (Baddeley 2003, p. 830). For occupational therapists interested in analysing the memory processes involved in a specific occupational performance event, for example when a person with memory impairment visits the shops, it is important to grasp these components and also more recent additions to the model. These are explored in the following paragraphs.

The 'phonological loop' functioned with language and sound, storing spoken and acoustic information (Baddeley 2003, p. 830). The phonological loop concept explained why, for example, it was harder to remember a list of multisyllabic words when compared with shorter words (Baddeley 2000). It also accounted for findings that it is harder to remember a short list of similar-sounding letters, such as T and V, when compared with dissimilar ones such as S and K (Baddeley 2000). The phonological loop was considered to interact with language, indicating that more 'fluid systems' interact with the 'crystallized systems', such as language, embedded in long-term memory (Baddeley 2015b).

The phonological loop could be divided into two components, a storage site and a control process, based on articulation of information using 'vocal or subvocal rehearsal' (Baddeley et al. 2001; Baddeley 2012, p. 5). It has been estimated that items in the phonological store decay after around two seconds, but that this rehearsal process can 'refresh' them, as long as all items are rehearsed within this time period (Gathercole and Hitch 1993). It is important to take these factors into account when presenting task instructions to a person with memory impairment, if the therapist is relying on written or spoken language.

The 'visuospatial sketchpad' was a restricted-capacity store for visual and spatial and, possibly, kinaesthetic information (Baddeley 2000, 2003, 2007). According to the model, aspects such as colour, location and shape are placed in separate silos, but are bound together by attention (Baddeley 2003). The visuospatial sketchpad was considered to interact with visual semantics, stored in long-term memory, another example of a more 'fluid' system interacting with a 'crystallized' memory system in long-term memory (Baddeley 2015b). The visuospatial sketchpad could also be divided into a region for storage, the 'visual cache', and an area in which information is retrieved in a dynamic manner, the 'inner scribe' (Baddeley 2003, p. 834). Again, the therapist should be aware of these factors; for example, the person with impairments in the visuospatial sketchpad may have difficulty remembering the location of items during a hospital-based kitchen task.

The 'central executive' was a controller that comprised two processes. The first was a process based on habits and guided by environmental cues; this was relatively automatic and therefore did not necessitate much attention (Baddeley 2003, p. 835). It may be noted that this is very similar to Kielhofner's (2008) description of 'habituation' and also Yerxa's (2000) comments about the energy-conserving aspects of 'habits' in occupational performance. Habit formation has been associated with the cerebral basal nuclei, which are discussed in detail in Box 1.3 later in the chapter. Second, a process called the 'supervisory attentional system', with restricted attentional capacity, could intervene to choose a course of action or identify solutions in situations where pre-existing habits were inadequate (Baddeley 2003, p. 835; Baddeley 2007). The central executive could also be involved in focusing on a task, shifting attention to another task or splitting attention between concurrent tasks (Baddeley 2003, 2015b). In addition, the supervisory attentional system is important in divided attention tasks, which are challenging for people with ATD (Baddeley 2015b). It has been found, for example, that people with ATD deteriorated in performance of concurrent tasks over a 12-month period, indicating that performance was linked to the disease progress (Baddeley et al. 2001).

At the start of the new millennium, a further temporary store with restricted capacity, the 'episodic buffer', was added to the multicomponent model of working memory (Baddeley 2000, p. 421; Baddeley 2003). The episodic buffer integrates information coded in multiple ways using a 'multidimensional code', which might include verbal, visual and semantic items that are drawn from various sources, which could encompass working memory itself, but also long-term memory and perception (Baddeley 2000, p. 421; Baddeley 2015b). The buffer acts as a 'workspace' in which this varied information can be bound together into a coherent episode that may be accessed consciously by the central executive (Baddeley 2000, 2003, 2015b). For example, it could facilitate the binding of different items of visual information into an integral percept or the placement of words into meaningful 'chunks' that permit sentences to be understood (Baddeley 2003, 2015b, p. 82). In addition, the central executive can attend to specific items in the buffer and construct novel representations with the information, which is thought to assist in solving problems (Baddeley 2000). These ideas are applied in more detail in Chapter 5.

The different components of the working memory model have been associated with functions of particular regions of the brain. These are discussed in more detail in Box 1.2.

As mentioned already, it has been suggested that working memory may also hold information about kinaesthesis, a term that refers to sensations of movement (Bastian 1887; Schmidt and Lee 2005). In addition, it will be recalled that, according to Baddeley (2012), verbal information may be rehearsed vocally or subvocally within the phonological loop. Jaroslawska et al. (2018) presented experimental data that seems to confirm both that working memory has a kinaesthetic component and that it might deploy similar rehearsal, albeit tapping motor control mechanisms.

These researchers note that people given a sequence of motor commands execute the actions more accurately than they can repeat them verbally (Jaroslawska et al. 2018). They conducted three experiments in each of which 16 young adults performed a sequence of fine or gross motor tasks. In the first, participants executed a series of actions on objects of different colours. The tasks were increasingly complex and delivered via spoken instruction. In addition, there were three interference conditions: suppression of articulatory rehearsal; counting backwards; and simultaneous performance of a sequence of hand movements, designed to suppress motor rehearsal (Jaroslawska et al. 2018). The authors measured the number of actions performed accurately with the required objects (Jaroslawska et al. 2018).

They found that performance of recalled sequences was better than recall of the verbal instructions, but that *all* of the suppression activities resulted in impaired recall, although this was less marked in the motor recall condition. Their second experiment used the same design but with a series of gross upper-limb movements as the motor suppression task (Jaroslawska et al. 2018). They found that backwards counting and motor suppression were linked to impaired performance in all of the recall tasks (Jaroslawska et al. 2018). Experiment three involved repeat measures of three suppression conditions: no suppression, articulatory and motor. There were also two formats for recall: verbal and action (Jaroslawska et al. 2018). The authors found that there was significantly better recall for the action format, but that there were no differences between the action and verbal formats in the motor suppression condition (Jaroslawska et al. 2018).

Overall, Jaroslawska et al. (2018, p. 2446) propose that the 'action advantage' might be a result of short-term storage of 'kinaesthetic representations' of movements to be performed and that working memory may utilise cognitive systems mediating motor control. They propose that these findings may need to be incorporated into the multicomponent model of working memory (Jaroslawska et al. 2018). These insights seem to justify occupational therapists' focus on assessing memory via performance of purposeful activities, rather than reliance on evaluations based on language and visual images, as is the case in many standardised cognitive screening tools, which fail to assess the kinaesthetic aspect of working memory.

Prospective Memory

Memory has also been subdivided into 'retrospective memory', for items from the past, and 'prospective memory', which involves making plans or commitments, retaining them while performing 'ongoing activities' and executing them at an appropriate time or on a particular cue (Eysenck 2015, p. 362; Graf 2012, p. 8). Prospective memory has been linked to activity in specific brain regions that are outlined in Box 1.2. Occupational therapists are involved in the assessment and treatment of people with memory impairments that may affect everyday commitments, such as remembering to take medication or attend appointments, and this memory system is therefore of great significance.

Zogg et al. 2012 have outlined a five-stage conceptual model of prospective memory. First, an intention is formed, along with a particular cue. The cue could be an event, for example encountering a specific person, or a predetermined time. This cue will trigger the retrieval of the intention. Prospective memory is improved if cues are processed in a manner relevant to the plan, because this association supports retrieval. For example, a medicine bottle placed on the table may be a more effective reminder than a note to take medication (Dismukes 2010; Graf 2012). Second, there is a delay, which could last up to a number of weeks, during which other activities are performed and the intention–cue dyad is in abeyance, although there may be ongoing monitoring for occurrence of the cue (Zogg et al. 2012). Third, there is cue recognition and self-retrieval of the intention (Einstein and McDaniel 2005; Zogg et al. 2012). Fourth, the intention is recollected from prospective memory. Fifth, the intention is executed (Zogg et al. 2012). These concepts may be useful in guiding occupational therapists when assisting people in identify cueing strategies for remembering commitments at an appropriate time.

Prospective memory can be divided into episodic and habitual subtypes: episodic prospective memory involves remembering to execute one-off intentions, while habitual prospective memory concerns tasks that must be performed repeatedly, such as taking prescribed medication (Graf 2012). In addition, prospective memory may be involved when remembering to resume a task that has been interrupted, and remembering to switch attention between tasks (Dismukes 2010).

Impaired prospective memory can lead to errors in everyday life with potentially serious consequences, for example neglecting to switch off an oven at the required time, and lapses in prospective memory have even been implicated in aviation accidents (Dismukes 2010). A close relationship has also been established between prospective memory capacity, as measured in laboratory tests, and medication adherence in people with human immunodeficiency virus and those with diabetes (Zogg et al. 2012). So, prospective memory impairments are potentially hazardous and should be considered during occupational therapy assessment.

BOX 1.2   LOBES OF THE CEREBRUM

The brain is divided into two cerebral hemispheres. The outermost part is the cerebral cortex. The largest and, in evolutionary terms, most recent part is called the neocortex, while the archicortex and paleocortex are older (Crossman et al. 2020). The surface of the neocortex is marked by folds called gyri, or gyrus in the singular, with grooves between them. The deepest grooves are termed fissures and the shallower ones are called sulci, or sulcus in the singular (Tortora and Derrickson 2011).

Each cerebral hemisphere is subdivided into four lobes with specialist functions. There are also a number of association areas, which are concerned with interpreting incoming sensory information and formulating appropriate motor responses (Martini 2018).

The lobes and key regions of the cerebral hemispheres are shown in Figure 1.2.

The frontal lobe is anterior to the central sulcus (Tortora and Derrickson 2011). This contains the primary motor cortex and premotor cortex, which are involved in motor control. Anterior to these is the extensive prefrontal cortex. This communicates with the parietal, occipital and temporal cortices (discussed later) via white-matter tracts called association fibres (Crossman et al. 2020; Tortora and Derrickson 2011). The prefrontal cortex is involved with high-level cognitive activity, including judgement, intellect, prediction and planning, learning and recall (Crossman et al. 2020; Tortora and Derrickson 2011).

The frontal lobes play an important role in the multicomponent model of working memory and also in prospective memory. For example, storage in the phonological loop has been linked to left hemisphere Brodmann area (BA) 40, while rehearsal has been linked to left BA 44, also known as Broca's area, a region involved in the motor production of speech (Baddeley 2000, 2007; Tortora and Derrickson 2011). In addition, the central executive has been associated with activation in the frontal lobes, while the

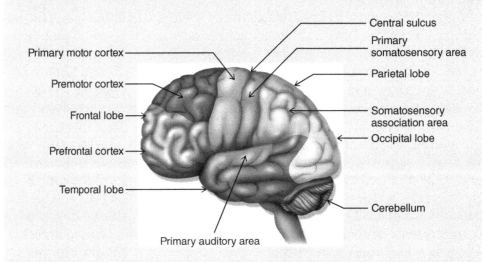

Figure 1.2 Lobes and key regions of the cerebral hemispheres (sagittal view of left hemisphere).

Source: RFBSIP/Adobe Stock.

right frontal lobe may be the neural substrate of the episodic buffer (Baddeley 2000, 2007; Berlingeri et al. 2008). Prospective memory, meanwhile, may depend on frontal brain regions as well as on the medial temporal lobes and the hippocampus (Zogg et al. 2012).

The parietal lobe is located posterior to the frontal lobe, superior to the temporal lobe and anterior to the occipital lobe. The parietal lobe contains the primary somatosensory area, which receives nerve impulses related to somatic sensations including touch, temperature, pain and proprioception, and allows conscious perception of these (Tortora and Derrickson 2011).

Posterior to the primary somatosensory area is the parietal association cortex, also called the somatosensory association area, which includes the inferior parietal lobule, an interface between the primary somatosensory area, the visual association areas of the occipital lobes, and auditory association area of the temporal lobes (Crossman et al. 2020; Tortora and Derrickson 2011). This area is involved in storage of somatic sensory memories and permits comparison of sensory inputs with experience from the past, allowing recognition of objects by touch (Tortora and Derrickson 2011).

The temporal lobes have a special role in declarative memory. The lateral aspect of the temporal lobe subdivides into superior, middle and inferior gyri (Crossman et al. 2020). The superior gyrus contains the primary auditory area, which is involved in the perception of sound (Crossman et al. 2020). Posterior to this is the auditory association cortex, where sounds are processed at a higher level, in the dominant, usually the left, hemisphere. This area includes Wernicke's area, which is involved in word recognition and the creation of thought from words (Crossman et al. 2020; Dronkers et al. 2000; Tortora and Derrickson 2011). There is minor variation in terminology and some authors state that Wernicke's area also spreads out to include part of the parietal cortex (Tortora and Derrickson 2011). As shown earlier, the inferior medial part of the temporal lobe is the location of the hippocampus, part of the archicortex, as well as the amygdala, and both of these structures are part of the limbic system, which is described further on (Crossman et al. 2020).

The inferior temporal cortex is considered as the region in which the highest level of processing of visual information takes place, allowing recognition of items on the basis of this visual input (Eichenbaum 2012). It is also thought to be the location of the silo in which long-term memories for visual items are stored (Eichenbaum 2012). This means that damage to this area can lead to 'visual agnosia', a failure to recognise visually presented items. Visual agnosia can be 'apperceptive', resulting from impaired perception, or 'associative', resulting from failure to recognise objects visually, despite having intact 'visual representations' (Eichenbaum 2012, p. 208; Gazzaniga et al. 2009, p. 226). A key message here is that cortical areas that are involved in analysing specific classes of information, in this case visual, are also involved in the long-term storage of that information (Eichenbaum 2012). For example, it has been shown that when people study a series of visual images and accompanying sounds, such as a picture of a dog with the sound of barking, and are subsequently asked to remember the appearance or sound of the object, visual regions and auditory regions were activated according to the modality of the recollection (Eichenbaum 2012). This phenomenon depends on the capacity of cortical neurons and networks to reinitiate their standard sensory response patterns once the stimulus is unavailable, thereby facilitating representation in memory (Eichenbaum 2012). Eichenbaum comments:

> *memory should be conceived as intimately intertwined with information processing in the cortex, indeed so much so that memory and information processing are inherently indistinguishable . . . the mechanisms of the cerebral cortex involve a combination of information processing and memory to constitute neural networks that contain the structure of our knowledge about the world. (Eichenbaum 2012, p. 216)*

Furthermore, there is a degree of hemispheric specialisation. The right temporal lobe may be important when reconstruction of autobiographical items and when memory for events require visual imagery or imagery in other sensory modalities. The left temporal lobe may be important in the storing of distant semantic or word-based material (Kopelman 2002).

The occipital lobe contains the primary visual cortex, which is where nerve impulses related to vision are first perceived (Crossman et al. 2020). The occipital lobe also contains the visual association cortices, which are engaged in recognition and interpretation of visual stimuli (Crossman et al. 2020). In the multicomponent working memory model, the visuospatial sketchpad is thought to depend on right hemisphere regions, including the temporo-parietal lobe (BA 40) and the right occipital lobe (BA 19) (Baddeley 2000; Baddeley 2007).

To continue the examination of the structure of the brain, Box 1.3 explores the basal nuclei and Box 1.4 describes the limbic system.

BOX 1.3   THE BASAL NUCLEI

The basal nuclei is a group of three paired nuclei named the caudate nucleus, putamen and globus pallidus, which are located deep to the cerebral cortex (Crossman et al. 2020). The caudate nucleus and putamen are often labelled collectively as the striatum or neostriatum; the putamen and globus pallidus are also sometimes described collectively as the lentiform nucleus (Crossman et al. 2020). Again, there is some variation in terminology and two other nuclei, the subthalamic and substantia nigra, are sometimes included within the basal nuclei (Crossman et al. 2020). In addition, the basal nuclei are often referred to in clinical practice as the basal ganglia, although, because a ganglion is a group of nerve cells located in the peripheral nervous system and a nucleus is located in the central nervous system, basal nuclei is a more anatomically correct term (Tortora and Derrickson 2011).

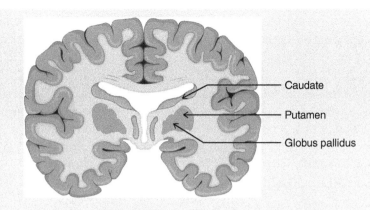

Figure 1.3 Basal nuclei (anterior coronal view of cerebrum).
Source: Design Praxis/Adobe Stock.

The component parts of the basal nuclei are shown in Figure 1.3.

The basal nuclei are considered to be involved in initiation of movements and behaviours needed in specific situations, and also inhibition of inappropriate actions (Crossman et al. 2020). The basal nuclei are known to be involved in learned behavioural responses to 'antecedent stimuli'; an example would be switching on a light switch in response to entering a darkened room (Yin and Knowlton 2006, p. 464). They are involved in the formation of habits and have a role in 'instrumental behaviours', which are actions required to produce a specific response (Yin and Knowlton 2006, p. 464). Crucially, these learned repertoires depend on the memory of the value placed on the desired response and also awareness of the relationship between the action and the outcome (Yin and Knowlton 2006).

The basal nuclei, specifically the dorsal region of the striatum, are involved in non-declarative procedural learning (Yin and Knowlton 2006). Yin and Knowlton (2006), for example, show that patients with Parkinson's disease, which affects the basal nuclei, are able to learn a task involving prediction of an outcome when presented with a stimulus that involves learning the linkage between the stimulus and the outcome, performing as well as without neurological impairment do. However, the evidence suggests that people with Parkinson's disease rely for this on medial temporal lobe mechanisms, which are involved in declarative memory, while individuals without neurological impairment are able to learn the task using the basal nuclei (Yin and Knowlton 2006). In addition, people with Huntington's disease, which also affects the basal nuclei, have been shown to be impaired on tasks involving procedural learning of motor skills (Eichenbaum 2012). Yin and Knowlton (2006) comment that it is likely that most learning involves a combination of habitual and declarative mechanisms, and that the relative contributions of these memory systems may be a function of the quantity of training involved, the difficulty of the learned associations involved and the integrity of the basal nuclei and medial temporal lobes. Indeed, they maintain that behaviour is likely a result of basal nuclei–cortical interaction, rather than a product of either region alone (Yin and Knowlton 2006).

It has also been found that when learning a new motor skill, the caudate nucleus and prefrontal cortex, labelled the 'associate network', are active.

However, once the skill is learned thoroughly and becomes more habitual, then the activation pattern during performance changes to the putamen and motor cortices, described as the 'sensorimotor network' (Yin and Knowlton 2006, p. 472). In addition, there are stronger connections between higher-order association areas of the prefrontal cortex with the caudate, and stronger connections between more dorsal motor regions of the cortex and the putamen (Crossman et al. 2020). One final point here is that another subcortical structure, the cerebellum (shown in Figure 1.2), is involved in the fine-tuning of learned motor responses in procedural memory (Eichenbaum 2012).

BOX 1.4   THE LIMBIC SYSTEM

The limbic system is a very ancient part of the cerebrum, located in the rim on the medial aspect of the cerebral hemisphere, from which it derives its name ('limbus' means rim in Latin) (Gazzaniga et al. 2009; Crossman et al. 2020). An earlier conception of the existence of a specific emotional system in the brain was proposed by James Papez in 1937, and the system has therefore also been known as the 'Papez circuit' (Eichenbaum 2012; Zogg et al. 2012). Papez included the cingulate cortex, the hippocampal region, the mammillary bodies of the hypothalamus and the thalamic nuclei (Eichenbaum 2012). A more contemporary view of the limbic system includes extra areas in addition to those proposed by Papez: the amygdala, septum and prefrontal cortex (Eichenbaum 2012).

The components of the limbic system are shown in Figure 1.4.

It is important to stress that there is some disagreement about the precise components of the limbic system and even whether the title is still valid (Eichenbaum 2012; Gazzaniga et al. 2009). However, authors generally include the parahippocampal gyrus and hippocampus, already discussed (Tortora and Derrickson 2011). In addition, it includes the amygdala,

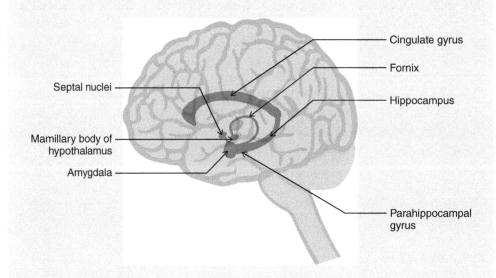

Figure 1.4 The limbic system (left sagittal view).
Source: joshya/Adobe Stock.

which has connections with the inferior temporal association area, the thalamus, olfactory tract and septum (Crossman et al. 2020). Furthermore, the amygdala receives inputs, via the thalamus, from visceral organs (Eichenbaum 2012). Overall, the amygdala receives and integrates information from multiple modalities (Eichenbaum 2012).

The limbic system permits fast responses to potential danger, so that sensory information passes by the neocortex and transmits directly to the limbic system, and relatively automated behaviours, such as fight or flight, are then initiated via the basal nuclei (Crossman et al. 2020). This is sometimes called a 'low road' for information processing, which allows 'quick but dirty' communication of sensory information from the thalamus to the amygdala, allowing for a rapid response (Gazzaniga et al. 2009, p. 372). Opposed to this is the 'high road', via which sensory inputs from the thalamus are first processed at the cortical level, before relay to the amygdala (Gazzaniga et al. 2009, p. 372). It will be shown later in this book that disorders in this area may underpin the problems encountered by people living with post-traumatic stress disorder (Brewin 2001).

The learning and memory of emotional responses underpinned by the amygdala may be implicit, non-declarative learning, meaning that the person does not have conscious awareness of the learning (Gazzaniga et al. 2009). Alternatively, the learning and memory can be explicit and declarative; here, the amygdala may work with the hippocampus to give a memory emotional salience, enhancing the force of the memory by its effect on storage (Gazzaniga et al. 2009). At the same time, explicit learning, perhaps about the dangers involved in a particular action and based on the hippocampus, may activate the amygdala so that, in future contemplation of this action, there will be generation of a fear response, reinforcing the message that it could bring unwelcome consequences (Gazzaniga et al. 2009).

Some evidence for the role of the amygdala comes from the studies of Henry Molaison, who had the amygdala removed bilaterally during surgery (Eichenbaum 2012). He showed lack of awareness of satiety and would continue eating even when he had just had a meal, blunted awareness of pain and a lack of interest in sex, despite being aware of sexuality at a declarative level (Corkin 2013; Eichenbaum 2012).

Other limbic system nuclei include the septum that communicates with the habenular nucleus of the epithalamus; this latter nucleus is involved in linking emotional responses and remembered aromas (Crossman et al. 2020; Tortora and Derrickson 2011). The orbitofrontal cortex is part of the frontal lobe and also has strong connections to the limbic system. For example, the orbitofrontal cortex connects to the inferior temporal cortex by means of the uncinate fasciculus, which will be discussed in relation to memory later in the book (Crossman et al. 2020). Fronto-temporal dementia, also discussed later in the book, involves atrophy in the prefrontal cortex and the amygdala (Crossman et al. 2020).

The limbic system communicates extensively with the association areas of the neocortex, meaning that goal-focused actions can be linked to more instinctual behaviour and homeostatic mechanisms, imbuing memory with these primitive characteristics (Crossman et al. 2020). Crossman et al.

(2020) provide an account in which sensory information is first detected in a specific modality, for example via vision or audition, and is then processed at higher levels in the parieto-occipital association areas, followed by the frontal and inferior temporal association cortices, until it achieves independence from sensory modality and can be processed in a semantic manner. The information then enters the limbic system via an indirect route to the hippocampal formation, which was discussed in Box 1.1, or directly to the amygdala (Crossman et al. 2020). Purposeful actions depend on the learned associations between past actions and outcomes, including emotional responses to rewards and sanctions, and in that sense depend on the memory properties of the limbic system (Crossman et al. 2020).

Towards a Culturally Situated Understanding of Memory

A school of psychology developed in the Soviet Union in the 1930s that stressed that cognitive processes change with social and historical development (Luria 1976). In addition, consciousness was not a passive property of the individual mind, but was shaped by the ways in which humans reacted to and acted on their environment in specific social and historical contexts (Luria 1976). The child's mental processes, for example, are shaped by those of previous generations via language, tools and the products of social labour (Luria 1976). Luria (1976, p. 164), stated:

> *The basic categories of human mental life can be understood as*
> *products of social history – they are subject to change when the basic*
> *forms of social practice are altered and thus are social in nature.*
> *(Luria 1976, p. 164)*

Luria (1976) worked with Vygotsky to analyse the mental operations of people living in Uzbekistan and Kirghizia during the social and economic changes resulting from the Russian Revolution of 1917. Key here were changed working practices, moving from small village life and high levels of illiteracy to collective agricultural and industrial production (Luria 1976). According to Luria (1976, p. 15), an important shift was that from 'graphical-functional' activity, in which cognition was orientated towards the objects of labour, to mediated thought, distinguished by higher levels of abstraction, with the emergence of thought guided not just by the practical task in hand but by language and logic.

For these thinkers, memory in non-literate societies was predominantly 'natural memory', influenced by the perception of external stimuli; however, the use of memory aids and the emergence of writing meant that memory became more 'culturally-elaborated' (Vygotsky and Cole 1978). At this stage, memory incorporates stimuli generated by the person themselves, described as 'signs' (Vygotsky and Cole 1978, p. 39).

Vygotsky and Cole (1978) believed this to be a feature of individual development as well. Vygotsky's research group found in experiments that children aged 5 or 6 could not use stimulus cards to help them in a memory task, but that children between the ages of 8 and 13 were able to do so. Vygotsky and Cole (1978) argued that tool use and language, which are both cultural phenomena and both emerge in infancy, provide the basis for further psychological development. Throughout development, they argued, there is then an interaction between biological processes and more complex psychological processes, which are of 'sociocultural origin' (Vygotsky and Cole 1978, p. 46). The young child at 5 or 6 was unable to use external signs to support memory, but at a later stage signs could be used to aid memory retrieval (Vygotsky and Cole 1978). Where aids were used at the younger age, it was found that the child only made use of them when the sign had some direct representation of the item of to be recalled, so the sign was not being used as a *symbol* (Vygotsky and Cole 1978). They argued that memory in early childhood was the foundation of other psychological processes, so that thinking *is* remembering (Vygotsky and Cole 1978). For example, if asked to describe a snail the child will give a concrete description of the qualities of a snail that they have observed, based on memory, rather a description of the abstract concept (Vygotsky and Cole 1978). However, during adolescence, when logical concepts are internalised, 'to recall means to think' and recognition involves identifying the part of the concept that the 'task indicates has to be found' (Vygotsky and Cole 1978, p. 51). In particular, mature human memory makes use of signs, an exemplar of which is tying a knot in a handkerchief to remember something, so that remembering becomes an 'external activity' (Vygotsky and Cole 1978, p. 51).

Conclusion

This chapter has surveyed the evidence linking learning and memory to experience-dependent neural plasticity. The potential role of long-term potentiation as a mechanism underpinning memory formation was discussed. It was shown how, remarkably, this phenomenon, which was identified in the 1970s, seemed to confirm the predictions of Hebb's postulate about learning and memory originally put forward in the 1940s.

There was a brief discussion of the history of thinking on memory. It was shown that the shift from behaviourism to an information processing approach, the so-called 'cognitive revolution' in the United States, opened up new vistas in memory research. At the same time, there were other traditions of thinking on memory, for example that represented by Bartlett in Britain and Luria and Vygotsky in the Soviet Union.

It was shown how a person's occupational history can influence neural plasticity and, in particular, brain regions know to be involved in memory. This should be a concern for practitioners guided by occupational justice principles. These issues are discussed further in Chapter 2.

The case of Henry Molaison was discussed in some detail. The space given to this history is justified by this case's lasting contributions to memory theory, in particular the understanding of the role of the medial temporal lobes and the hippocampal memory system. In addition, the categorisation of memory domains into non-declarative and declarative, or procedural and semantic, owes much to the research that was done with Molaison. Again, it may be useful to pause for thought here: it is hard to think of another example of a single case generating so many widely accepted and influential theories.

A detailed historical account of some contemporary concepts of memory was given. These included Tulving's tripartite hierarchy of procedural, semantic and episodic memory. Also there was discussion of the multicomponent model of working memory. One advantage of the latter model is that it acknowledges a central role for attention, in the form of the central executive. In addition, it is concerned with goal-directed task performance, and therefore has relevance for occupational therapists.

It was shown how these concepts can be applied to typical assessment situations in which the occupational therapist may be involved with persons with memory impairment. Furthermore, there was an explanation of concepts of prospective memory, with examples of application to occupational performance.

An outline of the structure and functions of key cerebral regions in relation to memory performance was provided. In particular, there was a detailed description of the hippocampal region, which is especially relevant to discussions of memory.

Finally, there was a brief overview of the socio-historical school of psychology. It is hoped that overall, occupational therapists may be encouraged to look beyond the, undoubtedly seminal, work undertaken in North America and consider other traditions of thinking on memory and cognition in general. These may be less well known, but they fit well with aspects of occupational therapy theory.

Points for Discussion

1. Steve is a senior occupational therapist on an acute stroke unit. He is training newly qualified therapists to use an electric whole-body hoist. Explain how he can use chunking to support the trainees to remember how to complete this task.
2. Maryam is a patient who has memory impairments following a TBI. She reports difficulty remembering to pick up her children from nursery each day. In addition, she states that she forgot a one-off meet-up with an old friend. Which memory systems would underpin these errors? Also, state some appropriate cues that might help Maryam.
3. Charles has ATD and impaired episodic memory. What suggestions could the occupational therapist make to his family to support retrieval of episodic memories?

Activities

1. Chunk the tasks involved in the activities of washing and dressing.
2. Chunk the tasks involved in completing grocery shopping.
3. Use the concept of 'depth of processing' when presenting a complex kitchen task to a service user with memory impairment.
4. Reflect on a critical incident using Gibbs' Reflective Cycle; discuss how episodic memory supports this process.

5. See if you can remember this sequence of random numbers:

996297

682701

788688

177753

884523

961890

Now construct an array of numbers that is made up of the dates of birth of people close to you and telephone numbers that you know. What do you notice about how many you can remember in comparison with the random numbers? Can you explain any differences you notice?

References

Amaral, D.G. and Strick, P.L. (2013). The organisation of the central nervous system. In: *Principles of Neural Science*, 5e (ed. E.R. Kandel, J.H. Schwartz, T.M. Jessell, et al.), 337–369. New York: McGraw Hill Education.

Aristotle and McKeon, R. (1941). *The Basic Works of Aristotle*. New York: Random House.

Atkinson, R.C. and Shiffrin, R.M. (1968). Human memory: a proposed system and its control processes. *Psychology of Learning and Motivation* 2:89–195.

Baddeley, A. (2000). The episodic buffer: a new component of working memory? *Trends in Cognitive Sciences* 4 (11): 417–423.

Baddeley, A. (2003). Working memory: looking back and looking forward. *Nature Reviews Neuroscience* 4 (10): 829–839.

Baddeley, A.D. (2007). *Working Memory, Thought, and Action*. Oxford: Oxford University Press.

Baddeley, A. (2012). Working memory: theories, models, and controversies. *Annual Review of Psychology* 63 (1): 1–29.

Baddeley, A. (2015a). Learning. In: *Memory* (ed. A. Baddeley, M.W. Eysenck, and M.C. Anderson), 107–135. London: Psychology Press.

Baddeley, A. (2015b). Working memory. In: *Memory* (ed. A. Baddeley, M.W. Eysenck, and M.C. Anderson), 67–105. London: Psychology Press.

Baddeley, A.D. and Hitch, G. (2017). Working memory. In: *Exploring Working Memory: Selected Works of Alan Baddeley* (ed. A. Baddeley), 43–79. London: Taylor and Francis.

Baddeley, A., Chincotta, D., and Adlam, A. (2001). Working memory and the control of action: evidence from task switching. *Journal of Experimental Psychology. General* 130 (4): 641–657.

Bartlett, F.C. (1995). *Remembering: A Study in Experimental and Social Psychology*. Cambridge: Cambridge University Press.

Bastian, H.C. (1887). The 'muscular sense'; its nature and cortical localisation. *Brain* 10 (1): 1–89.

Bauer, P.J., DeBoer, T., and Lukowski, A.F. (2007). In the language of multiple memory systems, defining and describing developments in long-term explicit memory. In: *Short- and Long-Term Memory in Infancy and Early Childhood: Taking the First Steps Toward Remembering* (ed. L.M. Oakes and P.J. Bauer), 240–270. Oxford: Oxford University Press.

Bear, M.F., Connors, B.W., and Paradiso, M.A. (2016). *Neuroscience: Exploring the Brain*, 4e. Philadelphia, PA: Wolters Kluwer.

Berlingeri, M., Bottini, G., Basilico, S. et al. (2008). Anatomy of the episodic buffer: a voxel-based morphometry study in patients with dementia. *Behavioural Neurology* 19 (1–2): 29–34.

Bliss, T.V. and Collingridge, G.L. (1993). A synaptic model of memory: long-term potentiation in the hippocampus. *Nature* 361 (6407): 31–39.

Bliss, T.V. and Lømo, T. (1973). Long-lasting potentiation of synaptic transmission in the dentate area of the anaesthetized rabbit following stimulation of the perforant path. *Journal of Physiology* 232 (2): 331–356.

Brewin, C.R. (2001). A cognitive neuroscience account of posttraumatic stress disorder and its treatment. *Behaviour Research and Therapy* 39 (4): 373–393.

Chatzikostopoulos, A., Moraitu, D., Tsolaki, M. et al. (2022). Episodic memory in amnestic mild cognitive impairment (aMCI) and Alzheimer's disease dementia (ADD): using the 'Doors and People' tool to differentiate between early aMCI—late aMCI—mild ADD diagnostic groups. *Diagnostics* 12 (7): 1768.

Corkin, S. (1968). Acquisition of motor skill after bilateral medial temporal-lobe excision. *Neuropsychologia* 6 (3): 255–265.

Corkin, S. (2002). What's new with the amnesic patient H.M.? *Nature Reviews Neuroscience* 3 (2): 153–160.

Corkin, S. (2013). *Permanent Present Tense: The Man with No Memory, and What He Taught the World*. London: Penguin.

Craik, F.I.M. and Lockhart, R.S. (1972). Levels of processing: a framework for memory research. *Journal of Verbal Learning and Verbal Behavior* 11 (6): 671–684.

Craik, F.I. and Tulving, E. (1975). Depth of processing and the retention of words in episodic memory. *Journal of Experimental Psychology. General* 104 (3): 268–294.

Crossman, A.R., Neary, D., and Crossman, B. (2020). *Neuroanatomy: An Illustrated Colour Text*, 6e. Amsterdam: Elsevier.

DeFelipe, J. (2006). Brain plasticity and mental processes: Cajal again. *Nature Reviews Neuroscience* 7 (10): 811–817.

Dismukes, R.K. (2010). Remembrance of things future: prospective memory in laboratory, workplace, and everyday settings. *Reviews of Human Factors and Ergonomics* 6 (1): 79–122.

Dronkers, N.F., Pinker, S., and Damasio, A. (2000). Language and the aphasias. In: *Principles of Neural Science*, 4e (ed. E.R. Kandel, J.H. Schwartz, and T.M. Jessell), 1169–1187. New York: McGraw Hill.

Eichenbaum, H. (2002). *The Cognitive Neuroscience of Memory: An Introduction*. Oxford: Oxford University Press.

Eichenbaum, H. (2012). *The Cognitive Neuroscience of Memory: An Introduction*, 2e. Oxford: Oxford University Press.

Einstein, G.O. and McDaniel, M.A. (2005). Prospective memory: multiple retrieval processes. *Current Directions in Psychological Science* 14 (6): 286–290.

Eluvathingal, T.J., Chugani, H.T., Behen, M.E. et al. (2006). Abnormal brain connectivity in children after early severe socioemotional deprivation: a diffusion tensor imaging study. *Pediatrics* 117 (6): 2093–2100.

Eysenck, M.W. (2015). Prospective memory. In: *Memory* (ed. A. Baddeley, M.W. Eysenck, and M.C. Anderson), 361–378. London: Psychology Press.

Farah, M.J. (2010). *Neuroethics: An Introduction with Readings*. Cambridge, MA: MIT Press.

Gabrieli, J.D.E., Corkin, S., Mickel, S.F., and Growdon, J.H. (1993). Intact acquisition and long-term retention of mirror-tracing skill in Alzheimer's disease and in global amnesia. *Behavioral Neuroscience* 107 (6): 899–910.

Gathercole, S.E. and Hitch, G.J. (1993). Developmental changes in short-term memory: a revised working memory perspective. In: *Theories of Memory* (ed. A. Collins, S.E. Gathercole, M.A. Conway, and P.E. Morris), 189–210. Hove: Erlbaum.

Gazzaniga, M.S., Ivry, R.B., and Mangun, G.R. (1998). *Cognitive Neuroscience: The Biology of the Mind*. New York: W.W. Norton.

Gazzaniga, M.S., Ivry, R.B., and Mangun, G.R. (2009). *Cognitive Neuroscience: The Biology of the Mind*, 3e. New York: Norton.

Gluck, M.A., Mercado, E., and Myers, C.E. (2008). *Learning and Memory: From Brain to Behavior*. New York: Worth Publishers.

Graf, P. (2012). Prospective memory: faulty brain, flaky person. *Canadian Psychology/Psychologie Canadienne* 53 (1): 7.

Hagedorn, R. (1992). *Occupational Therapy: Foundations for Practice: Models, Frames of Reference and Core Skills*. Edinburgh: Churchill Livingstone.

Hagedorn, R. (2000). *Tools for Practice in Occupational Therapy: A Structured Approach to Core Skills and Processes*. Edinburgh: Churchill Livingstone.

Hargreaves, J. and Page, L. (2013). *Reflective Practice*. Oxford: Wiley.

Hassabis, D. and Maguire, E.A. (2007). Deconstructing episodic memory with construction. *Trends in Cognitive Sciences* 11 (7): 299–306.

Hebb, D.O. (1949). *The Organization of Behavior: A Neuropsychological Theory*. New York: Wiley.

Hitch, D., Pépin, G., and Stagnitti, K. (2014). In the footsteps of Wilcock, part two: the interdependent nature of doing, being, becoming, and belonging. *Occupational Therapy in Health Care* 28 (3): 247–263.

James, W. (1890). *The Principles of Psychology*. New York: Holt.

Jaroslawska, A.J., Gathercole, S.E., and Holmes, J. (2018). Following instructions in a dual-task paradigm: evidence for a temporary motor store in working memory. *Quarterly Journal of Experimental Psychology* 71 (11): 2439–2449.

Kandel, E.R., Kupfermann, I., and Iverson, S. (2000). Learning and memory. In: *Principles of Neural Science*, 4e (ed. E.R. Kandel, J.H. Schwartz, and T.M. Jessell), 1227–1246. New York: McGraw Hill.

Kielhofner, G. (1995). *A Model of Human Occupation: Theory and Application*, 2e. Baltimore, MD: Williams & Wilkins.

Kielhofner, G. (2008). *A Model of Human Occupation: Theory and Application*, 4e. Baltimore, MD: Lippincott Williams & Wilkins.

Kopelman, M.D. (2002). Disorders of memory. *Brain* 125 (10): 2152–2190.

Lamprecht, R. and LeDoux, J. (2004). Structural plasticity and memory. *Nature Reviews Neuroscience* 5 (1): 45–54.

Law, M., Cooper, B., Strong, S. et al. (1996). The person-environment-occupation model: a transactive approach to occupational performance. *Canadian Journal of Occupational Therapy* 63 (1): 9–23.

Luria, A.R. (1966). *Higher Cortical Functions in Man*. London: Tavistock.

Luria, A.R. (1973). *The Working Brain: An Introduction to Neuropsychology*. New York: Basic Books.

Luria, A.R. (1976). *Cognitive Development: Its Cultural and Social Foundations*. Cambridge, MA: Harvard University Press.

Maguire, E.A., Gadian, D.G., Johnsrude, I.S. et al. (2000). Navigation-related structural change in the hippocampi of taxi drivers. *Proceedings of the National Academy of Sciences* 97 (8): 4398–4403.

Maguire, E.A., Woollett, K., and Spiers, H.J. (2006). London taxi drivers and bus drivers: a structural MRI and neuropsychological analysis. *Hippocampus* 16 (12): 1091–1101.

Malenka, R.C. (2003). The long-term potential of LTP. *Nature Reviews Neuroscience* 4 (11): 923–926.

Martini, F. (2018). *Fundamentals of Anatomy and Physiology*, 11e. Harlow: Pearson.

Melton, A.W. (1963). Implications of short-term memory for a general theory of memory. *Journal of Verbal Learning and Verbal Behavior* 2 (1): 1–21.

Miller, G.A. (1956). The magical number seven, plus or minus two: some limits on our capacity for processing information. *Psychological Review* 63 (2): 81.

Miller, G.A. (2003). The cognitive revolution: a historical perspective. *Trends in Cognitive Sciences* 7 (3): 141–144.

Miller, G.A., Galanter, E., and Pribram, K.H. (1960). *Plans and the Structure of Behaviour*. London: Holt, Rinehart & Winston.

Milner, B., Corkin, S., and Teuber, H.-L. (1968). Further analysis of the hippocampal amnesic syndrome: 14-year follow-up study of HM. *Neuropsychologia* 6 (3): 215–234.

Padurariu, M., Ciobica, A., Mavroudis, I. et al. (2012). Hippocampal neuronal loss in the CA1 and CA3 areas of Alzheimer's disease patients. *Psychiatria Danubina* 24 (2): 152–158.

Postle, B.R. and Corkin, S. (1998). Impaired word-stem completion priming but intact perceptual identification priming with novel words: evidence from the amnesic patient HM. *Neuropsychologia* 36 (5): 421–440.

Radomski, M.V. (2002). Assessing abilities and capacities: cognition. In: *Occupational Therapy for Physical Dysfunction*, 5e (ed. C.A. Trombly and M.V. Radomski), 197–211. Baltimore, MD: Lippincott Williams & Wilkins.

Rose, S.P.R. (1992). *The Making of Memory*. London: Bantam.

Rosenbaum, R.S., Köhler, S., Schacter, D.L. et al. (2005). The case of K.C.: contributions of a memory-impaired person to memory theory. *Neuropsychologia* 43 (7): 989–1021.

Sanes, J.R. and Jessell, T.M. (2013). Experience and the refinement of synaptic connections. In: *Principles of Neural Science*, 5e (ed. E.R. Kandel, J.H. Schwartz, T.M. Jessell, et al.), 1259–1283. New York: McGraw Hill Education.

Schacter, D.L. (2008). *Searching for Memory: The Brain, the Mind, and the Past*. New York: Basic Books.

Schacter, D.L. and Wagner, A.D. (2013). Learning and memory. In: *Principles of Neural Science*, 5e (ed. E.R. Kandel, J.H. Schwartz, T.M. Jessell, et al.), 1441–1460. New York: McGraw Hill Education.

Schacter, D.L., Addis, D.R., and Buckner, R.L. (2007). Remembering the past to imagine the future: the prospective brain. *Nature Reviews Neuroscience* 8 (9): 657–661.

Schmidt, R.A. and Lee, T.D. (2005). *Motor Control and Learning: A Behavioral Emphasis*. Champaign, IL: Human Kinetics.

Scoville, W. (1968). Amnesia after bilateral medial temporal-lobe excision: introduction to case HM. *Neuropsychologia* 6 (3): 211–213.

Scoville, W.B. and Milner, B. (1957). Loss of recent memory after bilateral hippocampal lesions. *Journal of Neurology, Neurosurgery, and Psychiatry* 20 (1): 11.

Shallice, T. and Warrington, E.K. (1970). Independent functioning of verbal memory stores: a neuropsychological study. *Quarterly Journal of Experimental Psychology* 22 (2): 261–273.

Siegelbaum, S.A. and Kandel, E.R. (2013). Overview of synaptic transmission. In: *Principles of Neural Science*, 5e (ed. E.R. Kandel, J.H. Schwartz, T.M. Jessell, et al.), 177–188. New York: McGraw Hill Education.

Squire, L.R. (2009). The legacy of patient H.M. for neuroscience. *Neuron* 61 (1): 6–9.

Tortora, G.J. and Derrickson, B. (2011). *Principles of Anatomy and Physiology*, 13e. Hoboken, NJ: Wiley.

Trombly, C.A. (2002). Conceptual foundations for practice. In: *Occupational Therapy for Physical Dysfunction*, 5e (ed. C.A. Trombly and M.V. Radomski), 1–15. Baltimore, MD: Lippincott Williams & Wilkins.

Tulving, E. (1983). *Elements of Episodic Memory*. Oxford: Clarendon Press.

Tulving, E. (1985a). How many memory systems are there? *American Psychologist* 40 (4): 385–398.

Tulving, E. (1985b). Memory and consciousness. *Canadian Psychology/Psychologie Canadienne* 26 (1): 1.

Tulving, E. (2002). Episodic memory: from mind to brain. *Annual Review of Psychology* 53 (1): 1–25.

Tulving, E. and Madigan, S.A. (1970). Memory and verbal learning. *Annual Review of Psychology* 21 (1): 437–484.

Vygotsky, L.S. and Cole, M. (1978). *Mind in Society: Development of Higher Psychological Processes*. Cambridge, MA: Harvard University Press.

Wilcock, A.A. (2006). *An Occupational Perspective of Health*, 2e. Thorofare, NJ: Slack.

Yerxa, E.J. (2000). Confessions of an occupational therapist who became a detective. *British Journal of Occupational Therapy* 63 (5): 192–199.

Yin, H.H. and Knowlton, B.J. (2006). The role of the basal ganglia in habit formation. *Nature Reviews Neuroscience* 7 (6): 464–476.

Zogg, J.B., Woods, S.P., Sauceda, J.A. et al. (2012). The role of prospective memory in medication adherence: a review of an emerging literature. *Journal of Behavioral Medicine* 35 (1): 47–62.

2 Memory and Occupation Across the Lifespan

Earlier theorists on memory suggested that infants were largely incapable of memory. However, innovative research methods have led to findings that even newborn babies show evidence of remembering complex stimuli presented prior to birth and in the first months of life.

Evidence is offered in this chapter that the task of crawling is linked to memory development as the infant explores their environment. It is also shown that the concept of 'infantile amnesia' has been used to explore the onset of conscious memory in children. In particular, researchers have explored how this may be affected by socio-cultural factors.

The chapter demonstrates that the multicomponent model of working memory, outlined in Chapter 1, can help explain the development of mathematics, reading and writing skills. Conversely, evidence is presented that working memory impairments may underpin some specific learning disorders.

Forms of memory may develop at different rates. For instance, procedural memory may mature earlier than declarative memory, as explained in this chapter. Declarative memory develops throughout childhood and adolescence. However, this may be affected by negative life events.

In addition, the concept of 'relational memory' is introduced. Some authors have argued that episodic and semantic memory, which were covered in Chapter 1, are fundamentally forms of relational memory.

Just as infantile locomotion seems to spur the development of memory, so reduced mobility in older people has been correlated with impaired cognition in later life. This chapter also shows that the different parts of the multicomponent working memory model may be affected in different ways in dementia. In particular, people with Alzheimer's type dementia (ATD) may have difficulty in dual tasks requiring divided attention that depend on the central executive.

Anthropological data shows that cognitive decline may be a general feature of human development after the age of 40. In addition, prospective memory performance may decline with age.

The impact of socio-economic status (SES) on memory performance in children is examined. It is shown that children from lower SES families tend to perform more poorly on tests of memory in a range of domains. This links to research demonstrating neural plasticity in memory-linked brain areas in animals raised in 'enriched environments'. The interaction of SES and risk of dementia is described in depth. Finally, the chapter includes a table showing key aspects of memory development throughout the lifespan.

Memory in Infancy

Up until the 1980s, the dominant view was that infants up to the age of 2 years dwelt in a world of immediate experience, with no sense of future or past (Bauer et al. 2010). These beliefs were influenced by the work of Piaget, who stressed that the capacity for using symbols was required for representation of items not immediately present to sensation (Bauer et al. 2010).

Such views were also a function of limitations in methods for evaluation of infant memory (Bauer 2002). Bauer et al. (2010) point out that the earlier research on young children's memory had relied on verbally based approaches and, when children were unable to repeat lists of words or pictures at the same level as older children, it was assumed that they were incapable of memorisation. Researchers have now been able to develop techniques that allow valid appraisal of infant memory. Some of these are discussed in this section.

DeCasper and Spence (1986) produced remarkable evidence that learning can take place prior to birth. The first part of their sample was 33 pregnant women in the third trimester of pregnancy, around 7.5 months. Each woman was allocated one of three stories to read to their foetus twice per day. Once the babies were born, 16 infants were eventually included in the study (DeCasper and Spence 1986). The babies were placed in their cradles and provided with an artificial nipple that was attached to apparatus that measured the rate and force of their sucking. A baseline sucking pattern was established for each. The infant then had to exceed this baseline pattern in order to activate a recording of the story that their mother had read to them in utero; if they did not achieve this then they heard a different story (DeCasper and Spence 1986). There were also 12 newborns in a control group who were tested under the same procedure but had not had the stories read to them before birth.

The study found that for the infants who had been read to, the familiar story was significantly more reinforcing of sucking behaviour. Also, it made no difference if the recording was of the baby's mother's voice or that of another woman (DeCasper and Spence 1986). The infants in the control group showed no effect. The authors concluded that the babies must have 'learned and remembered' something about the target stories and speculate that they may have been alert to variables such as the beat of syllables or the temporal sequence of the story (DeCasper and Spence 1986).

Another example of research into memory in infants is the work of Bahrick and Pickens (1995). These researchers conducted a series of experiments testing memory for motion in babies. Their first experiment tested 72 babies, who were required to view a film of cylinders containing marbles moving in an arc pattern. The babies were then shown the film again, alongside another film showing the item moving in a novel pattern. An examiner observed them and recorded each time they fixed their gaze on either of the two screens (Bahrick and Pickens 1995). There were three groups: the first was three months old at testing and was observed one minute after viewing the original film; the second was also three months old and was observed one day after the original viewing;

and the third group was four months old when observed one month after the first viewing. Bahrick and Pickens (1995) found that the infants showed a significant preference for the original film, both at one minute and one month after the initial viewing.

Bahrick and Pickens (1995) conducted a second experiment, in which 74 three-month-old babies initially viewed one of four films, each of which showed one of two different objects moving in a circular or left-to-right horizontal path. The test condition consisted of viewing the film the infant had seen in the initial viewing, alongside a film of the familiar object moving along a previously unseen path. The infants were divided into groups for testing at one minute, one day, two weeks and one month after the initial viewing (Bahrick and Pickens 1995). It was found that, while the babies showed a significant preference for the novel item after one minute, they showed a significant preference for the familiar item one month later (Bahrick and Pickens 1995).

In a third experiment, the procedure was the same as for the second, with the exception that only 16 infants were involved and they were tested three months after the initial viewing, so they were six months old when tested (Bahrick and Pickens 1995). It was found that there was still a significant preference for the familiar stimulus after three months (Bahrick and Pickens 1995). The authors argue that there is therefore evidence that infant memory for motion persists across one to three months. However, they also state that it is not possible, on the basis of their data, to confirm whether this is implicit or declarative memory, or whether such infant memory is equivalent to the long-term memory that emerges in later life (Bahrick and Pickens 1995).

Bauer et al. (2003) conducted research with infants using a 'deferred imitation' approach. This involves showing babies a series of actions using toys and other props and then seeing if they can imitate these after a delay. It is considered to be a test of declarative memory performance in infants (Bauer et al. 2003, 2010; Herbert et al. 2007). In the study, 57 nine-month-olds were shown three action sequences over three sessions. They were tested to see if they recognised the sequences immediately and then one week after the event; their ability to imitate was then tested one month later when they were shown the learned tasks alongside three new tasks. The researchers also recorded event-related potentials (ERPs), providing an electrophysiological measure of brain activity during the experiment (Bauer et al. 2003). After one month, the babies were shown the original action sequences again, alongside three new ones. The researchers found that 46% of the infants were able to perform at least one of the four sequences correctly, and that, from this group, the original sequences were significantly more likely to be performed correctly, which the authors took as evidence of recall memory (Bauer et al. 2003).

The ERP data showed that all infants recalled the original task immediately after presentation. However, after one week it was found that for those infants who subsequently performed at least one sequence correctly a month later, there were significant differences in ERP responses when viewing the original task, as compared to viewing a novel one (Bauer et al. 2003). It was also found that ERPs indicating recognition of the task at one week were significant predictors of ability to recognise the original tasks after one month (Bauer et al. 2003). Overall, the authors maintain that the variance in successful task performance at one month could be explained by differences in storage and consolidation, rather than initial encoding (Bauer et al. 2003). They also suggest that this might be explained by differences in the level of development in the dentate gyrus of the hippocampus, a region that undergoes a great deal of change towards the end of the first year of life (Bauer et al. 2003).

Implicit Memory in Infancy

Another experimental approach to testing memory in infancy is the 'mobile conjugate reinforcement paradigm' (Bauer et al. 2010, p. 157). Here, a mobile is placed above the infant's cot. The mobile can be activated by pulling on a ribbon that is attached to the baby's leg. The baby learns over a few minutes that they can operate it by kicking their leg. The mobile and ribbon are then removed, but the mobile is returned after a delay; if the baby's kicking is now above that recorded at baseline this is taken as evidence of memory (Bauer et al. 2010). It has been found that infants at two months old remember the mobile for as many as three days and at six months old for as many as fourteen days (Bauer et al. 2010). These memories are highly specific: babies between two and three months old, for example, fail to remember if even a small detail of the mobile or cot is changed. This inflexibility suggests that this is a form of implicit rather than declarative memory (Bauer et al. 2010).

Ecological Model of Infant Memory: The Task of Crawling and the Development of Memory

A key theme in conceptual practice models developed by occupational therapy theorists is the conception of humans as dynamic open systems that change through time and both shape, and are shaped by, the environment (Howe and Briggs 1982; Kielhofner 1995; Case-Smith and O'Brien 2009; Law et al. 1996). This 'reciprocity' (Bronfenbrenner 1977, p. 519) between the person, their occupations and the environment is instantiated as the infant starts to crawl from around seven months (Sharma and Cockerill 2014).

Crawling is an example of a motor 'transition' in the person's life (Case-Smith in Case-Smith and O'Brien, 2009, p. 46). Here, there is mutually reinforcing motor development, cognition and exploration of the environment (O'Brien and Williams in Case-Smith and O'Brien 2009). Researchers have examined the impact of this transition on learning and memory and some of this work is discussed in this section.

Herbert et al. (2007) were interested in exploring the impact of crawling on deferred retention. The authors state that learning in this paradigm is marked by the same specificity found in other aspects of memory in babies: if one aspect of the stimulus or context changes, then six-month-old infants cannot imitate after the delay, although this specificity declines with age, and at one year babies can demonstrate deferred imitation in a different context to the original learning (Herbert et al. 2007).

These authors deployed the technique of deferred imitation (Herbert et al. 2007, p. 184). In their study, 64 nine-month-old babies, both crawling and non-crawling, observed the demonstrator performing a task in which pressing a button on a toy cow or duck produced a 'moo' or 'quack' sound, respectively. The babies were then assigned to one of two groups: deferred imitation where the demonstration stimulus and context were the same; and deferred imitation where the demonstration stimulus and context were changed. While all infants demonstrated retention when the demonstration stimulus and context were the same, only those who were crawling demonstrated retention when the stimulus and context were different. The authors concluded that the onset of crawling is linked to greater flexibility in memory retrieval. They suggest that the increased experiences the infant has as a result of autonomous locomotion propel their cognitive skills to a higher level (Herbert et al. 2007).

The links between infant locomotor ability and spatial memory were investigated by Clearfield (2004). In an initial experiment, babies were divided into three groups: 8-month-old beginning crawlers; 11-month-old crawling experts; and 14-month-old walkers (Clearfield 2004). An adapted version of the Morris water maze task was used, in which the infants were placed in an octagonal arena. The child's mother was located in another part of the arena and the child, after viewing their mother's location, was turned to face another segment of the arena. The mother would then hide and the baby's task was to find where she was hidden (Clearfield 2004).

Overall, 8-month-olds had significantly less success than 12- or 14-month-olds. However, it was also found that the experience of both forms of locomotion had an effect, meaning that infants with six weeks or less experience of walking *or* crawling could not find their mothers and all 8-month-olds with less than seven weeks of crawling experience failed to find their mothers.

In a second experiment, another sample of infants was divided into the same groups as for the first experiment (Clearfield 2004). The procedure was the same, except this time a visual cue was placed at the mother's location before she hid (Clearfield 2004). The results were similar to experiment one: the 8-month-olds had significantly less success, while those with six weeks or less experience of walking or crawling failed to find their parent.

Clearfield (2004) argues that the results as outlined suggest that spatial memory and learning do not consist of abstract concepts held in the brain, but develop as we move through our environment. Further, she suggests that the 'soft assembly' of memory, locomotion capability and perception underpins the behaviour needed to complete the task, and that this is an example of 'embodied cognition', whereby the required knowledge is put together during task performance (Clearfield 2004, pp. 236, 239). This would explain why one component of the 'soft assembly', namely experience of crawling or walking, could disrupt task performance at different developmental stages (Clearfield 2004). Overall, the results of this study and that of Herbert et al. (2007) provide evidence that supports occupational therapists' dynamical systems approaches to analysing the interaction of learning and memory, occupation and the environment.

Autobiographical Memory in Infants

Infantile Amnesia

Autobiographical memory is memory for particular events and for information relating to oneself (Baddeley 2015). It draws on both semantic memory, for example knowledge of an address we once lived at, and episodic memory, for example memory of a specific event from school (Baddeley 2015). The term 'infantile amnesia' refers to the episodic aspect of autobiographical memory, and was first used by Freud (1991, p. 315) to describe the phenomenon of people having 'a few unintelligible and fragmentary recollections' of life events from before 6–8 years old. In keeping with his psychoanalytic perspective, he remarked that this occurred not because of incapacity to remember, as children otherwise show evidence of cognitive and affective ability, but from the 'repression' of memories of the 'sexual impulses of childhood' (Freud 1991, pp. 315–316). Later accounts of infantile amnesia stressed that young children were unable to reliably encode, store and retrieve information because they lacked language capability and were unable to form 'mental representations' (Pillemer 1998; Bauer 2002, p. 127; Bauer et al. 2003). Pillemer (1998), for example, argues that amnesia occurs because the child does not have the cognitive or linguistic skill to understand events and integrate them into a life narrative schema.

The age of onset of infantile amnesia has also been revised, with more contemporary authors suggesting that our earliest memories are from around 3–4 years of age and that even major life events are rarely remembered if they occur before 2 years of age (Pillemer 1998). In addition, what is remembered becomes vaguer the further back the events occurred, with memories from before 2 years old being less detailed than those from 3 years, and those from 3 years being less detailed than those from 4 or 5 years old (Bauer et al. 2010; Pillemer 1998). This strengthening of autobiographical detail in the pre-school child's memory results in an enhanced sense of themselves in time, as a person with a past and a future (Bauer et al. 2010). It is also recognised that there is considerable interindividual variability in the age of onset of infantile amnesia (Pillemer 1998). Research has focused on explaining this variability and some of the findings have relevance for occupational therapy practice and theory. These are explored in this section.

The social environment has an impact on children's memory development (Bauer et al. 2010). Pillemer (1998) argues, for example, that a key factor is children's conversations with their parents about the past at around 2 years old and that adults offer cues that aid this development, facilitating autobiographical memory. One variable here is the *way* in which parents involve their children in talk about the past; parents who give rich and detailed descriptions are said to use an 'elaborative' style and those who simply ask limited factual questions are said to have a 'restrictive' or 'low elaborative' style (Bauer et al. 2010, p. 167).

Bauer et al. (2010, p. 167) suggest that, from a 'social-constructivist' position, the elaborative style provides children with a framework of narrative into which details of an event can be placed. The development of this framework also allows children to build their own individual history, the foundation of 'autobiographical memory' (Bauer et al. 2010, p. 167).

In experiments where mothers of children aged between 20 and 29 months have been instructed to provide more elaborate memory narratives, it was found that the children subsequently gave more detailed and full accounts of personal incidents than those in a control group (Bauer et al. 2010). In 3-year-old children from backgrounds with few economic resources, similar effects have been found up to one year after the training (Bauer et al. 2010). Furthermore, it has been found that the relationship quality between parent and child affects the degree of elaboration (Bauer et al. 2010).

The child's sex has also been identified as a factor in autobiographical memory, with parents tending to use more emotional language with girls in conversations about the past; it has also been found that girls tend to give more complex and complete personal narratives than boys in the same age groups and that women's earliest memories tend to date back further than men's (Bauer et al. 2010). In addition, it has been found that adolescents with mothers who used a more elaborative style when they were younger tended to report earlier primary memories, with a mean of 2.7 years, compared to those whose mothers used a more restrictive style, who had a mean of around 3.33 years (Bauer et al. 2010). These findings support occupational therapists' emphasis on reciprocity between the person, environment and occupation as being crucial in human development (Law et al. 1996; Wilcock 2006).

Reese et al. (1993) evaluated the reminiscence styles of 19 mother–child dyads. Measurements were taken at four points in the child's life: at 50, 46, 58 and 70 months old. The mothers were directed to discuss three shared memory events. Analysis of the transcribed conversations was used to identify 'elaborations', moments when the mother progressed to a theme related to the initial memory or asked their child a question in order to elicit further information about the event; or 'repetitions', where the mother's questions drew a response from the child but added no new information (Reese et al. 1993). In addition, children's utterances were classed as 'memory responses', where they shifted the conversation to a different aspect of the reminiscence or added information about the event; or 'memory placeholders', where children simply reiterated earlier statements and provided nothing new (Reese et al. 1993).

It was found that children of mothers who used many elaborations provided significantly more memory responses than memory placeholders, whereas there was no difference in the quantity of memory responses or placeholders for children whose mothers provided few elaborations (Reese et al. 1993). The study also revealed that there was a significant positive correlation between the number of elaborations given by mothers at 40 months and children's memory responses at 58 and 70 months (Reese et al. 1993). Furthermore, the sole predictor of the amount of children's memory responses at 70 months was the quantity of such responses at 58 months. The authors argue, therefore, that it was the mothers' elaborations that were shaping this later behaviour (Reese et al. 1993).

Reese et al. (1993) also noted that, at 58 and 70 months, the relationship works both ways, as more memory responses from the child elicit more elaborations from the mother. They also found a sex imbalance, in that mothers made more elaborative interactions with girls and girls subsequently provided significantly higher numbers of memory responses at 58 and 70 months (Reese et al. 1993). The authors argue that a key conclusion of their study is that mothers and their children create memories together and that the elaborative mothers collaborated with their children in this regard (Reese et al. 1993).

Wang (2003) offers a definition of autobiographical memory as memory relating to the self that is expressible in spoken or written language as a result of intentional recall; infantile amnesia, then, describes a state in which these memories are no longer accessible linguistically. Wang (2003) comments on the usefulness of comparing North American and East Asian children, arguing that the long-standing religious, political and philosophical variations between the two regions lead to marked contrasts in social behaviour, emotion and cognition. In this sense, cross-cultural studies of infantile amnesia are a powerful way of assessing the impact of environment on children's memory.

Wang (2003) notes differences in the age of onset of infantile amnesia between white American, European and East Asian children, with children from the first two groups reporting their earliest memories dating from 3.5 years old, which is six months earlier than Chinese or Korean children. In addition, this author reports that American children's earliest memories are often elaborate, specific and focused on themselves, while Chinese children's earliest recollections are often 'skeletal, generic, centred on relationships and emotionally unexpressive' (Wang 2003, p. 65).

Wang (2003) outlines five potential explanations for infantile amnesia. First, it is argued that the mental equipment required for adult social roles cannot accommodate the 'memory schemata' of young children, meaning that these early memories are inaccessible, while the development of adult cognitive functions affects perception, sensation, language and emotion. Wang (2003) draws on evidence about differences in North American middle-class families' approaches to child rearing and those of Chinese families. In the former, she argues, the child is considered to have agency from birth, while in the latter the child is not considered to have autonomy until around 4–6 years old; prior to this the child is in an 'age of innocence', while after this they are subject to strict discipline in preparation for their social and family roles (Wang 2003, p. 68). It may be, she suggests, that this leads to an abrupt break in cognitive function and could explain the more marked amnesia for early memories found in Chinese children. In addition, the author presents evidence that children who have migrated and have adapted to a new culture, for example from China or Hispanic countries to the United States, report earliest memories from 12 to 17 months later when compared to 'monocultural' children from these backgrounds, suggesting that the shift in culture makes older memories harder to access (Wang 2003, p. 68).

A second explanation centres on the development between 18 and 24 months of a 'cognitive self' that allows categorisation of experience into things that have happened to 'me' and facilitates the person's awareness that they have particular cognitive capabilities (Gathercole and Hitch 1993; Wang 2003, p. 69). From this perspective, earlier memories cannot be integrated into the person's autobiography and therefore cannot be accessed. Wang (2003) suggests, however, that, in addition to this sense of self, the social influences on the child, such as their interaction with parents, is of great importance for autobiographical memory. In addition, she argues that East Asian culture tends to define the self in relation to the wider society, as opposed to the more individualistic definition of Western culture, and that this also explains the differences in the earliest autobiographical memories between children from these societies described earlier (Wang 2003).

Third is the argument that parent–child interactions give children the narrative skills that underpin autobiographical memory and that events occurring before these skills emerge are inaccessible (Wang 2003). Wang (2003) presents evidence that American mothers tend to involve their 3-year-old children in elaborate discussions of past events, while Chinese mothers tend to ask their 3-year-olds about the past in order to elicit factual responses without further elaboration. In addition, American parents tend to explore the child's feelings, views and roles in co-narration about the past, while East Asian parents use these conversations to reinforce social mores and expectations, which she describes as being in line with 'Confucian ethics' (Wang 2003, p. 72). These differences are then reflected in children's descriptions of autobiographical memories.

A fourth, functional explanation of childhood amnesia suggests that memories that do not fit and serve adult schemata may be forgotten or 'reconstructed' in such a way that they become useful for the person (Wang 2003, p. 72). Wang (2003) also stresses that autobiographical memory may develop in ways that are functional to Western societies, which, she argues, emphasise individual autonomy, and to East Asian cultures, which, she suggests, place importance on the self in relation to others. In the former, memories may be elaborate and orientated to the self; in the latter, they may be more generic and focused on social convention (Wang 2003). In addition, autobiographical memory acquisition and style may be a function of identity formation in these societies, with Western culture valuing individual life stories, and East Asian culture stressing that identity is linked to membership of a social group, while these differing uses of memory may also lead to contrasting narrative styles when retelling the past (Wang 2003).

Finally, it may be the case that societies characterised by stability and predictability rather than excitement and change may actually provide their members with less to remember (Wang 2003). Wang (2003, p. 74) cites evidence that urban Chinese children can recall their earliest memories as dating back one year earlier than children raised in the country, and argues that the 'repose and redundancy associated with the countryside . . . render a life with boredom and no story'. (Compare this with writers in the English Romantic tradition, such as Wordsworth, who provide accounts of rural childhood memories that are full of precisely observed and dramatic detail.) The author also comments that social and economic changes in China may lead to more similarity in the earliest age of memory in Chinese and American children (Wang 2003, p. 74). The impact of social and economic factors on memory development is expored in Box 2.1.

Wang (2003) argues that the culture of a particular society gives a shared meaning system that shapes participation in life happenings, as well as interpretation and subsequent remembering and recounting of those events. Furthermore, she maintains that these 'cultural models' will affect the encoding, reconstruction and narration of these memories at the point of retrieval (Wang 2003, p. 76). In addition, the representation and narration of memories are interconnected, so that each retelling of memory 'rewrites' the original memory trace (Wang 2003, p. 77). In relation to East Asia, Wang (2003) suggests

BOX 2.1   OCCUPATIONAL DEPRIVATION, OCCUPATIONAL JUSTICE AND THE DEVELOPMENT OF MEMORY

The effect of 'occupational deprivation' (Wilcock 2006, p. 164) on human development has been a concern of occupational therapy theorists. Similarly, the impact of inequality on brain and memory development has been a focus for researchers from different scientific backgrounds. In this section, we look at research on how these factors affect memory in children and also on the incidence of dementia in older people.

Hackman and Farah (2009) reviewed research on the impact of SES and brain development. They identified evidence that infants from lower SES backgrounds performed worse on working memory. In addition, they found that middle-school children in the United States, equivalent to years seven to nine in the United Kingdom, showed decrements in memory, working memory and cognitive control tasks that were related to lower SES (Hackman and Farah 2009). Furthermore, the authors refer to their own research using fMRI showing that children between 6 and 9 years old from lower SES backgrounds had a strong positive relation between levels of activation in the left fusiform gyrus and phonological awareness, which is the capacity to recognise spoken aspects of a sentence, such as rhyming and alliteration, a relationship not present in children from higher SES backgrounds (Hackman and Farah 2009). The authors suggest that more affluent children may be 'buffered' by being raised in a more enriched environment, presumably meaning that less brain activity is needed to perform these tasks.

Hackman and Farah (2009) maintain that, while the bulk of psychology research participants are from middle SES backgrounds, some researchers have manipulated the power and status of their sample as part of the research design. These studies show that reduced power is linked to impaired attention, making it harder to focus and ignore distraction (Hackman and Farah 2009). The authors point to analogies with the well-documented social gradient in general health status and suggest that the higher stress levels that may be linked to lower SES can affect brain development. In particular, it has been found that stress levels can have an impact on the development of the hippocampus and the prefrontal cortex (Hackman and Farah 2009; Wilkinson and Pickett 2010). Hackman and Farah 2009 also suggest that cognitive performance is shaped by epigenetic factors, meaning that the expression of specific genes is linked to environmental influences.

Researchers have found that in the United States, socio-economic disparities between Black and white people explained much of the higher risk for dementia among older Black people (Yaffe et al. 2013). It is therefore of interest that Farah et al. (2006) conducted a study comparing the performance of 30 African American children from low SES backgrounds with 30 African American children from middle SES families. Both groups had a mean age of 11.7 years. Representative employment of parents of low SES included working in nail bars or healthcare assistants, while that of middle SES parents included owning small businesses or working as a 'surgical technician' (Farah et al. 2006, p. 170).

Farah et al. (2006) administered a battery of cognitive tests and found significantly different scores for tests of working memory known to be underpinned by lateral prefrontal activity, while the strongest effect was found for memory tasks supported by the medial temporal system. Children of middle SES scored higher than low SES children in both cases. The authors suggest that one reason for this disparity may be the relatively greater enriched environments of middle SES children, which could include more access to toys and books and visits to more locations (Farah et al. 2006). In addition, they emphasise the point made earlier that higher levels of stress, which may be experienced more in low SES homes, can influence development of the hippocampus and memory capacity (Farah et al. 2006).

that the industrial transformation occurring in these societies and the concomitant spread of Western influence may lead to changes in autobiographical memory.

Wang et al. (2000) conducted research with 41 mother–child dyads: 21 were white American, with an average child age of 3.3 years, and 20 were Chinese, with an average child age of 3.4 years. The mother was asked to talk to her child about any shared incident that had taken place in the previous month and also discuss a picture book story. The conversations were recorded and the transcripts were coded. Codes included a number of categories. 'Elaborations' indicated where mother or child shifted the conversation onto a new facet of the event or provided extra information about it. 'Repetitions' occurred where the theme was repeated with no new information added. 'Evaluations' negated or gave confirmation to an earlier statement. 'Affect' indicated emotional responses. 'Didactic' comments occurred where the mother or child used the topic to talk about expected social norms and moral principles. 'Autonomy' encompassed statements about the child's needs, opinions or preferences. Finally, 'metacognitive' statements related to knowing, remembering and cognitive capability (Wang et al. 2000, p. 163).

The researchers found that American mothers made significantly more evaluative and autonomy comments, while Chinese mothers made significantly more didactic comments (Wang et al. 2000). There was no difference in the mothers' use of elaborations; however, it was found that American children made significantly more elaborative comments and also significantly more statements of autonomy (Wang et al. 2000). In addition, there were significant positive correlations between American children's and mothers' elaborative responses and Chinese mothers' and children's repetition responses. The authors suggest that these correlations indicate that mothers from different cultures create differing 'narrative environments' for their children when talking about the past (Wang et al. 2000).

These authors argue that the differences in conversation reflect different cultural functions of autobiographical memory. The American style was focused on autonomy and autobiography, while the Chinese style functioned to reinforce behavioural expectations and connection to the wider community (Wang et al. 2000). It is, perhaps, important to take into account that this study used a comparatively small sample and also that no differences were found in the amount of elaboration used by mothers from either culture. However, the results provide some support for the notion that environment has an impact on children's memory development.

Wang et al. (2007) tested this hypothesis further. They took a sample of 101 university students from the United States, 104 from England and 97 from China. The participants were given five minutes to write down as many memories as they could from 5 years old and under. They were also required to rate the memories on a number of dimensions, including the source of the memory; that is, whether they actually experienced it or learnt about it from another (Wang et al. 2007).

It was found that there were significant differences in the numbers of memories recalled between US and Chinese students, English and Chinese students, and English and US students. Overall, students from the United States had more memories, English students fewer and Chinese students the fewest (Wang et al. 2007). In addition, the earliest age for first memories that were not derived from others differed, with an average of 32.37 months for US students, 31 months for English and 37.6 months for Chinese. Again, these differences were statistically significant. It is worth noting, however, while that the authors argue that England falls somewhere between China and the United States in terms of cultural stress on personal autonomy, their results show that English students were able to remember further back than US students, which partially contradicts their hypothesis. The authors also found that women across all cultures produced significantly more memories than men, and relate this to the evidence discussed earlier that parents tend to engage in more elaborate memory talk with girls (Wang et al. 2007). In conclusion, the authors argue that, since factors such as language development, the emergence of a cognitive self and brain development are fairly invariant, then the differing results are related to cultural factors, notably an emphasis in Chinese culture on 'community' and 'dependence' and in the United States a focus on autonomy and 'agency' (Wang et al. 2007).

Episodic Memory in Children

Other researchers have focused on the emergence of episodic autobiographical memory in children. Pillemer et al. (1994) investigated the memory capacity of groups of children with a mean age of 3.5 or 4.5 years. A fire alarm had gone off in the child study centre that the children were working in and they were initially questioned about their memories of this two weeks later. The questions focused on areas such as their ongoing activities when the emergency occurred, where they were at the time and so on (Pillemer et al. 1994). It will be recalled that research shows that earliest memories can be dated to around 3.5 years (Pillemer et al. 1994).

Pillemer et al. (1994) found that the 4.5-year-old group gave richer and more accurate descriptions of the event, with greater appreciation of causality. For example, 95% of the older group correctly placed themselves inside the building when the alarm went off, compared with 55% of the younger children (Pillemer et al. 1994). Moreover, 75% of the older children talked about the feeling of urgency on evacuation, but only 33% of 3.5-year-olds did so, while 44% of the 4.5-year-olds mentioned, unprompted, the reasons the alarm had gone off, compared with only one 3.5-year-old (Pillemer et al. 1994).

Seven years later, 12 of the 3.5-year-old group and 16 of the 4.5-year-old group were interviewed about their memories of the event (Pillemer et al. 1994). It was found that 82% of the younger children were unable to provide even a 'fragmentary memory' of the event, while 57% of the older children were able to (Pillemer et al. 1994). When given a forced choice, 86% of the older children correctly identified the location and only 54% of the younger children did so (Pillemer et al. 1994). The authors do not use the term episodic memory, but it would be fair to conclude that the older group was more likely to have richer episodic memories of the event.

Hamond and Fivush (1991) investigated young children's memories of a trip to Disneyworld. There were 48 children divided into two groups: the younger group had a mean age of 37 months, the older group a mean age of 49 months. The children were interviewed either 6 months after the trip or 18 months after. This meant that younger children interviewed 6 months after were an average of 44 months old when interviewed and those interviewed 18 months after were an average of 54 months old when interviewed. Meanwhile, older children interviewed 6 months after were, on average, 55 months old and those interviewed 18 months after were an average of 66 months old (Hamond and Fivush 1991).

Hamond and Fivush (1991, pp. 437, 439) classed the children's responses as 'propositions', such as 'I saw Mickey Mouse', or 'elaborations', which were adjectives or adverbs, for example a statement that a child saw 'big Dumbos' counted as one proposition and one elaboration (Hamond and Fivush 1991, pp. 437, 439). Adult carers were also interviewed in order to provide a detailed account of what had happened. In addition, the adults were asked to rate how much they talked to their children about the visit (Hamond and Fivush 1991). One unanticipated result was that neither the age of the children nor the length of time since the visit made any difference to the general results: all children recalled about 40 propositions (Hamond and Fivush 1991). It was found, however, that older children included significantly more elaborations in their descriptions (Hamond and Fivush 1991). Also, all children were significantly more likely to include information spontaneously 6 months after the visit than 18 months later (Hamond and Fivush 1991). It was noted, in addition, that children who talked with their families more about the trip subsequently gave more information in the interview, although this result did not reach significance (Hamond and Fivush 1991). The authors argue that older children's enhanced ability to recall information spontaneously may be a function of greater retrieval ability, while their greater use of elaborations may indicate improved retrieval or greater verbal capacity (Hamond and Fivush 1991).

Source Memory and Infantile Amnesia

'Source memory' refers to the ability to remember the origin of learned information (Schacter 2008). Drummey and Newcombe (2002) argue that episodic memory and autonoetic consciousness (discussed in Chapter 1) are important components of autobiographical memory, and a corollary of this is the importance of recognising the source of the memory, for example in relation to where and when the event occurred. Furthermore, since infantile amnesia concerns episodic memory, findings about source memory should give insight into the phenomenon (Drummey and Newcombe 2002).

Drummey and Newcombe (2002) investigated the presence of source memory in 4-, 6- and 8-year-old children. They gave 167 children a series of facts to remember that were presented either by the experimenter directly, or via a puppet. One week later the children were tested on their memory of the facts and also asked where they had learnt them from.

A stable increase in fact retention was noted as the children's age increased, indicating a steady improvement in semantic memory with age (Drummey and Newcombe 2002). However, 4-year-olds showed significantly poorer performance than 6- and 8-year-olds in the source memory task, and 60% of their errors involved attribution to sources such as parents or teachers, who were not even involved in the experiment. However, there was no difference in source memory performance between 6- and 8-year-olds, suggesting a sudden change in source memory between 4 and 6 years old (Drummey and Newcombe 2002).

The researchers posit that the errors in source memory prior to this age may underpin infantile amnesia (Drummey and Newcombe 2002). In addition, they present evidence that source memory may be reliant on the prefrontal cortex, and also that this region is still developing throughout childhood (Drummey and Newcombe 2002). The immaturity of this region may, therefore, contribute to infantile amnesia (Drummey and Newcombe 2002).

Working Memory from Ages 5 to 12

Working memory in childhood is a major concern for occupational therapists working in paediatrics. For example, in school, phonological working memory underpins the ability to follow complex instructions, recall lists of similar-sounding words and remember and write complex sentences and paragraphs (Alloway and Alloway 2015). Visual–spatial working memory is essential for mental arithmetic, completing number sequences or telling a story using pictures (Alloway and Alloway 2015). Some more examples are discussed in this section.

Multiplication tables are taught in schools so as to be embedded in long-term memory. When working on a multiplication problem, the child needs to extract this information from the long-term store for support. At the same time, they need to grasp place-value in order to understand the value of the individual digits in the numbers included in the multiplication problem written in the book, which requires visuospatial processing (Luria 1973). So the child needs to work with items from long-term memory and the visuospatial sketchpad simultaneously to solve the problem. Similarly, reading is taught in English schools via phonics, which is based on the *sounds* of letters. However, some words, for example 'night', are not phonetic and the child is required to commit these to long-term memory as part of a bank of 'tricky words'. Here, the child needs to retrieve these 'tricky words' from the long-term store at the same time as using the phonological loop while reading. In addition, working memory is one of the cognitive abilities underpinning handwriting skills (Schneck and Case-Smith 2015).

Working memory impairments may affect the child's ability to learn. Visual–spatial working memory problems in particular are a feature of attention deficit/hyperactivity disorder (Hilton 2015; Alloway and Alloway 2015). In addition, problems with phonological working memory have a role in dyslexia, as the child may have difficulty remembering and simultaneously processing spoken or written instructions (Alloway and Alloway 2015). Similarly, visual–spatial working memory impairments may lead to dyscalculia, as the child may be unable to draw on long-term memory items, for example of multiplication tables, in order to solve problems in the 'mental workspace' afforded by the working memory system (Alloway and Alloway 2015). A clear understanding of this memory system is therefore vital for occupational therapists. Two pieces of large-scale research that focused on clarifying aspects of the multicomponent working memory model in school-aged children are described in some detail here.

Gathercole et al. (2004) conducted an experiment with two aims. First, they wished to investigate whether the developmental improvements in performance on tasks linked to separate working memory subsystems occurred at the same rate. Second, they wanted to know if the structure of working memory changes throughout childhood (Gathercole et al. 2004). They pointed out, for example, that some evidence suggests that the phonological loop and visuospatial sketchpad may not be clearly demarcated in very young children; rather, task performance in these areas may be facilitated by the central executive (Gathercole et al. 2004).

It may be the case, therefore, that the multicomponent system with distinct domains may be in place only later in development (Gathercole et al. 2004). On the other hand, it could be that the central executive plays an increasingly important role in supporting the phonological loop and visuospatial sketchpad throughout childhood and adolescence, as the frontal brain regions supporting executive processes mature (Gathercole et al. 2004). This may mean, for example, that the connection between ratings of central executive and subsystem functions may strengthen with development; alternatively, an independent central executive may only fully emerge in later childhood, with young children relying more on domain-specific subsystems (Gathercole et al. 2004).

Gathercole et al. (2004) tested over 700 children from 4 to 15 years old using tasks thought to tap the different domains of the multicomponent model. Three tasks assessed phonological storage and three complex memory, which involved simultaneous storage and processing (Gathercole et al. 2004). An example of a complex memory task is listening recall: children were required to judge the truth or falsehood of a series of sentences and then state the last item mentioned in each sentence in the correct order (Gathercole et al. 2004). The assumption was that complex memory tasks implicate both the central executive for processing and the phonological loop for storage (Gathercole et al. 2004). A further three tasks tested the separate visual and spatial holding capacity of the visuospatial sketchpad (Gathercole et al. 2004).

Gathercole et al. (2004) found a linear improvement on all tests from 4 to 15 years, with performance evening out between 14 and 15 years of age. One exception was a test of memory for visual patterns, where there was a dip in performance at 11 years, followed by a slight rise at 14 and 15 years (Gathercole et al. 2004). The authors tested the degree to which their data fitted with the three-part multicomponent model as compared to a two-part model consisting of a verbal holding and more complex verbal performance component (Gathercole et al. 2004). The data for 4- and 5-year-olds was excluded from this analysis as they had only been tested on one complex memory task, and there was therefore insufficient data (Gathercole et al. 2004).

Gathercole et al. (2004) found that the three-part model fitted the data best, and that the fit was statistically significant for all of the age groups from 6 to 15 (Gathercole et al. 2004). The two-part model, on the other hand, differed significantly from the data. In addition, the authors argue that this close fit for the three-part model could not be explained by the surface similarity of the tasks, but by the underlying cognitive capacities underpinning task performance (Gathercole et al. 2004). For example, the visuospatial tasks involved both tapping blocks and tracing mazes, which were very different, and yet the data fitted to the factor in the model associated with the visuospatial sketchpad (Gathercole et al. 2004).

They noted, in addition, the weaker connections between the visuospatial and phonological aspects that they found both fitted with the predictions made in the multicomponent model and also provided evidence that the neural mechanisms underlying these components are anatomically distinct (Gathercole et al. 2004). The researchers established too that the factor in their analysis that was equivalent to the central executive connected closely with the visuospatial and phonological factors, as would be predicted by the multicomponent model (Gathercole et al. 2004).

Overall, Gathercole et al. (2004) argued that their findings show that the segments of the multicomponent model are present by the age of 6 years and that there is a linear expansion of capacity in these components from 4 to 15 years. In addition, they state that, while the visuospatial and phonological components are fairly independent, the central executive maintains a closer relationship with both, and that this arrangement is maintained throughout child development (Gathercole et al. 2004).

Alloway et al. (2006) report results from tests carried out on 708 children with an age range from 4 to 11 years. The authors had two aims: first, to examine the structure of verbal and visuospatial working memory in this age group; second, to test a model of working memory in which a non-domain-specific central executive controls and monitors separate domain-specific visuospatial and verbal components, as predicted in the multicomponent working memory model (Alloway et al. 2006).

Twelve tests from the Automated Working Memory Assessment (AWMA) were used (Alloway and Alloway 2015). Six of the tests required simultaneous storage and processing and were regarded by the authors as tests of working memory (Alloway et al. 2006). An example is the 'odd one out' test, in which the child had to identify an odd shape in a series of arrays, and then, at the end of the sequence, indicate the location of each odd shape and also the order in which it was presented (Alloway et al. 2006, p. 1703). The other six tests involved only storage of verbal or visual material and were regarded as short-term memory tests only (Alloway et al. 2006).

Four different models were tested using confirmatory factor analysis. The authors found that the scores for both the working memory and short-term memory tasks increased consistently throughout the age span, and argue that this shows that the components of the multicomponent model are in place from the age of 4 years (Alloway et al. 2006). They also found that the multicomponent model made the best fit with the data (Alloway et al. 2006). In addition, there was a stronger connection between the non-domain-specific construct in the model and the domain-specific visuospatial construct in the 4–6-year-old children, suggesting that this age group relied more on executive functions when performing visuospatial tasks (Alloway et al. 2006). The authors propose that this is an example of 'developmental fractionation', meaning that the apparatuses underpinning cognition can develop at different tempos (Alloway et al. 2006, p. 1713; Pickering et al. 2001). On the basis of this evidence, it seems that the different elements of the multicomponent working memory model are present in school-aged children, suggesting that occupational therapists working with this population should be familiar with the model and its implications for occupational performance.

Another insight from this research is that visuospatial tasks may be 'static' or 'dynamic' in nature (Alloway et al. 2006, p. 1713). Dynamic visuospatial tasks require active perceptual and motor tracking of stimuli and may require more central executive resources in the 4–6-year-old group (Alloway et al. 2006). An example of a dynamic spatial task is the Corsi block test, in which the person is required to recall sequences of increasing numbers of taps on identical blocks, while a static task example is the visual patterns test, in which the participants are required to recall patterns of shaded squares on a matrix (Alloway et al. 2006).

Pickering et al. (2001) presented visual pattern tasks to children in static and dynamic formats. In the static condition, the child was shown a matrix with some squares filled in in black. They were then shown a blank copy of the matrix and asked to indicate the location of the filled-in squares from the previously viewed matrix. The number of filled-in squares increased with each trial (Pickering et al. 2001). In the dynamic task, the matrix was presented on a computer screen and squares were filled in one after the other for half a second each; the child was then asked to indicate the sequence in which they had been filled in (Pickering et al. 2001). Children scored significantly better on the static task, indicating that the dynamic task was more taxing (Pickering et al. 2001). For occupational therapists working with children with working memory impairments, it may therefore be important to consider whether the tasks are static or dynamic in nature, as part of task and activity analysis.

The phonological storage component of the phonological loop appears to be developed between 3 and 5 years of age (Gathercole and Hitch 1993). However, the articulatory rehearsal mechanism of the loop is not developed until around 7 years old (Gathercole and Hitch 1993). Despite this, the visuospatial sketchpad appears to be functioning in younger children, as they are able to remember items that are associated with a visual image (Gathercole and Hitch 1993). However, 5-year-olds rely more on the visuospatial sketchpad to support immediate visual memory than older children, while 10-year-olds are able to recode items phonologically to support memory (Gathercole and Hitch 1993). These areas are explored further in Chapter 5.

Development of Declarative and Procedural Memory

Bauer et al. (2010, p. 155) explain that memory systems can be classed as 'declarative' or 'non-declarative'. Declarative memory involves explicit knowledge of dates, places, names and other facts about the world. Non-declarative memory encompasses skills that do not require conscious awareness and also the capacity to learn new abilities (Bauer et al. 2010). Non-declarative learning is manifest through changed behaviour or skilled performance in the absence of the person being aware of the events leading to this change (Bauer et al. 2010).

Brain areas that underpin non-declarative memory include the neocortex, the cerebellum, and the striatum, all of which were discussed in Chapter 1. These areas mature at an early stage, meaning that non-declarative memory can also develop early in the child's life (Bauer et al. 2010). Declarative memory, however, depends on areas such as the medial temporal lobe and other cortical regions, also as described in Chapter 1 (Bauer et al. 2010). The medial temporal lobe matures early on, but other cortical regions take longer to develop fully. Bauer et al. (2010) state that the different regions begin to work in concert from about the age of 1 year, but that this process continues to develop over several years, with concomitant changes in declarative memory capacity. In this section, evidence about the development of declarative memory in children is explored.

Flores-Lázaro et al. (2017) argue that children start to develop cognitive learning strategies at around 7 years old and that these develop throughout middle childhood, from 6 to 11 years, reaching an optimum level at about 11 or 12 years old. These strategies can include linking items semantically, which occurs at around 10 years; grouping words so that they are repeated in the same order that they were delivered; and organising words subjectively, for example into things one likes (Flores-Lázaro et al. 2017). The development of these cognitive strategies means that middle childhood is the strongest period for the development of declarative memory, which is in turn associated with improved use of executive function and development of the prefrontal cortex (Flores-Lázaro et al. 2017).

Mabbott et al. (2009) evaluated the relationship between the development of white matter tracts and declarative memory performance in later childhood and adolescence. The authors comment that declarative memory is linked to connectivity between the temporal and prefrontal regions and that the uncinate fasciculus, discussed in Chapter 1, is a key white matter tract facilitating communication between these areas (Mabbott et al. 2009). In addition, declarative memory in infancy, which, as shown earlier, is assessed using novel stimulus preference and recognition tasks, predominantly involves the medial temporal lobe. The more complex declarative memory that emerges from 3 to 7 years old is underpinned by the growth of the temporal lobe and prefrontal cortex, as well as further development of the hippocampus (Mabbott et al. 2009). During late childhood and adolescence, as mentioned earlier, cognitive control processes also advance (Mabbott et al. 2009).

Mabbott et al. (2009) used diffusion tensor imaging (DTI) to examine the uncinate fasciculus as well as other brain regions, including the parietal lobes and cerebellums, of 22 9–15-year-olds (Mabbott et al. 2009). DTI gauges the diffusion of water in tissues and provides a measure of white matter integrity (Mabbott et al. 2009). Visual–perceptual memory performance was also tested using the Rey–Osterrieth complex figure assessment, and auditory–verbal memory was assessed using a cued and free-recall word list test (Mabbott et al. 2009).

Mabbott et al. (2009) made a number of findings. First, they identified age-linked increases in white matter integrity in the frontal, temporal and parietal regions (Mabbott et al. 2009). Second, they found that greater integrity of the left uncinate fasciculus predicted better auditory–verbal memory performance, which they suggest may be a function of increased 'packing' of the white matter strands and also greater levels of myelination, both of which may enhance neural transmission in the fasciculus (Mabbott et al. 2009). Third, higher performance in visual–perceptual memory was predicted by greater integrity in the temporal and occipital white matter bilaterally (Mabbott et al. 2009). The authors suggest that their results point to the importance of white matter tract development in the progress of age-related declarative memory performance (Mabbott et al. 2009).

Another perspective on the role of the hippocampus and declarative memory is concerned with 'relational memory' (Townsend et al. 2010). In this view, declarative memory is seen as involving analysis of the relationships between different memorised items (Eichenbaum 2012). For example, episodic memory requires association of information with a particular time and space, while semantic memory involves integration of items into a matrix of other knowledge (Eichenbaum 2012). Procedural memory, however, is not relational, as there is no requirement to relate it to a specific context or earlier experience (Eichenbaum 2012).

The hippocampus has been found to be crucial to the encoding and retrieving of relational information; people with amnesia following medial temporal lobe lesions have specific difficulties in this area, for example (Townsend et al. 2010). In particular, the hippocampus is thought to be involved in 'allocentric' learning, which is place learning that is independent of the person's viewpoint but depends on the location of objects in external space, as opposed to 'egocentric' learning, which has the person's own location as the reference point (Jeannerod 1988; Townsend et al. 2010, p. 739).

There is an association here with occupation, as children show evidence of basic allocentric place learning at around 16 months, which can be linked to crawling and walking, although mature place learning may not emerge until 5–10 years of age (Townsend et al. 2010). This also aligns with the view that the hippocampus supports the development of 'cognitive maps' and knowledge of spatial relations, linking items and their surroundings (Nadel 1991; Gazzaniga et al. 2009; Townsend et al. 2010; Eichenbaum 2012). The hippocampus has been found to contain 'place cells' indicating an organism's location and the entorhinal cortex is known to contain 'grid cells' that calculate the direction and distance of travel (Schafer and Schiller 2020, p. 32). In that sense the cognitive maps in the hippocampus and entorhinal cortex may also support relational memory (Schafer and Schiller 2020).

Townsend et al. (2010) explored the role of the medial temporal lobe in memory in middle childhood and adulthood with reference to place learning and the application of relational information. They used two tasks. The first was 'place learning', in which the person encodes and then recalls a location in space using awareness of location and distance from landmarks. The second was 'transitive interference', where the participant first views pairs of stimuli and learns by trial and error to recognise the stimulus that takes precedence, following which they view the same stimuli regrouped into different pairs and, on the basis of their learning in the first trial, infer which one takes precedence (Townsend et al. 2010, p. 740).

There were three groups of 30 children, aged 6, 8 and 10 years old; in addition there were two groups of adults: a place learning group with a mean age of 42 years and a transitive interference group with a mean age of 29.5 years (Townsend et al. 2010). Participants were first asked to locate a target hidden in a virtual environment and remember its location. They were then required to relocate the target, navigating from a range of different starting points. In this trial, 6-year-olds were significantly slower than other groups; 8-year-olds were significantly slower than 10-year-olds and adults; and 10-year-olds performed at the same level as adults (Townsend et al. 2010). Following this, landmark cues close to the hidden target were removed, meaning that participants needed to rely on their memory of the environment for navigation. In this second trial, 6- and 8-year-olds were significantly slower than the other groups, while 10-year-olds and adults performed at similar levels, showing an improvement in place learning for the older children (Townsend et al. 2010).

In the second-level transitive interference task, which was based on inference from the first level of learning, it was found that 6- and 8-year-olds performed at the same level as each other and also that there were no significant differences between the 10-year-olds and the adults; in addition, the 6- and 8-year-olds performed significantly worse than the adults (Townsend et al. 2010). This was taken as evidence of an improvement in relational memory in the older children, with performance equivalent to adults (Townsend et al. 2010). The authors suggest that mature, flexible relational memory that allows inferences to be drawn from stimuli may be underpinned by interacting mechanisms in the medial temporal lobe and prefrontal cortex (Townsend et al. 2010).

DiGiulio et al. (1994) conducted an investigation into the development of procedural and declarative memory in children. A sample of 88 children was divided into two groups, one 8 years old and one 12 years old (DiGiulio et al. 1994). The children were tested using 'Gollin figures', which consist of a series of five broken line drawings of familiar objects with progressively more detail added in each picture, the fifth picture being nearly complete (DiGiulio et al. 1994). In addition, they were tested with 'degraded words', which follow the same principle: a series of words is shown with the letters more complete in each successive picture (DiGiulio et al. 1994).

First, the children were shown, and asked to name, the most complete of each of the Gollin figures, the fifth picture in each sequence; this was intended as a 'priming' stage, facilitating subsequent recognition, which is viewed as a form of procedural memory (DiGiulio et al. 1994). They were then shown the incomplete pictures in random order and asked to identify them at different levels of completeness (DiGiulio et al. 1994). Following this, their declarative memory was tested by asking them to remember as many of the pictures as possible, in any order. They were also shown the degraded words at the different levels and asked to identify them.

It was found that the priming effects were similar for both age groups, meaning that prior exposure to the nearly complete Gollin figure gave the same advantage for all children (DiGiulio et al. 1994). The 12-year-old group, however, had significantly different declarative memory scores. The authors present this as evidence that procedural memory develops earlier than declarative. They argue that this is likely to be underpinned by slower maturation of the hippocampus, diencephalon and temporal region, while procedural memory may be supported by cortico-striatal connections (DiGiulio et al. 1994).

Ofen et al. (2007) investigated the role of the prefrontal cortex and the medial temporal lobe in declarative memory in a sample of 49 people, aged 8–24 years. Participants were asked to view pictures of indoor and outdoor scenes while their brains were scanned with functional magnetic resonance imaging (fMRI; Ofen et al. 2007). They then viewed the scenes again, outside the scanner, and the viewed scenes were mixed with others that had not been viewed before. They were asked first to judge which scenes had been previously observed. Second, they were asked to rate these earlier scenes according to whether their memory of them was clear and vivid, or whether the scene was merely familiar to them (Ofen et al. 2007).

Ofen et al. (2007) found that levels of activity in the prefrontal cortex and the medial temporal lobe had been higher for earlier viewed scenes that were later remembered compared with those that were forgotten. The researchers also found significant increases of activity with age in particular prefrontal cortical regions, left Brodmann area (BA) 46 and right BA 9; however, there was no significant correlation between age and brain activity in the medial temporal lobe, including the hippocampus (Ofen et al. 2007). So, formation of memories was linked to age-related activation levels in the prefrontal cortex but not in the medial temporal lobe (Ofen et al. 2007).

Ofen et al. (2007) also found a significant correlation with age-related activation and clear remembering of previously viewed scenes and the number of correct recognition judgements – that is, accurate identification of previously seen and rejection of previously unseen views – that increased significantly with age (Ofen et al. 2007). There was a significant positive correlation between age and recognition accuracy for clearly and vividly remembered views, though this was not the case for the merely familiar. In addition, the number of vivid recognition responses was positively correlated with age (Ofen et al. 2007).

Ofen et al. (2007) comment that their results show that the ability to encode vivid and detailed episodic memories increases with age. They conclude that the development of declarative memory is based on ongoing development of the dorsolateral prefrontal cortex between 8 and 24 years and the medial temporal lobe, which is completely developed by the age of 8 (Ofen et al. 2007, p. 1201).

Finn et al. (2016) point out that, in keeping with the findings outlined here, declarative and working memory abilities develop throughout childhood and early adulthood. They wished to find out if this also applied to procedural memory. They tested 32 children, aged 10, and 29 adults, aged 24, on a series of tasks. Declarative memory was tested via a verbal learning test, while working memory was evaluated using a task where the participants had to remember the order in which a number of targets had appeared as part of different arrays of shapes (Finn et al. 2016). Procedural memory was tested using rotary pursuit, which involved using a stylus to track a rotating target, learning to trace a star in a mirror, learning an artificial grammar and a task whereby the participants learnt to predict a weather scenario by viewing different pairs of cards (Finn et al. 2016).

Finn et al. (2016) found that adults performed significantly better on the declarative and working memory tasks, but that there was no difference in performance on the procedural memory tests (Finn et al. 2016). The authors conclude that, while declarative and working memory continue to develop throughout childhood and early adulthood, procedural memory is already at adult levels by the age of 10 (Finn et al. 2016). They argue that declarative and procedural memory are therefore two distinct systems. In addition, they argue that this dissociation is underpinned by the neural regions involved: declarative memory depends on the medial temporal lobes and structures of the diencephalon, while procedural memory depends on basal nuclei, cerebellum and neocortical regions (Finn et al. 2016).

Environmental Factors Affecting Declarative Memory

Negative and stressful life events may have impacts on the development of the hippocampus and lead to impaired declarative memory performance. Van der Heijden et al. (2011) tested 255 children between 6 and 12 years old on a verbal declarative memory test, the Auditory Verbal Learning Test (AVLT), which tests 'immediate memory span', learning of new material and recognition. They also tested visual declarative memory using the Rey Visual Design Learning Test, and procedural memory using a mirror drawing task. The children's carers were asked to complete a questionnaire on whether the children had experienced negative and stressful events, such as divorce or bereavement.

It was found that children who had experienced negative and stressful events performed on average 9% lower on verbal declarative memory than others (van der Heijden et al. 2011). In addition, experience of these events had a strong negative relation to two scores on AVLT, the total of correctly remembered words over a number of trials, and delayed recall (van der Heijden et al. 2011). However, no relation was noted for non-verbal declarative and procedural memory.

The authors suggest that these results may be explained by impaired hippocampal development, possibly linked to increased cortisol levels at the time when stressful life events were occurring (van der Heijden et al. 2011). They argue that these conclusions are reinforced by the fact that they had controlled for other factors, such as parenting approach and impaired sleep, so that these could not explain the results. The authors adduce evidence from other researchers showing that stress leads to heightened release of cortisol via the hypothalamus–adrenal–pituitary axis, which has been shown to impede plasticity of hippocampal synapses (van der Heijden et al. 2011). In addition, there is evidence that adults who have experienced stressful happenings as children have reduced hippocampal volume and also that adults living with chronic daily stress have impaired performance on memory tasks implicating the hippocampus (van der Heijden et al. 2011). One anomalous finding in this study is that there was no impairment in the performance of non-verbal declarative memory, and the authors admit that there is no clear explanation for this (van der Heijden et al. 2011). Nonetheless, this study appears to confirm that the environment has impacts on both neural and cognitive development, as emphasised in occupational therapy conceptual practice models.

Memory in Adolescence

Development of the Neocortex and Hippocampus

It was noted in Chapter 1 that primary sensory regions of the cerebrum send information to neocortical association areas specialised for vision, audition and somatosensory modalities (Bauer et al. 2007). These association areas then send the information encoded in these modalities to association areas at the limbic–temporal, posterior and anterior parietal regions; these are 'polymodal' in relation to sensory inputs, and are the loci for storage of long-term memory (Bauer et al. 2007, p. 248).

The association regions of the neocortex develop relatively late. For example, most of the neocortex has six distinct layers, but in the association areas these are only clearly present at two months before birth (Bauer et al. 2010).

Another feature of neural development is 'synaptogenesis', the development of new synapses, which takes both before and after birth (Gazzaniga et al. 2009). With maturation these synapses are 'pruned' back, which allows more granular tuning of the nervous system for specialist functions (Gazzaniga et al. 2009).

In the prefrontal cortex, synaptic density increases rapidly from 8 months old, reaching a high point between 15 and 20 months old. The region reaches an adult form at 24 months old; however, further pruning then takes place at puberty, with adult density only being reached in adolescence or early adulthood (Bauer et al. 2007, 2010). Furthermore, myelination in the prefrontal cortex continues into adolescence, while the final complement of some neurotransmitters in the region is not arrived at until one's 20s or 30s (Bauer et al. 2007). Given the role of higher association areas and the prefrontal cortex in declarative and working memory, it should be clear that this later development also has impacts on these memory systems.

It was also shown in Chapter 1 that the hippocampus plays a crucial role in declarative memory. It is therefore important to understand the development of this structure when considering changes in declarative memory with age. This is explored in this section.

The hippocampus matures very early, with most neurons in place prior to birth, while by 6 months the synaptic density and quantity have reached adult levels, as has the level of glucose consumption in the temporal cortex as a whole (Bauer et al. 2007, 2010). However, the dentate gyrus, which connects the cortex and hippocampus, does not reach its adult form until 12–15 months (Bauer et al. 2007, 2010). The dentate gyrus peak synaptic density comes between 16 and 20 months, following which synapses are pruned back, reaching an adult level at around 4–5 years (Bauer et al. 2007, 2010). Overall, these different rates of progress mean that hippocampal development is not complete until around 5 years (Townsend et al. 2010).

The later development of the dentate gyrus may affect memory development. As shown in Chapter 1, inputs from polymodal association areas converge on the entorhinal cortex and are then relayed to the dentate gyrus; this mechanism is the likely underpinning of declarative memory and the immaturity of the dentate may therefore affect this memory system (Bauer et al. 2007).

Bauer et al. (2007) state that these different stages of development make predictions about the growth of declarative memory feasible. First, declarative memory would emerge somewhere at a late stage of the infant's first 12 months, with the augmentation of synaptic density in the dentate and prefrontal regions (Bauer et al. 2007). There would then be dramatic declarative memory development in the following 12 months as synaptogenesis continues from months 20 to 24, and slowed but continuous progress in the following years as synapses in the dentate gyrus and prefrontal cortex are pruned back (Bauer et al. 2007).

Development of Prospective Memory in Adolescence

Executive functions develop throughout childhood and adolescence, linked to the development of the prefrontal cortex (Altgassen et al. 2017). Prospective memory is underpinned by a number of executive functions, including monitoring for the prospective memory cue, which was discussed in Chapter 1; inhibition of other stimuli, which allows focus on the task to be remembered; and task switching (Altgassen et al. 2017). This means that prospective memory also develops throughout childhood and adolescence, and is an important component of achieving independence (Altgassen et al. 2017).

Robey et al. (2014) suggest that prospective memory ability may also increase as a response to environmental changes, such as increased school or work demands. It has been found that the ability to plan and switch between tasks, both executive functions, may explain some of the variation in prospective memory ability in 7–12-year-olds (Robey et al. 2014). Moreover, attentional control and the skill of switching attention between tasks have been shown to explain some of the variance in prospective memory in adolescents (Robey et al. 2014). Working memory and retrospective memory ability have also been demonstrated to affect prospective memory performance in children up to 12 years old (Robey et al. 2014).

The Use of Memory Strategies

Memory strategies are defined as tasks used for a cognitive intention that are effortful, may be conscious, and are controlled by the person (Schneider 2010). The capacity to use such strategies, which can be deployed at the point of encoding or retrieval, emerges between 5 and 10 years of age, while before this children may lack the mental ability and knowledge to use them (Schneider 2010).

Schneider (2010) shows that there is considerable interindividual variation in the use of memory strategies, with some children better able to use them than others. Also, while some children are able to *learn* a strategy for organising information, they may have subsequent difficulty *using* it, a phenomenon called 'utilisation deficiency' (Schneider 2010, p. 243). It has been found too that children may use more than one memory strategy simultaneously (Schneider 2010). Furthermore, it has been argued that the storage capacity of memory is constant throughout life but what changes, and what underpins the improvements noted in memory performance with age, is the ability to use strategies (Gathercole and Hitch 1993). The application of memory strategies, in this view, releases storage capacity, so that the amount that can be remembered increases (Gathercole and Hitch 1993).

Pressley et al. (1989, p. 858) proposed a 'good information processor model', which outlines the characteristics that underpin intellectual success in learners. In addition to an absence of neurological impairment, the person should be able to deploy appropriate strategies, such as chunking, which can expand the capacity of short-term memory, or activating beliefs that motivate (Pressley et al. 1989). They should also be capable of attention to the task and be able to screen out distractors (Pressley et al. 1989). In addition, they should have extensive information stored in long-term memory on which they can draw to support performance, for example via chunking (Pressley et al. 1989). Overall, the person is 'planful' with regard to action and thought, and their plans are subordinate to their goals (Pressley et al. 1989, p. 862). One study examining the changing use of strategies in children as they develop, and its association with memory performance, is discussed next.

Schneider et al. (2004) conducted a longitudinal study of children's memory performance in relation to their use of memory strategies. Initially, 102 children with a mean age of 6.5 years were tested on a range of memory tasks, including recall, short-term and working memory (Schneider et al. 2004). The researchers also measured the degree of sorting the children did while studying the items in the recall task and the amount of clustering evidenced during recall (Schneider et al. 2004). The children were interviewed about their use of memory strategies while addressing the tasks and their responses were used to score their knowledge of metamemory. They were measured at the start, after six months and after another six months; 99 children finished the study (Schneider et al. 2004).

It was found that the use of sorting and recall scores changed significantly between measurements two and three, and that the measurement point had a significant effect on both scores. The correlation between recall and sorting scores strengthened between measurements one and three; the metamemory scores also correlated significantly with the recall scores at the third measurement, suggesting that the use of strategies had increased (Schneider et al. 2004). Generally, children who used strategies scored significantly higher in the memory tests, especially at the second time point (Schneider et al. 2004). Also, children who used two strategies scored significantly higher than those who used one strategy or none.

The researchers found a lot of variation in the use of strategies: 57 children did not use strategies at the first two measurement points; 28 children started strategising at the second point; and 4 used strategy at the first point but not after this point (Schneider et al. 2004). The results show that, while the use of strategies increases with age and this is linked to improved memory performance, there is considerable interindividual variation in their use.

The Growth of 'Metamemory'

Flavell (1971, p. 276) observed that young children may 'assimilate' information but they do not do this consciously, with future recall in mind, so learning and retrieval are 'incidental'. He commented that 'memorizing is like storing nuts for the winter; it has a planful quality about it that ordinary perceiving and remembering do not have', and was beyond the capabilities of a typical 4-year-old (Flavell 1971). Flavell (1971, p. 277) suggested that memory development may consist of the enhancement of 'metamemory', which he described as using intelligence to organise and store, and search for and retrieve, information, in addition to intelligently and knowingly monitoring these 'operations'. This concept is explored here.

Metamemory is the understanding that information can be acquired voluntarily and stored for later retrieval; it involves cognizance of one's own memory (Gathercole and Hitch 1993; Schneider 2010). Metamemory may involve strategies such as rehearsal, mediation with language and linking items in a cluster. It also involves evaluations of how easy it will be to remember one item compared to another, whether one will be able to remember something later, or if one already knows the information (Gathercole and Hitch 1993; Schneider 2010). Metamemory develops with age, and improvements in this area have been linked to improvements in general memory performance (DiGiulio et al. 1994; Gathercole and Hitch 1993).

Declarative Metamemory

'Declarative metacognitive knowledge' refers to the child's explicit knowledge about factors affecting performance, such as age, the difficulties of the task and knowledge about strategies (Schneider 2010, p. 362). Cognisance of these strategies increases throughout the school career and, as knowledge increases, use of the strategies tends to increase as well (Schneider 2010).

Although metamemory is considered to be developed by around 12 years old, children's knowledge here is often partial and it has been found that even adolescents and adults may not be aware of more complex techniques that are available (Gathercole and Hitch 1993; Schneider 2010). Furthermore, increased depth of knowledge in specific areas can lead to improved memory performance in those domains, affecting the quantity of information the child can recall, as well as enhancing their knowledge of strategies and metacognitive knowledge (Schneider 2010). These effects can mean that a child who is an expert in a knowledge area can perform at the same level as an adult expert, both in terms of the quantity of information and in the mental representation of the information (Schneider 2010).

Overall, Schneider (2010, p. 365) points to the interaction of several factors influencing childhood memory performance, and refers to the 'model of good information processing', meaning the interaction of neural capacity, strategy, knowledge and motivation. This latter factor is considered to be key in the retention of domain-specific knowledge (Schneider 2010). The emphasis on the importance of motivation in learning and memory fits well with conceptual practice models used by occupational therapists, including the Canadian Model of Occupational Performance and Engagement (Sumsion et al. 2011) and the Model of Human Occupation (Kielhofner 1995).

Procedural Metamemory

'Procedural metacognitive knowledge' refers to children's 'self-regulation' and 'self-monitoring' during memory tasks, and is done subconsciously (Schneider 2002, p. 244). There is some uncertainty about the progress of such procedural knowledge throughout childhood and its development is less clear than that for declarative metacognition (Schneider 2002). However, it has been shown that even primary school-age children are able to self-monitor and that improvement in procedural metacognition with age is linked to children's increased ability to use this self-monitoring to regulate their behaviour (Schneider 2002).

Memory in the Ageing Person

The Centrality of Occupation

Just as crawling has been linked to neural development and the emergence of memory skills in the infant, so the activity of walking has been linked to memory in the older person. Atkinson et al. (2007) explored the relationship between gait speed decline and cognitive function in a sample of 2349 people with an average age of 75.6, recruited via the Health, Ageing and Body Composition study in the United States. General cognitive status was evaluated using a modified version of the Mini-Mental State Examination (MMSE), while executive function was assessed using a clock drawing task and executive function interview (Atkinson et al. 2007). Normal gait speed was tested for the participants over 20 metres.

Atkinson et al. (2007) found that one standard deviation (SD) reduction in cognitive test scores was associated with greater reduction in gait speed over a three-year period. For example, one SD reduction in modified MMSE scores was associated with a decline of 0.016 m/s in gait speed. These relationships were all statistically significant. Once comorbidities were taken into account the effect size was reduced, but remained significant for modified MMSE and clock drawing scores, although the relationship with scores on the executive function interview was no longer significant (Atkinson et al. 2007). The authors conclude that general cognitive status and executive function predict decline in gait speed. They suggest that this may be because gait speed maintenance requires cognitive skills such as memory; alternatively, cognitive performance and gait speed may be affected in common by conditions such as vascular disease or other lesions (Atkinson et al. 2007).

Working Memory in Alzheimer's Type Dementia

ATD affects as much as 11% of the population over the age of 65 (Tortora and Derrickson 2011). It is likely, therefore, that many older patients encountered by occupational therapists may have the condition. It has been noted that the putative domains of the multicomponent working memory may be vulnerable to the disease (Baddeley 2007). Some of this evidence is discussed in the following paragraphs.

Filgueiras et al. (2013) conducted a systematic review investigating the impact of ATD on the different components of the multicomponent working memory model. They found, overall, that impairment in central executive and episodic buffer was reported in all their selected studies, and that the phonological loop and visuospatial sketchpad were generally the last areas affected (Filgueiras et al. 2013).

Huntley and Howard (2010) also conducted a review of research on the impact of ATD on the different components of the multicomponent working memory model. They found evidence that dual-task performance, thought to rely on the central executive, was impaired in mild–moderate ATD and may even be affected at a preclinical stage of 'mild cognitive impairment' (MCI; Huntley and Howard 2010). They state that the central executive may be affected by frontal lobe degeneration and deficits in connectivity between brain regions in ATD.

Huntley and Howard (2010) also note that ATD patients have difficulties 'chunking' information, which may point to malfunction in the episodic buffer, although they concede that further evidence is needed to support the claim of episodic buffer impairment (Huntley and Howard 2010, p. 126). For the phonological loop, the authors identified evidence that people with early-stage ATD have problems with verbal memory, although this may be a function of an impaired central executive, rather than the phonological loop per se (Huntley and Howard 2010). Neither did they identify strong evidence for visuospatial sketchpad impairments in ATD (Huntley and Howard 2010). The following paragraphs present evidence from two studies looking at the vulnerability of the central executive and episodic buffer, respectively, in ATD.

Baddeley et al. (1991) evaluated the impact of dual-task performance on people with ATD. They wished to test the hypothesis that this population was particularly vulnerable to central executive impairments. In the first experiment, 28 people with ATD were required to maintain a light pen on a randomly moving square that moved faster throughout the test. A peak level of challenge was identified for each person when they were no longer able to keep the pen in place and this level of difficulty was then used for subsequent testing (Baddeley et al. 1991). They first performed the tracking task on its own and then alongside each of three different activities in a dual-task condition. First, 'articulatory suppression' involved counting from one to five repeatedly at a fixed rate; second, reaction time to random tones was tested using a foot switch; and third, the person was asked to repeat a series of digits (Baddeley et al. 1991, p. 2523).

The group was tested again at 6 and 12 months, although only 15 people completed the test at the final measurement. In addition, a control group of 18 non-impaired elderly people was used (Baddeley et al. 1991). It was found that there were significant effects both of task and test session for all of the dual-task conditions, with performance deteriorating with the additional task and also in each subsequent test for the ATD group, but not for the control group, who maintained steady performance in all conditions (Baddeley et al. 1991).

A second experiment involved participants selecting the category of a target item as the range of categories from which to choose was increased.

For example, an animal name was presented on a screen and the person had to select which category it belonged to from a number of category names (Baddeley et al. 1991). The targets and categories were presented for a maximum of four seconds and the participants had to press a key to indicate their selection (Baddeley et al. 1991). Performance was measured by average response time and number of correct answers. There were 30 people with ATD in the study along with 30 elderly controls without memory impairment.

In this second experiment, the ATD group showed significant deterioration in performance when the number of categories was increased from one to two and from one to four, but not from two to four (Baddeley et al. 1991). There was, however, no effect of condition on the control group, who performed at a steady rate as the categories increased (Baddeley et al. 1991). In addition, the ATD participants showed significantly longer response times and greater lengthening of response times as categories increased (Baddeley et al. 1991).

At 7.4 months, 15 of the ATD and 14 of the participants without memory impairment were then retested. It was found that the accuracy of the ATD group's performance deteriorated significantly as categories increased, while the performance of the group without mental impairment did not change (Baddeley et al. 1991). The authors argue that their results show that reduced ability of the central executive to 'direct and control attentional resources' may be a central feature of ATD-related impairment, in keeping with the notion of the central executive as a 'supervisory attentional system' (Baddeley et al. 1991, p. 2538).

Berlingeri et al. (2008) investigated the neural substrate of the episodic buffer in people with ATD. Their methods were based on research findings that immediate recall of a short story that outstripped the capacity of short-term memory relied on, and was vulnerable to, impairments in the episodic buffer. They divided a sample of 21 people with ATD into 10 who could recall some elements of a story immediately after hearing it and 11 who remembered nothing (Berlingeri et al. 2008). They also included a control group of 22 neurologically intact individuals. The researchers conducted MRI voxel-based morphometry analysis, which allows visualisation of anatomical structure, along with a series of neuropsychological tests.

Berlingeri et al. (2008) found that the 11 participants who remembered nothing had significantly higher levels of atrophy in the left anterior hippocampus. The authors therefore propose this as a substrate for the episodic buffer, a finding that they suggest complements rather than contradicts earlier findings that the right frontal cortex is involved in the episodic buffer (Berlingeri et al. 2008).

Selective Impairment of Divided Attention: Implications for Occupational Performance

Andiel and Liu (1995) present evidence that people over the age of 70 may have difficulty in tasks that involve simultaneous storage and processing of information. At the same time, they may have non-impaired immediate memory, as measured via digit span (Andiel and Liu 1995). Furthermore, the researchers show that ATD may have an impact on the central executive (Andiel and Liu 1995). Functional difficulties might include difficulty in drawing inferences; this means that the therapists should be careful to make any instructions quite literal and easy to follow.

Baddeley et al. (2001) investigated the impact of ATD on the performance of tasks involving focused attention, the ability to screen out distracting stimuli; and divided attention, the ability to attend to two tasks simultaneously. The latter is considered a key function of the central executive. The authors were interested in comparing the 'cognitive slowing hypothesis' (Baddeley et al. 2001, p. 1493), which suggests that declining task performance from youth to age is caused by a general reduction in information processing speed, with their own hypothesis that people with ATD experience a specific deficit in central executive–based tasks.

Baddeley et al.'s (2001) sample consisted of three groups: ATD patients; second, age-, education- and occupation level-matched healthy controls; and healthy controls between 20 and 50 years old, who were also matched with the other groups for education and occupation. They conducted four experiments with two difficulty levels in each. The first was a simple reaction time task, where participants needed to press a button when circles appeared on a screen, or a more challenging choice reaction time task, where they pressed the button if circles rather than squares appeared (Baddeley et al. 2001). In experiment two, participants had to cross out the letter Z, presented either against a background of curved letters or, more challengingly, against a background of angular letters (Baddeley et al. 2001). Experiment three involved crossing out a sequence of boxes while reciting a list of digits read by the examiner; the number of boxes crossed out correctly in two minutes was measured, along with the length of digit span and number of errors in repetition (Baddeley et al. 2001). Experiment four necessitated crossing out target pictures while simultaneously identifying the name 'Bristol' from a list of other British cities read out loud by the tester; here, performance was measured by the number of lines of pictures done in two minutes, with the number of mistakes and the number of times that 'Bristol' was identified correctly (Baddeley et al. 2001).

The results for experiment one showed that shifting from the simple reaction time to the choice reaction time conditions affected both the elderly control group and the ATD group similarly. The authors argue that this goes against the general slowing hypothesis, which would predict greater slowing for the ATD group (Baddeley et al. 2001). In experiment two, it was found that there was a significant interaction effect of age and condition, meaning that the older groups performed worse on the more difficult visual search task, although the authors stated that it was more difficult to identify a specific effect of ATD in these (Baddeley et al. 2001). In experiment three, there was no significant difference between the performance of the healthy elderly and younger control groups, whereas combining the scores on both tasks into a single figure showed that the ATD group scored significantly lower than the healthy elderly group (Baddeley et al. 2001). In experiment four, there was a significant effect of condition, with a higher number of errors for the dual task. When the young control group was taken out of the analysis, there was an interaction effect of group and condition, indicating that the performance of the ATD was significantly worse than the healthy elderly (Baddeley et al. 2001). Also, when results for the two tasks in experiment four were combined into a single figure, it was found that the ATD group was significantly more impaired (Baddeley et al. 2001). Overall, the authors argue that there is a specific impairment for people with ATD when performing two tasks simultaneously, indicating a deficit in divided attention for this group.

Cognitive Decline with Age in Pre-industrial and Industrial Societies

Gurven et al. (2017) provide an anthropological perspective on cognitive development and decline. They studied the pre-industrial Tsimane people of Bolivia, who live by foraging and horticulture. The authors ran a battery of cognitive tests on 919 Tsimane, 33% of whom had not been to school and 60% of whom had two or fewer years of schooling (Gurven et al. 2017). Attention was tested via digit span, verbal declarative memory via repeating lists of Tsimane words after a delay, and semantic fluency via generation of lists of words in particular classifications. Working memory was assessed via spatial span, where the examiner tapped a sequence of boxes in a picture and the participant had to repeat the pattern (Gurven et al. 2017).

The results mirrored those that would be found in an industrialised population: performance on all the tests was significantly poorer in those over 40 (Gurven et al. 2017). It was also found that a higher level of schooling was associated with better performance throughout the age range, but did not prevent decline after age 40 (Gurven et al. 2017).

The authors explain their results in relation to patterns of human occupation. Our large brains, longer lifespan and investment in younger generations may be adaptations to archaic subsistence on resources that were difficult to access, such as hunted animals and 'extracted roots' (Gurven et al. 2017). They suggest, therefore, that natural selection has adapted humans to develop 'fluid' capacities, which require effort, such as the ability to solve problems in new situations, and 'crystallised' capacities, which involve the application of acquired skills and knowledge (Gurven et al. 2017, p. 2). According to these authors, a pattern of decline in fluid ability from the 30s onward, with crystallised ability continuing to improve into one's 50s, seems to be general in all human societies (Gurven et al. 2017).

Some support for these findings comes from the work of Singh-Manoux et al. (2012), who examined a cohort of middle-aged civil servants in the United Kingdom, recruited via the 'Whitehall II cohort' study. The authors point out that the study was fairly heterogeneous, for example there was a 10-fold difference between the salaries at those at the top of the cohort and those at the bottom, and two-thirds of the cohort were male (Singh-Manoux et al. 2012). They divided the sample into five age categories: 45–49, 50–54, 55–59, 60–64 and 65–70 (Singh-Manoux et al. 2012). All participants were tested on memory, reasoning and vocabulary, and semantic and phonemic fluency, three times over 10 years. Memory was tested with a 20-item list of words to be remembered in any order within two minutes (Singh-Manoux et al. 2012).

It was found that all scores except for vocabulary dropped significantly for all age groups over the test period. This was even the case for those aged 45–49 at the start of the study. Men in this group, for example, showed a 2.9% drop in memory scores, while women in the group showed a 2.5% drop (Singh-Manoux et al. 2012). The authors comment that this may underestimate the results that would be found in the general population as, despite the gaps in salary, all members of the cohort were in stable white-collar roles (Singh-Manoux et al. 2012). They also found that adjusting for educational attainment levels made little difference to these results. These results suggest that some of the middle-aged and older patients encountered in occupational therapy practice may have some degree of memory impairment, even in the absence of a diagnosis of dementia.

Changes in Prospective Memory: Implications for Occupational Performance

Gryffydd et al. (2022) state that prospective memory impairments are a common complaint in older adults and may affect activities of daily living. In addition, they explain that prospective memory utilises retrospective memory mechanisms, when recalling the required task following a delay, and also executive function, in that attention must be diverted from a current activity in order to perform the intended task.

Gryffydd et al. (2022, p. 105) investigated the relationship between self-reported prospective memory problems and performance on clinical and 'naturalistic' tasks. Their sample consisted of 43 adults over 65, with a mean age of 73.63, who were living in the community. The Prospective and Retrospective Memory Questionnaire (PRMQ) allowed the participants to provide a self-assessment of their usual performance in these areas, while the Cambridge Prospective Memory Test was used in the clinical setting (Gryffydd et al. 2022). The participants were also asked to text, telephone or email the researchers at specific times during the week, giving a 'naturalistic measure' of prospective memory performance (Gryffydd et al. 2022, p. 106). In addition, a neuropsychological test of attention switching was conducted.

It was found that self-reported prospective memory impairments showed a negative significant correlation with the naturalistic test, meaning that lower scores on the self-assessment were associated with higher numbers of errors in the real-world task (Gryffydd et al. 2022). However, there was no significant correlation between self-rated scores and the clinical task (Gryffydd et al. 2022). Also, the scores on retrospective memory and attention switching did not predict performance on prospective memory (Gryffydd et al. 2022).The authors suggest, therefore, that the inclusion of realistic activities, such as the telephone task, may be important in assessment of prospective memory, as, in this case, they were significantly correlated with self-reported difficulties (Gryffydd et al. 2022). This echoes the demands of occupational therapy researchers for ecologically valid assessments of memory, which are discussed further in Chapter 4 (Hartman-Maeir et al. 2009).

Crook-Rumsey et al. (2022) argue that prospective memory errors are frequently the first reported symptoms of dementia, and investigated the impact of MCI on prospective memory in older adults. MCI is a bridging condition between normal ageing and a diagnosis of dementia, and the authors point out that the presence of MCI is a major risk factor for subsequent dementia, increasing the likelihood of a dementia diagnosis by 10 times (Crook-Rumsey et al. 2022).

The sample in their final analysis consisted of 29 young adults, 36 healthy older adults and 23 older adults with MCI. The participants performed an 'ongoing working memory task' (Crook-Rumsey et al. 2022, p. 111), where they needed to press a button if a presented word was in the same semantic group as a previously presented word. They also performed a perceptual prospective memory task, which used the same procedure as the working memory task but also required the person to remember to press a button if a word was displayed in upper case. In addition, there was a conceptual prospective memory condition, which used the same working memory task procedure, but with the addition that the person needed to press a button if the presented word belonged to the category of animals with four legs (Crook-Rumsey et al. 2022). At the same time, levels of electroencephalographic (EEG) activation were measured (Crook-Rumsey et al. 2022).

The MCI groups performed significantly worse on the working memory task than the young and healthy older adults. Crook-Rumsey et al. (2022) also state that the MCI group performed worse on the conceptual prospective memory task than the healthy older group; however, this difference was not statistically significant. In addition, all groups performed significantly more poorly on the conceptual prospective memory task compared with the perceptual prospective task. So, there is no evidence here that the MCI group had a specific impairment related to prospective memory performance.

The EEG results showed that the MCI group had lower amplitudes in regions linked to sense of familiarity and knowing in episodic memory, and that impairments in these areas might be a feature of MCI (Crook-Rumsey et al. 2022). In addition, it was noted that another EEG event-related potential that may be linked to shifting between working memory and prospective memory tasks was higher in the young adults in lateral frontal regions throughout both prospective memory tasks when compared with the other groups (Crook-Rumsey et al. 2022). Overall, the authors suggest that their results indicate that reduced working memory and attention may play a part in the prospective impairments noted in those with MCI (Crook-Rumsey et al. 2022).

Varley et al. (2021) point out that prospective memory may be either time based, for example 'switch off the oven in one hour', or event based, for example 'buy eggs when I next go to the shop'. However, they argue that studies have tended to confuse these by including cues that are both time and event based, for example remembering to view a clock as a cue to do something at a certain time (Varley et al. 2021). In their study, they therefore controlled for this by having the timer completely hidden in one condition.

Their sample was a group of younger adults with a mean age of 19 and older adults with a mean age of 71. All participants performed an ongoing arithmetic task, presented on a computer monitor. In addition, they performed a prospective memory task, which consisted of remembering to press the keyboard space bar after one minute, in one of four conditions. First, an hourglass timer was presented on a monitor but could only be viewed by pressing a particular key. Second, the timer was accessible by simply shifting the focus of vision. Third, the timer was completely inaccessible and the person needed to rely on their internal time sense. The fourth condition was event based: the participant needed to remember to press the space bar when the answer to an arithmetic question was 'three' (Varley et al. 2021).

It was found that younger adults' timing was significantly more precise in conditions where the timer was visible when a key was pressed or with a shift of vision. However, there was no difference between the young and old groups when the timer was hidden and they relied on their own internal time sense, or in the event-based condition (Varley et al. 2021). The authors suggest that their results indicate that the internal 'temporal processing' that supports time-based prospective memory performance over a short period is not affected by age (Varley et al. 2021, p. 622).

Evidence from the 'Enriched Environments' Paradigm

'Enriched environments' is an experimental approach in which one group of animals, often rats, is kept in cages with opportunities to socialise, run on a wheel, play with toys, forage, run through tunnels and so on (van Praag et al. 2000, p. 191). A control group, meanwhile, is housed in a standard cage (van Praag et al. 2000). Hebb, whom we encountered in Chapter 1, first proposed that such an enriched environment might facilitate neural plasticity (van Praag et al. 2000).

Evidence does indeed show that enriched environments are associated with improved spatial learning and memory performance, as well as greater numbers of higher-order dendrites in rats (van Praag et al. 2000). In addition, enrichment has been linked to an increase in the number of dendritic spines in CA1 and CA3 hippocampal regions, while female rats from enriched environments had a greater number of dendrites on each neuron in the dentate gyrus, part of the hippocampal region (van Praag et al. 2000).

In birds, enriched environments have been associated with heightened levels of nerve growth factor and brain-derived neurotropic growth factor, both of which have been linked to synaptic plasticity and learning (van Praag et al. 2000). There is also evidence that enriched environments may lead to increased levels of acetylcholine, while exercise is associated with a raised presence of noradrenaline and serotonin; all of these neurotransmitters have been linked to learning and memory (van Praag et al. 2000).

Nithianantharajah and Hannan (2006, p. 703) link the neural plasticity associated with experience of an enriched environment to the concept of 'cognitive reserve'. This is based on evidence that higher levels of mental and physical activity may be a protective factor against dementia and also the progress of the condition, following diagnosis (Nithianantharajah and Hannan 2006). They propose that this may be an equivalent of the effects of enrichment observed in the laboratory.

Findings from non-human animals are not always applicable to humans. However, given that mechanisms of neural plasticity are likely to be the same in all species, findings such as these may help explain some of the variation in memory outcomes for children from different SES backgrounds.

Kempermann (2019) presents evidence that environmental enrichment in animals leads to higher brain size and weight, and is effective into advanced old age. Kempermann (2019) shows that much of the enriched environment research has focused on the birth of new neurons in the hippocampus, which could underpin spatial learning and other aspects of cognition. As outlined earlier, enriched environments have been linked especially to the birth of new neurons in the dentate gyrus of the hippocampal region (Kempermann 2019).

Kempermann (2019) also shows that early evidence from this research was an important influence on the Head Start programme in the United States, which aimed to provide early enrichment experiences for children from poorer resourced backgrounds (Kempermann 2019). Head Start was, in turn, an inspiration for the Sure Start programme in the United Kingdom (Toynbee and Walker 2010). This is an interesting example of evidence from neuroscience informing social policy.

Kempermann (2019) notes that the mechanisms by which enriched environments work appear to be multifactorial and encompass increased physical action, social mingling, and cognitive and mental spurring. Thus it is a complex phenomenon that demonstrates 'emergent properties', suggesting that the outcomes of enriched environments may be difficult to predict (Kempermann 2019, p. 237). This means that there are methodological challenges in trying to understand the precise paths by which the intervention works that call for 'interfield and interlevel integration' (Kempermann 2019, p. 237).

An example of the challenges comes from attempts to model ATD in animals. The research here is predicated on the idea that environmental factors including cognitive and physical activity and educational status are known to affect the risk of having ATD (Kempermann 2019). Despite this, a clear picture of the effects of environment in animal models of ATD has not emerged, though this may be a result of methodological limitations in the studies (Kempermann 2019). Kempermann (2019) does suggest, however, that enriched environments may provide a useful approach in neurorehabilitation.

The Socio-economic Gradient in Dementia

Yaffe et al. (2013) conducted a prospective cohort study of 2457 people with a mean age of 73.6 years, 41.5% of whom were Black, assessing the likelihood of developing dementia over a 12-year period. The study was conducted in the United States. At baseline, all were free of dementia and a number of baseline measurements were taken, including SES, presence of diabetes mellitus, hypertension, presence of the ε4 variant of apolipoprotein E, cognitive status, alcohol consumption and smoking, and physical activity levels (Yaffe et al. 2013). SES was measured using a number of factors, including yearly income, educational attainment level and literacy level; it was found at baseline that Black participants had significantly lower SES than whites (Yaffe et al. 2013).

Over the 12-year period 18.3% of the cohort were diagnosed with dementia and it was found that Black people were significantly more likely to be diagnosed than whites (Yaffe et al. 2013). The hazard ratio of getting dementia was 1.44 for Black participants, meaning that they were 1.44 times more likely to be diagnosed over the period (Yaffe et al. 2013). Further analysis showed that SES explained 80% of the excess hazard for Black people, and the presence of four factors associated with low SES was linked to a 1.32 hazard ratio in both Black and white people, meaning those in this category were 1.32 times more likely to receive a dementia diagnosis (Yaffe et al. 2013).

The authors argue that 'these results suggest that black-white disparities in risk of dementia may be largely attributed to socioeconomic differences' (Yaffe et al. 2013, p. 3). The authors posit that this is an effect of 'allostatic load', meaning multiple system dysfunction stemming from the cumulative impact of stress and life happenings (Yaffe et al. 2013, p. 3). The effects of this can include inflammation and cardiovascular and metabolic dysfunction, have been shown to impair neurogenesis in the non-human hippocampus and are linked to smaller hippocampal volume in humans (Yaffe et al. 2013, p. 3). On the other hand, the authors suggest that the higher educational attainment levels linked to higher SES may provide greater cognitive reserve, acting as a buffer against dementia (Yaffe et al. 2013).

Galvin et al. (2021) used a community dwelling sample of 374 with a mean age of 69.2 years. The participants lived in New York and were divided into white, Hispanic and African American subgroups. Cognitive status was measured using the Montreal Cognitive Assessment (MoCA) and AD8, a brief self-report questionnaire that screens for dementia (Galvin et al. 2021). In addition, SES was measured using the Hollingshead index.

Galvin et al. (2021) found that white participants had significantly higher MoCA and AD8 scores, as well as significantly more years in education (Galvin et al. 2021). The sample was then broken down into clusters: the first cluster were older and had lower SES; the second cluster were younger and had middle SES; and the third cluster were older and had higher SES (Galvin et al. 2021). It was found that the first cluster had the worst overall health outcomes. However, cluster three had the best health outcomes and had MoCA scores similar to the younger participants (Galvin et al. 2021). In each cluster, whites had higher SES and better health generally, and MoCA scores were significantly higher for whites within all clusters, although there were no significant differences on AD8 scores (Galvin et al. 2021).

The authors suggest that the lower cognitive status scores of the African American and Hispanic groups could be explained by the concept of white participants having higher 'peak cognitive reserve', indicated by a higher occupational status and greater levels of attainment in education, and therefore a marker of SES inequality (Galvin et al. 2021, p. 1572). In addition, they suggest that, in the US context, higher SES may bring better access to healthcare, while race may affect the quality of services offered (Galvin et al. 2021).

Babulal et al. (2023) point out that Black/African American people have twice the risk for dementia, and Hispanic people have 1.5 times the risk, compared with the non-Hispanic white population. These researchers used data on 6958 people over the age of 50 from the United States (Babulal et al. 2023). All were free of cognitive impairment at baseline and were also free of neuropsychiatric symptoms, a term that is interchangeable with 'behavioural or psychological symptoms' in dementia (Babulal et al. 2023, p. 1). All had had a minimum of one follow-up with repeated screening (Babulal et al. 2023).

Babulal et al. (2023) calculated a hazard ratio for each of 12 neuropsychiatric symptoms. This ratio assessed the effect of race and neuropsychiatric symptoms on subsequent cognitive impairment, by comparing these with the hazard ratios for non-Hispanic white people (Babulal et al. 2023). It was found that Black/African American people were significantly more likely to transition to impaired cognitive status when assessed on each of the 12 neuropsychiatric symptoms. This group had a 15–23% higher hazard ratio when one neuropsychiatric symptom was present. This was followed by Hispanic people, who had a significantly higher hazard ratio for progression to impaired cognition when six neuropsychiatric symptoms were present, with a hazard ratio of 24–28%, and Asian people, who had a significantly higher hazard ratio (39–40%) for two neuropsychiatric symptoms (Babulal et al. 2023). The authors make the following point:

> *Race and ethnicity are fundamental to identity but are rudimentary proxies for social and environmental determinants of health dimensions like education, socioeconomic status, structural racism, discrimination, outdoor and indoor pollution, and area-level deprivation—all of which increase the risk for both NPS [neuropsychiatric symptoms] and dementia.*
>
> *(Babulal et al. 2023, p. 7)*

With respect to the intersection of race, social class and environment, reporting has shown that in the United States, Black, Hispanic and Asian people are more likely to be exposed to a range of environmental pollutants, including those from coal-produced electricity, large diesel vehicles and agriculture (Thompson 2019; Lloyd 2021). In the United Kingdom, these injustices have been highlighted by the case of Ella Kissi-Debrah, a 9-year-old girl from London who died following an asthma attack and who became the first person internationally to have air contamination recorded as a cause of their death (Carrington 2023). With regard to internal pollutants, Awaab Ishak died at the age of 2 of respiratory disease following extended exposure to mould in his home in Rochdale in 2020 (Williams 2022).

Bukhbinder et al. (2023) point out that Mexican Americans experience cognitive impairment at a younger age but are diagnosed with dementia later than non-Hispanic white people. They suggest that this may be because of reduced access to healthcare services, but may also reflect differing cultural beliefs. In addition, risk factors for dementia, such as obesity and diabetes, occur more frequently in the Mexican American population (Bukhbinder et al. 2023).

Appel et al. (2022) investigated the separate and combined effects of SES and educational level on the risk of receiving a dementia diagnosis. The authors used a Danish national register of 1 210 720 people over 60 years of age who had not received a diagnosis up until 60. They were followed up on the register after a 10-year period, finishing in 2017. Educational levels were grouped into three categories: high, more than 12 years in education; middle, from 10 to 12 years; and low, equal to or less than 9 years in education (Appel et al. 2022). Dementia cases were measured using 'person years', which was calculated as the number of people in the study together with the number of years they were in the study.

It was found that each step down the educational level was linked to an additional 14.8 dementia cases per 100 000 person years, a trend that was statistically significant. Each step down occupational levels, which ranged from higher nonmanual management roles to unskilled manual work and self-employment, was linked to 10.9 additional cases per 100 000 person years, which was also a significant trend (Appel et al. 2022). It was found, however, that in the highest education group SES was usually not linked to higher dementia risk, although the link between dementia risk and occupation level applied to middle and lower educational groups (Appel et al. 2022). Indeed, the highest level of 78.3 additional dementia cases per 100 000 person years occurred in the low education group, giving a hazard ratio of 1.4 (Appel et al. 2022).

Appel et al. (2022) propose two key explanations for their findings. First, heavy manual workers may be exposed to environmental hazards such as pesticides or magnetic fields, as well as having higher levels of cardiovascular and other diseases, all of which could increase dementia risk (Appel et al. 2022). On the other hand, they suggest that the greater levels of autonomy and complexity in higher-level occupations provide mental stimulation that can build 'cognitive reserve', meaning that greater pathology is needed before symptoms of dementia become apparent (Appel et al. 2022, p. 184).

De Lange et al. (2021) investigated the interactions between SES, brain age, social isolation and subjective loneliness in 24 867 people in the United Kingdom, with a mean age of 63.86 years, based on information held in the UK Biobank national database. The Townsend Deprivation Index was used to measure SES, together with household income (de Lange et al. 2021). Social isolation was scored according to answers given to questions about quantity of social contacts. The UK Biobank also includes data from brain MRI scans and the authors used measurements of cortical thickness, volume and area from specific brain regions to calculate a 'brain age gap', based on subtraction of the brain age predicted by these measurements from the person's actual chronological age (de Lange et al. 2021, p. 3).

De Lange et al. (2021) found that higher scores for social isolation and lower SES, as well as other factors such as presence of hypertension and higher alcohol consumption, were significantly associated with raised brain age compared to actual chronological age (de Lange et al. 2021). Thus, the authors suggest that risk of dementia arises from the interaction of a number of factors; they also suggest that further work is needed on the impact of social isolation on brain health in the wake of the Covid-19 pandemic (de Lange et al. 2021). Again, this underlines the importance of environment in shaping memory performance, and fits with the approaches taken in occupational therapy conceptual practice models.

Table 2.1 summarises some key landmarks in memory development throughout the lifespan, alongside other important milestones.

Table 2.1 Memory though the lifespan.

Age	Memory development	Other developments
25 weeks gestational age (GA)		Brain and sense organs developed enough to perceive and learn about sounds
34–36 weeks GA	Demonstrates evidence of habituation to sounds Stops moving when sound played repeatedly Movement starts again when novel sound played	
Neonate (2–3 days after birth)	Demonstrates evidence of memory of patterns of stories read to them in utero	
2 months	Learns to activate mobile; remembers this for a few days without a cue and can remember 21 weeks later if given a visual cue Memory highly context dependent	
5.5 months		Rolls over
7 months		Sits up May start crawling
10 months	Remembers puppet following training two months previously	
1 year		Stands up May walk
18–24 months		'Cognitive self' emerges
1–2 years	Declarative memory, dependent on medial temporal lobe, emerges	Masters basic language
2 years	Narrative autobiographical memory emerges	
3–4 years	Memory span of 2–3 verbal items	
3–5 years	Coherent and detailed narrative autobiographical memory emerges Phonological store of phonological loop present	
3–7 years	More complex declarative memory still developing	Temporal and prefrontal cortex develop more as well as further development in hippocampus
4–5 years	Complex reading and grammar develop	
4–8 years	Children taught semantic facts by person or puppet: ▪ At 4 years remembered 23% of facts ▪ At 6 years remembered 32% of facts ▪ At 8 years remembered 51% of facts ▪ At 4 years remembered source in about 20% of cases ▪ At 6–8 years remembered source of facts (person or puppet) in about 40% of cases ▪ Episodic memory only properly present from 6 to 8 years	
5 years	Able to recall four blocks in a visual pattern	Hippocampus fully mature
5–6 years	Digit span of 3–4 (for English-speaking children)	
6 years	Components of multicomponent model of working memory present	Synaptogenesis increases in prefrontal cortex up to 6 years

(Continued)

Table 2.1 (Continued)

Age	Memory development	Other developments
7 years	Articulatory rehearsal aspect of phonological loop present Remembers 2.5 items in complex working memory task requiring central executive	
8 years		Medial temporal lobe completely developed
8–24 years	Declarative and working memory continue to develop	Dorsolateral prefrontal cortical regions involved in declarative memory continue to develop
9–10 years	Digit span of 5–6 (for English-speaking children) Procedural memory at adult levels	
9–15 years	Advanced memory skills, including cognitive control mechanism linked to frontal lobe development Declarative memory fully developed	Greater connectivity within temporal region and between frontal and temporal regions
10 years	Able to recode visually presented information phonologically Remembers 4.5 items in complex working memory task requiring central executive	
11 years	Recalls around 14 blocks in a visual pattern (equivalent to adult capacity)	
12 years	Memory span of 6 verbal items Metamemory developed, with knowledge of strategies to support learning and memory	
14–15 years	Digit span of 7 (for English-speaking children)	
15 years	Remembers 5.5 items in complex working memory task requiring central executive	
18 years	Remembers 6.5 items in complex working memory task requiring central executive	
Mid-40s	Decline in verbal memory ability	Decline in effortful cognitive processing (fluid) ability Pilots aged 40–60 have fewer accidents than younger pilots
Over 60	Increased difficulty in learning rotary pursuit task (procedural memory)	Elderly people with active social lives and who exercise have better cognitive function
Elderly	Digit span 6–6.5 Working memory is one of the first systems to show age-related decline Older people can learn to use a computer, but learning is slower and they make more errors Some individuals with specialist skills continue to perform into old age: ■ Expert typists in their 60s and 70s can perform as well as typists in their 20s and 30s ■ Chess and bridge experts improve with age Semantic memory learnt in the past may be remembered Episodic memory from distant past may be retained	By 80, the brain has lost 5% of its weight Study of 3600 MRI scans of healthy brains of 65–97-year-olds found one-third had lesions consistent with small strokes Long-term potentiation may be less efficient in ageing, meaning that synapses and hence learning may be more unstable

Conclusion

The early view that infants were largely incapable of remembering has been challenged by evidence from innovative experiments. Remarkably, data has shown some level of infant memory for events occurring in utero.

It has been demonstrated that crawling appears to facilitate memory. This may occur as the infant begins to explore their environment. It has been shown that the social environment may also influence memory development. Some researchers, for example, have found a later age for the offset of infantile amnesia for children from different cultural backgrounds. One crucial factor here is the nature of parent–child interactions. This research confirms the importance of analysing the development of memory not as a discrete cognitive phenomenon, but rather in the context of task performance within specific environments. This fits with occupational therapy conceptual practice models, as will be discussed in Chapter 4.

It has been shown in this chapter that, building on concepts introduced in Chapter 1, different memory systems develop at different ages. The different parts of the multicomponent working memory system, for example, appear to mature at different rates. In addition relational memory, including declarative and episodic memory, continues to improve throughout childhood, while prospective memory develops into adolescence. Furthermore, children's ability to use memory strategies appears to improve with age. These insights are important for occupational therapists working with children, particularly in the school setting. It may be important, for example, to consider this data during task analysis with children at different ages.

A key theme was the impact of environmental factors on memory and brain development. For example, early negative life events have a deleterious effect on declarative memory. In addition, lower SES is linked to impaired memory performance in children.

Although some level of cognitive decline from the mid-40s onwards seems to be a general feature of human society, marked inequalities exist. People of lower SES, for example, have an increased risk of developing dementia. This suggests that socio-economic inequalities affect memory development throughout the lifespan. From a theoretical perspective, data such as this provides support for occupational therapy conceptual practice models that emphasise the impact of the environment on occupational performance.

Points for Discussion

1. Zara is an occupational therapist working with a 5-year-old boy called Archie. Archie's teacher has reported that he seldom speaks in class. For example, when the teacher asks the children what they did at the weekend or over the holidays, Archie does not usually say anything. Zara observes Archie at home interacting with his mother. Zara notes that Archie's mother usually asks him closed-ended questions about things he has done, which require only 'yes' or 'no' responses. Bearing in mind Archie's teacher's concerns, what advice could Zara offer to Archie's mother?

2. Archie's teacher, introduced in discussion point 1, reports that in conversation Archie is sometimes able to discuss what he has learnt in school. However, Archie seems confused about *where* he has learnt the information. For example, when discussing a topic covered in a history lesson, Archie states that he learnt about this from a man on television. Should Zara see this is a cause for concern? Explain your answer.

3. Dave is a 76-year-old man with MCI. He is attempting to teach himself to use a computer spreadsheet application. He complains that, while entering data into the spreadsheet, he often forgets the instructions he has just read and loses track of what he is doing. Impairments in which type of memory do you think might be causing Dave's difficulties?

Activities

1. Describe your earliest memory in as much detail as you can.
2. Describe memories from 5 to 10 years after this earliest memory in as much detail as you can.
3. What do you notice about the difference in your descriptions for activities 1 and 2?
4. Repeat this sequence of random numbers:

396

456

185

861

233

030

284

Now, see if you can repeat the numbers and then state the middle digit of each number in order. Record your score. Next, give this test to people of different ages and see if the scores vary according to age.

5. How would you explain any variations in the scores in activity 4?

References

Alloway, T.P. and Alloway, R.G. (2015). *Understanding Working Memory*, 2e. London: Sage.

Alloway, T.P., Gathercole, S.E., and Pickering, S.J. (2006). Verbal and visuospatial short-term and working memory in children: are they separable? *Child Development* 77 (6): 1698–1716.

Altgassen, M., Kretschmer, A., and Schnitzspahn, K.M. (2017). Future thinking instructions improve prospective memory performance in adolescents. *Child Neuropsychology* 23 (5): 536–553.

Andiel, C. and Liu, L. (1995). Working memory and older adults: implications for occupational therapy. *American Journal of Occupational Therapy* 49 (7): 681–686.

Appel, A.M., Brønnum-Hansen, H., Garde, A.H. et al. (2022). Socioeconomic position and late-onset dementia: a nationwide register-based study. *Journal of Aging and Health* 34 (2): 184–195.

Atkinson, H.H., Rosano, C., Simonsick, E.M. et al. (2007). Cognitive function, gait speed decline, and comorbidities: the health, aging and body composition study. *Journals of Gerontology Series A: Biological Sciences and Medical Sciences* 62 (8): 844–850.

Babulal, G.M., Zhu, Y., and Trani, J.-F. (2023). Racial and ethnic differences in neuropsychiatric symptoms and progression to incident cognitive impairment among community-dwelling participants. *Alzheimer's and Dementia* 19 (8): 3635–3643.

Baddeley, A.D. (2007). *Working Memory, Thought, and Action*. Oxford: Oxford University Press.

Baddeley, A. (2015). Autobiographical memory. In: *Memory* (ed. A. Baddeley, M.W. Eysenck, and M.C. Anderson), 299–326. London: Psychology Press.

Baddeley, A.D. et al. (1991). The decline of working memory in Alzheimer's disease: a longitudinal study. *Brain* 114 (6): 2521–2542.

Baddeley, A.D., Bressi, S., Della Sala, S. et al. (2001). Attentional control in Alzheimer's disease. *Brain* 124 (8): 1492–1508.

Bahrick, L.E. and Pickens, J.N. (1995). Infant memory for object motion across a period of three months: implications for a four-phase attention function. *Journal of Experimental Child Psychology* 59 (3): 343–371.

Bauer, P.J. (2002). Early memory development. In: *Blackwell Handbook of Childhood Cognitive Development* (ed. U. Goswami), 127–146. Oxford: Blackwell.

Bauer, P.J., Wiebe, S.A., Carver, L.J. et al. (2003). Developments in long-term explicit memory late in the first year of life: behavioral and electrophysiological indices. *Psychological Science* 14 (6): 629–635.

Bauer, P.J., DeBoer, T., and Lukowski, A.F. (2007). In the language of multiple memory systems, defining and describing developments in long-term explicit memory. In: *Short- and Long-Term Memory in Infancy and Early Childhood: Taking the First Steps Toward Remembering* (ed. L.M. Oakes and P.J. Bauer), 240–270. Oxford: Oxford University Press.

Bauer, P.J., Larkina, M., and Deocampo, J. (2010). Early memory development. In: *The Wiley-Blackwell Handbook of Childhood Cognitive Development*, 2e (ed. U. Goshwami), 153–179. Oxford: Wiley-Blackwell.

Berlingeri, M., Bottini, G., Basilico, S. et al. (2008). Anatomy of the episodic buffer: a voxel-based morphometry study in patients with dementia. *Behavioural Neurology* 19 (1–2): 29–34.

Bronfenbrenner, U. (1977). Toward an experimental ecology of human development. *American Psychologist* 32 (7): 513–531.

Bukhbinder, A.S., Hinojosa, M., Harris, K. et al. (2023). Population-based Mini-Mental State Examination norms in adults of Mexican heritage in the Cameron County Hispanic Cohort. *Journal of Alzheimer's Disease* 92 (4): 1323–1339.

Carrington, D. (2023). 'Remember me': Ella's law would be fitting legacy after London air pollution death, says mother. *The Guardian*, 10 February. https://www.theguardian.com/environment/2023/feb/10/ellas-law-rosamund-kissi-debrah-air-pollution-death-london (accessed 16 August 2023).

Case-Smith, J. and O'Brien, J.C. (2009). *Occupational Therapy for Children*. Maryland Heights, MO: Elsevier.

Clearfield, M.W. (2004). The role of crawling and walking experience in infant spatial memory. *Journal of Experimental Child Psychology* 89 (3): 214–241.

Crook-Rumsey, M., Howard, C.J., Hadjiefthyvoulou, F., and Sumich, A. (2022). Neurophysiological markers of prospective memory and working memory in typical ageing and mild cognitive impairment. *Clinical Neurophysiology* 133: 111–125.

DeCasper, A.J. and Spence, M.J. (1986). Prenatal maternal speech influences newborns' perception of speech sounds. *Infant Behavior and Development* 9 (2): 133–150.

DiGiulio, D.V., Seidenberg, M., O'Leary, D.S., and Raz, N. (1994). Procedural and declarative memory: a developmental study. *Brain and Cognition* 25 (1): 79–91.

Drummey, A.B. and Newcombe, N.S. (2002). Developmental changes in source memory. *Developmental Science* 5 (4): 502–513.

Eichenbaum, H. (2012). *The Cognitive Neuroscience of Memory: An Introduction*, 2e. Oxford: Oxford University Press.

Farah, M.J., Shera, D.M., Savage, J.H. et al. (2006). Childhood poverty: specific associations with neurocognitive development. *Brain Research* 1110 (1): 166–174.

Filgueiras, A., Landeira-Fernandez, J., and Charchat-Fichman, H. (2013). Working memory in Alzheimer disease: a 5-year systematic review of empirical evidences from Baddeley's working memory model. *Conexoes Psi* 1 (1): 57–76.

Finn, A.S., Kalra, P.B., Goetz, C. et al. (2016). Developmental dissociation between the maturation of procedural memory and declarative memory. *Journal of Experimental Child Psychology* 142: 212–220.

Flavell, J.H. (1971). First discussant's comments: what is memory development the development of? *Human Development* 14 (4): 272–278.

Flores-Lázaro, J.C., Salgado Soruco, M.A., and Stepanov, I.I. (2017). Children and adolescents' performance on a medium-length/nonsemantic word-list test. *Applied Neuropsychology: Child* 6 (2): 95–105.

Freud, S. (1991). *The Essentials of Psychoanalysis: The Definitive Collection of Sigmund Freud's Writing*. Harmondsworth: Penguin.

Galvin, J.E., Chrisphonte, S., and Chang, L.-C. (2021). Medical and social determinants of brain health and dementia in a multicultural community cohort of older adults. *Journal of Alzheimer's Disease* 84 (4): 1563–1576.

Gathercole, S.E. and Hitch, G.J. (1993). Developmental changes in short-term memory: a revised working memory perspective. In: *Theories of Memory* (ed. A. Collins, S.E. Gathercole, M.A. Conway, and P.E. Morris), 189–210. Hove: Erlbaum.

Gathercole, S.E., Pickering, S.J., Ambridge, B., and Wearing, H. (2004). The structure of working memory from 4 to 15 years of age. *Developmental Psychology* 40 (2): 177.

Gazzaniga, M.S., Ivry, R.B., and Mangun, G.R. (2009). *Cognitive Neuroscience: The Biology of the Mind*, 3e. New York: Norton.

Gryffydd, L., Mitra, B., Wright, B.J., and Kinsella, G.J. (2022). Assessing prospective memory in older age: the relationship between self-report and performance on clinic-based and naturalistic tasks. *Aging, Neuropsychology, and Cognition* 29 (1): 104–120.

Gurven, M., Fuerstenberg, E., Trumble, B. et al. (2017). Cognitive performance across the life course of Bolivian forager-farmers with limited schooling. *Developmental Psychology* 53 (1): 160.

Hackman, D.A. and Farah, M.J. (2009). Socioeconomic status and the developing brain. *Trends in Cognitive Sciences* 13 (2): 65–73.

Hamond, N.R. and Fivush, R. (1991). Memories of Mickey Mouse: young children recount their trip to Disneyworld. *Cognitive Development* 6 (4): 433–448.

Hartman-Maeir, A., Katz, N., and Baum, C.M. (2009). Cognitive functional evaluation (CFE) process for individuals with suspected cognitive disabilities. *Occupational Therapy in Health Care* 23 (1): 1–23.

van der Heijden, K.B., Suurland, J., Swaab, H., and de Sonneville, L.M.J. (2011). Relationship between the number of life events and memory capacity in children. *Child Neuropsychology* 17 (6): 580–598.

Herbert, J., Gross, J., and Hayne, H. (2007). Crawling is associated with more flexible memory retrieval by 9-month-old infants. *Developmental Science* 10 (2): 183–189.

Hilton, C.L. (2015). Interventions to promote social participation for children with mental health and behavioural disorders. In: *Occupational Therapy for Children and Adolescents* (ed. J. Case Smith and J. Clifford-O'Brien), 321–345. St Louis, MO: Mosby.

Howe, M.C. and Briggs, A.K. (1982). Ecological systems model for occupational therapy. *American Journal of Occupational Therapy* 36 (5): 322–327.

Huntley, J. and Howard, R. (2010). Working memory in early Alzheimer's disease: a neuropsychological review. *International Journal of Geriatric Psychiatry* 25 (2): 121–132.

Jeannerod, M. (1988). *The Neural and Behavioural Organization of Goal-Directed Movements*. Oxford: Clarendon Press/Oxford University Press.

Kempermann, G. (2019). Environmental enrichment, new neurons and the neurobiology of individuality. *Nature Reviews Neuroscience* 20 (4): 235–245.

Kielhofner, G. (1995). *A Model of Human Occupation: Theory and Application*, 2e. Baltimore, MD: Williams & Wilkins.

de Lange, A.-M.G., Kaufmann, T., Quintana, D.S. et al. (2021). Prominent health problems, socioeconomic deprivation, and higher brain age in lonely and isolated individuals: a population-based study. *Behavioural Brain Research* 414: 113510.

Law, M., Cooper, B., Strong, S. et al. (1996). The person-environment-occupation model: a transactive approach to occupational performance. *Canadian Journal of Occupational Therapy* 63 (1): 9–23.

Lloyd, R. (2021). People of color breathe more unhealthy air from nearly all polluting sources. *Scientific American*, 28 April. https://www.scientificamerican.com/article/people-of-color-breathe-more-unhealthy-air-from-nearly-all-polluting-sources (accessed 16 August 2023).

Luria, A.R. (1973). *The Working Brain: An Introduction to Neuropsychology*. New York: Basic Books.

Mabbott, D.J., Rovet, J., Noseworthy, M.D. et al. (2009). The relations between white matter and declarative memory in older children and adolescents. *Brain Research* 1294: 80–90.

Nadel, L. (1991). The hippocampus and space revisited. *Hippocampus* 1 (3): 221–229.

Nithianantharajah, J. and Hannan, A.J. (2006). Enriched environments, experience-dependent plasticity and disorders of the nervous system. *Nature Reviews Neuroscience* 7 (9): 697–709.

Ofen, N., Kao, Y.-C., Sokol-Hessner, P. et al. (2007). Development of the declarative memory system in the human brain. *Nature Neuroscience* 10 (9): 1198–1205.

Pickering, S.J., Gathercole, S.E., Hall, M., and Lloyd, S.A. (2001). Development of memory for pattern and path: further evidence for the fractionation of visuo-spatial memory. *Quarterly Journal of Experimental Psychology Section A* 54 (2): 397–420.

Pillemer, D.B. (1998). What is remembered about early childhood events? *Clinical Psychology Review* 18 (8): 895–913.

Pillemer, D.B., Picariello, M.L., and Pruett, J.C. (1994). Very long-term memories of a salient preschool event. *Applied Cognitive Psychology* 8 (2): 95–106.

van Praag, H., Kempermann, G., and Gage, F.H. (2000). Neural consequences of environmental enrichment. *Nature Reviews Neuroscience* 1 (3): 191–198.

Pressley, M., Borkowski, J.G., and Schneider, W. (1989). Good information processing: what it is and how education can promote it. *International Journal of Educational Research* 13 (8): 857–867.

Reese, E., Haden, C.A., and Fivush, R. (1993). Mother-child conversations about the past: relationships of style and memory over time. *Cognitive Development* 8 (4): 403–430.

Robey, A., Buckingham-Howes, S., Salmeron, B.J. et al. (2014). Relations among prospective memory, cognitive abilities, and brain structure in adolescents who vary in prenatal drug exposure. *Journal of Experimental Child Psychology* 127: 144–162.

Schacter, D.L. (2008). *Searching for Memory: The Brain, the Mind, and the Past*. New York: Basic Books.

Schafer, M. and Schiller, D. (2020). The brain's social road maps. *Scientific American* 322 (2): 31–35.

Schneck, C.M. and Case-Smith, J. (2015). Prewriting and handwriting skills. In: *Occupational Therapy for Children and Adolescents* (ed. J. Case-Smith and J. Clifford-O'Brien), 498–524. St Louis, MO: Mosby.

Schneider, W. (2002). Memory development in childhood. In: *Blackwell Handbook of Childhood Cognitive Development* (ed. U. Goswami), 236–256. Oxford: Blackwell.

Schneider, W. (2010). Memory development in childhood. In: *The Wiley-Blackwell Handbook of Childhood Cognitive Development* (ed. U. Goswami), 347–376. Oxford: Wiley-Blackwell.

Schneider, W., Kron, V., Hünnerkopf, M., and Krajewski, K. (2004). The development of young children's memory strategies: first findings from the Würzburg Longitudinal Memory Study. *Journal of Experimental Child Psychology* 88 (2): 193–209.

Sharma, A. and Cockerill, H. (2014). *From Birth to Five Years: Practical Developmental Examination*. London: Routledge.

Singh-Manoux, A., Kivimaki, M., Glymour, M.M. et al. (2012). Timing of onset of cognitive decline: results from Whitehall II prospective cohort study. *British Medical Journal* 344: d7622.

Sumsion, T., Tischler-Draper, L., and Heinicke, S. (2011). Applying the Canadian model of occupational performance. In: *Foundations for Practice in Occupational Therapy* (ed. E.A.S. Duncan), 81–91. London: Churchill Livingstone.

Thompson, A. (2019). Air inequality. *Scientific American* 8–10.

Tortora, G.J. and Derrickson, B. (2011). *Principles of Anatomy and Physiology*, 13e. Hoboken, NJ: Wiley.

Townsend, E.L., Richmond, J.L., Vogel-Farley, V.K., and Kathleen Thomas, K. (2010). Medial temporal lobe memory in childhood: developmental transitions. *Developmental Science* 13 (5): 738–751.

Toynbee, P. and Walker, D. (2010). *The Verdict: Did Labour Change Britain?* London: Granta.

Varley, D., Henry, J.D., Gibson, E. et al. (2021). An old problem revisited: how sensitive is time-based prospective memory to age-related differences? *Psychology and Aging* 36 (5): 616.

Wang, Q. (2003). Infantile amnesia reconsidered: a cross-cultural analysis. *Memory* 11 (1): 65–80.

Wang, Q., Leichtman, M.D., and Davies, K.I. (2000). Sharing memories and telling stories: American and Chinese mothers and their 3-year-olds. *Memory* 8 (3): 159–177.

Wang, Q., Conway, M., and Hou, Y.-B. (2007). Infantile amnesia: a cross-cultural investigation. *New Research in Cognitive Sciences* 1 (1): 95–104.

Wilcock, A.A. (2006). *An Occupational Perspective of Health*, 2e. Thorofare, NJ: Slack.

Wilkinson, R. and Pickett, K. (2010). *The Spirit Level: Why Equality Is Better for Everyone*. London: Penguin.

Williams, Z. (2022). The appalling death of Awaab Ishak shows how social housing tenants are treated as an underclass. *The Guardian*, 17 November. `https://www.theguardian.com/commentisfree/2022/nov/17/awaab-ishak-social-housing-tenants-underclass-black-mould` (accessed 16 August 2023)

Yaffe, K., Falvey, C., Harris, T.B. et al. (2013). Effect of socioeconomic disparities on incidence of dementia among biracial older adults: prospective study. *British Medical Journal* 347: f7051.

3 Memory Impairments

In this chapter amnesia is defined, including the subtypes of retrograde and anterograde amnesia. Key causes of amnesia include Korsakoff's syndrome, herpes encephalitis, hypoxia, vascular disorders, traumatic head injury and concussion.

The concept of post-traumatic amnesia (PTA) is introduced and there is a description of 'Ribot's law' of retrograde amnesia. The respective roles of damage in the hippocampal region and the neocortex in amnesia are discussed.

The 'standard consolidation model' of retrograde amnesia is explained, along with the newer 'multiple trace' hypothesis. It is shown that this newer model can inform occupational therapy assessment and that it also fits with views of memory that were encountered in Chapter 1.

Regarding anterograde amnesia, the early view that this results from a deficit in attention is explained. A more contemporary view is that anterograde amnesia actually represents a failure of consolidation. The chapter shows that amnesia may also result from a failure to relate items to each other, binding them into a unitary memory trace. This links back to the concept of 'relational memory' that was introduced in Chapter 2.

There is extensive discussion of Alzheimer's type dementia (ATD) and related dementias. It is shown that some authors have argued that changing occupational behaviours in young people may mean that current projections may underestimate the future incidence of these conditions.

The neuropathology underpinning Alzheimer's disease is explained. In addition, genetic and environmental risk factors are described. The role of acetylcholinesterase inhibitors and drugs inhibiting N-methyl-D-aspartate (NMDA) receptors is discussed. It is shown that these pharmacological treatments have only limited effectiveness and do not target the underlying disease process.

There is also a detailed account of the results of a randomised controlled trial of lecanemab, a drug that does tackle the underlying neuropathology in Alzheimer's disease. This is justified by the amount of publicity afforded to this trial at the time of writing.

The role of episodic memory impairment in Alzheimer's disease is explained. In addition, there are descriptions of the other principal causes of dementia.

Memory Impairment and Occupation: A Guide to Evaluation and Treatment, First Edition.
Jonathon O'Brien.
© 2024 John Wiley & Sons Ltd. Published 2024 by John Wiley & Sons Ltd.

These include vascular dementia, the fronto-temporal dementias (FTD) and Lewy body dementias (LBD).

Finally, there is a discussion of the memory impairments encountered in post-traumatic stress disorder (PTSD). In particular, the theoretical distinction between 'verbally accessible memory' (VAM), which is dependent on the medial temporal lobe, and 'situationally accessible memory' (SAM), which bypasses this region and may be typical of memory in PTSD, is outlined.

Amnesia

Kopelman (2002) defines amnesia as a disordered state of mind where learning and memory are disproportionately impaired relative to other areas of cognition. Amnesia affects declarative memory – that is, memories of episodes and information that can be consciously retrieved – while procedural memory for skills, and the ability to learn new skills, is intact (Eichenbaum 2012; Kopelman 2002). Kopelman (2002) cites the case of Henry Molaison as an example of this (see Chapter 1). It is important to point out that, in subcortical dementias such as Huntington's disease or Parkinson's disease, there may also be deficits in procedural learning (Kopelman 2002). However, putting these exceptions to one side, a key message is that the tasks and activities typically used in occupational therapy assessment and treatment may be relatively unimpaired, even in the presence of marked amnesia. However, the person may experience difficulty in work or educational settings requiring declarative memory as part of occupational performance.

There are also subtypes of amnesia. These include retrograde amnesia, which covers events happening prior to the causative injury or illness, and antero-grade amnesia, which describes loss of memory for things happening after the illness or injury (Bear et al. 2016). This section contains a description of some key causes of amnesia, while ATD and other causes of dementia are discussed further on in the chapter.

Korsakoff's syndrome is caused by a deficiency in thiamine, often resulting from excessive alcohol consumption (Kopelman 2002). There is a pattern of marked retrograde amnesia and also confabulation, a condition in which the person cannot distinguish false memories from events that actually happened (Worthington 2012). Memory impairments in the condition have been linked to damage in three main areas: first, the dorsomedial thalamic nucleus, which conveys inputs from the limbic system, including the amygdala, the basal nuclei and infero-temporal neocortex, to extensive regions of the frontal cortex; second, the mammillary bodies of the hypothalamus, which are connected to the hippocampus via the fornix; and third, the anterior thalamus, which receives inputs from the mammillary bodies of the hypothalamus and the hippocampus (Amaral and Strick 2013; Bear et al. 2016; Kopelman 2002; Tortora and Derrickson 2011). It has been suggested, therefore, that the condition may disrupt a memory circuit linking the frontal and medial temporal lobes (Kopelman 2002).

Amnesia may also be caused by herpes encephalitis, which causes extensive bilateral, and sometimes unilateral, damage to the temporal lobes as well as frontal lesions, and may also be associated with general atrophy of the cortex

(Kopelman 2002). Kopelman (2002) notes that the medial temporal lobes, including the hippocampus, amygdala, entorhinal, perirhinal and parahippocampal cortical areas, may be affected.

Of patients surviving herpes encephalitis, 70% have been found to have memory impairments (Wilson 2012). Retrograde amnesia may be extensive, with very little recollection of even remote memories, and lack of any episodic memories (Reed and Squire 1998). This may result from involvement of the lateral parts of the temporal cortex, which, as shown in Chapter 1, are a repository for long-term memory (Reed and Squire 1998). The pattern of amnesia is comparable to that in Korsakoff's syndrome, although the person may have greater insight into their impairments than in Korsakoff's and early memories may not be as spared (Kopelman 2002).

Warrington and Shallice (1984) describe two patients with a diagnosis of herpes simplex encephalitis. One, J.B.R., had extensive bilateral temporal lobe damage and marked retrograde and anterograde amnesia, while another, K.B., also had damage in these regions, but with more extensive lesions on the left side, and had profound anterograde amnesia (Warrington and Shallice 1984).

These people also had an unusual pattern of associative agnosia that affected identification of animate objects, such as animals, more than inanimate ones (Gazzaniga et al. 2009; Warrington and Shallice 1984). K.B. had more difficulty recognising food items than inanimate objects, a point worth remembering if working with patients with this condition on cooking activities (Warrington and Shallice 1984). Again, it can be seen that temporal lobe damage appears key to understanding the presence of amnesia and also, in these cases, associative agnosia.

Extreme hypoxia may be caused by failed attempts at suicide by hanging or breathing in carbon monoxide. There may be anterograde amnesia in these cases, stemming from concomitant damage to the thalamus and hippocampus (Kopelman 2002). For example, hypoxia has been linked to damage in the CA1 region of the hippocampus and the fornix, suggesting disruption to the networks connecting the hippocampus and the thalamus (Kopelman 2002).

Amnesia linked to vascular disorders is often associated with infarction of the medial temporal lobes, the thalamus and the retrosplenial cortex, which is located posteriorly to the hippocampus and receives inputs from the hippocampal formation (Kopelman 2002; Woolsey et al. 2003). It may also occur in subarachnoid haemorrhage (Kopelman 2002). Where damage is confined to the anterior region of the thalamus, this is associated with antero- rather than retrograde amnesia (Kopelman 2002). The hippocampus receives its blood supply from branches of the internal and external carotid arteries and bilateral damage to these structures leads to global amnesia, encompassing both retro- and anterograde amnesia, while unilateral damage leads to amnesia for specific types of information (Kopelman 2002).

Post-traumatic Amnesia

Traumatic head injury may also cause amnesia and is the most common cause of amnesia in people under the age of 25 (Kopelman 2002; Wilson 2012). Kopelman (2002, p. 2155) maintains that it is important to distinguish between different patterns of amnesia that can occur following trauma: retrograde amnesia, which is frequently short lasting; PTA; and 'islands' of preserved memory within the amnesia. Kosch et al. (2010) explain that PTA is the period following injury during which uninterrupted memory cannot be established and that duration of PTA has been used as an index of severity of traumatic brain injury (TBI) since 1932. PTA is discussed in more detail next.

Kosch et al. (2010) comment that the presence of diaschisis following from altered cholinergic function and diffuse axonal pathways may contribute to PTA (Kosch et al. 2010). Other authors show that PTA is frequently linked to diffuse axonal injury, secondary to impact causing rotation in the head, and the severity of the PTA is linked to the extent of injury and is also a predictor of the social, cognitive and psychiatric results (Baddeley 2015; Kopelman 2002).

PTA is distinguished by general cognitive disruption, delirium, retro- and anterograde amnesia, as well as agitation, sleep perturbation and delusion (Trevena-Peters et al. 2018). It is sometimes considered that active therapy treatment is not appropriate at this stage (Trevena-Peters et al. 2018).

Typically, the extent of PTA reduces in the period following the injury. An observed pattern of recovery is that personal information, followed by information about place and time, tends to return first (Baddeley 2015). However, once PTA reduces, there is generally a degree of residual retrograde amnesia, and this may be particularly marked in anterior temporal and frontal injury (Baddeley 2015; Kopelman 2002).

Kopelman (2002) points out that memory impairment can occur following mild concussion, after a blow to the head or abrupt halting of the head when in motion, such as in a road traffic accident. Mild concussion can lead to unconsciousness lasting from seconds to hours and is the most frequent cause of brain injury (Tortora and Derrickson 2011). In these cases, there may be recovery from amnesia after three months (Kopelman 2002).

Finally, Kopelman (2002) describes transient global amnesia, which affects mainly middle-aged and older men; it is characterised by marked anterograde amnesia and some retrograde amnesia, lasting between 4 and 11 hours. It is caused by reduced blood supply in the circuits linking the limbic and hippocampal regions. In addition, transient epileptic amnesia is a passing global amnesia resulting from epileptic seizures (Kopelman 2002).

A key feature of all these amnesias is that they are linked to harm in the medial temporal and/or diencephalic regions, or the basal forebrain inputs to these areas (Kopelman 2002). In the following sections, more detailed accounts of retrograde and anterograde amnesia are provided.

Retrograde Amnesia

Temporal Gradient in Retrograde Amnesia

Ribot (1882, p. 195) noted that the memory loss following brain injury extends back prior to the event itself, noting that 'forgetfulness is always retrograde'. He posited a 'law of regression or reversion' (Ribot 1882, p. 122), which stated that the memory impairment in brain disease fitted a pattern in which the most recent memories, being the least 'organised', were the most vulnerable, while earlier memories, being more organised, were more resistant. This hypothesis is now called 'Ribot's law' and has been accepted in the models of retrograde amnesia described next (Baddeley 2015; Eichenbaum 2012, p. 21).

Russell and Nathan (1946) stated that retrograde amnesia occurs for events that happened prior to injury, while the person was conscious. They argued that these events must have been registered by the senses but are not remembered. Russell and Nathan (1946) noted that the period of retrograde amnesia often reduces with time. For example, they recount the example of a soldier who had a head injury following an air raid in 1940. At first he remembered nothing about the six months before the event, but six months later he could remember what happened up to a few minutes preceding the injury (Russell and Nathan 1946). In addition, they show, like Ribot (1882), that restitution of memory is not a function of the *importance* of the events but of their *time*, so that earlier memories return first (Russell and Nathan 1946).

More recent authors have explored the phenomenon described by Ribot's law. Squire et al. (2001), for example, provided further evidence to support the view that retrograde amnesia is often 'temporally graded', so that earlier memories are more spared. They argue that this is linked to damage in the medial temporal lobe, for example in bilateral CA1 of the hippocampus, or areas of the broader hippocampal region, such as the dentate gyrus or entorhinal cortex.

Squire et al. (2001) show that, where retrograde amnesia does not show this temporal gradient so that remote and recent memories are equally affected, damage is in the neocortical lateral and anterior lobes. The authors suggest that this indicates that the medial temporal lobe structures underpinning recent memory have only a temporary function: memories depend on these initially but then become independent of them as time elapses (Squire et al. 2001).

Based on clinical case reports and also on animal studies, Squire et al. (2001) argue that the hippocampus is important for memory only for a limited period. However, the perirhinal and entorhinal regions are involved for longer, supporting the view that these two regions may mediate between the hippocampus and the long-term storage sites in association regions of the temporal and parietal neocortex, among other areas, which are the permanent repositories for long-term items (Squire et al. 2001). Overall, this means that memory consolidation must occur in a staged sequence (Squire et al. 2001).

Reed and Squire (1998) tested four patients experiencing varying levels of brain lesions. The aim was to determine the extent of retrograde and anterograde amnesia associated with different degrees of injury severity. Two patients had damage limited to the hippocampal formation, one as a result of anoxia following cardiac arrest and one of unknown origin. The third had more extensive damage to the bilateral regions of the temporal lobe, including the hippocampal formation but also the fusiform gyrus, part of the temporal neocortex, while the fourth had far-reaching damage to the medial temporal lobes bilaterally (Reed and Squire 1998; Gazzaniga et al. 2009). Patients three and four both had herpes simplex encephalitis. In addition, 13 age-matched, neurologically intact controls were included.

All the participants in Reed and Squire's (1998) study were evaluated on a range of measures. These included tests of vocabulary that entered the lexicon between 1985 and 1989, knowledge of public events occurring between 1940 and 1995, and images of famous faces from the same period. In addition, each person completed an autobiographical memory interview where questions covered recent events, early adulthood and childhood, with their answers being verified by two family members (Reed and Squire 1998).

One of the two patients with damage limited to the hippocampal formation was able to produce 10 autobiographical recollections, but 9 of these were from 10 to 13 years before the initiation of amnesia, suggesting that he had retrograde amnesia for autobiographical items extending to about 10 years prior to amnesia (Reed and Squire 1998). The other showed a similar pattern of impairment for recent happenings along with recall for earlier life events comparable with the neurologically intact controls (Reed and Squire 1998). In addition, these two patients' scores on most of the neuropsychological tests were comparable with the controls. Where they performed more poorly, this was for information from the period *after* they became amnesic, for example for famous faces and public events, and the scores were therefore explained with reference to anterograde amnesia, as their memory impairment meant that they would not have been able to learn this new information (Reed and Squire 1998).

Of the two patients with widespread damage to the temporal lobes, one scored zero for early adulthood and childhood autobiographical memory, while the other scored at the lower end of the normal range for early adult life but scored highly for childhood, results indicating severe retrograde amnesia for both participants (Reed and Squire 1998). In the latter case, the authors argue that the damage to the lateral temporal cortex was not as extensive, meaning that some memory was preserved (Reed and Squire 1998). Both of these patients also scored significantly worse on all the neuropsychological tests (Reed and Squire 1998).

Overall, the authors argue that these results suggest that the hippocampal formation is involved in the formation of new memories but not involved in the retrieval of older, established information (Reed and Squire 1998). When damage is confined to this region, retrograde amnesia is fairly limited. However, retrograde amnesia is more marked when damage extends to other regions of the temporal cortex, suggesting that these areas are the repository sites for older memories (Reed and Squire 1998).

Explaining Retrograde Amnesia

Explanatory models of retrograde amnesia in episodic and semantic memory have traditionally been based on a two-stage process (Winocur et al. 2010). Winocur et al. (2010, p. 2339) describe such models as 'standard consolidation theory' (SCT), dating back to the early work of Ribot (1882) and the research conducted with Henry Molaison (Scoville and Milner 1957).

In this standard consolidation approach, researchers have posited two time-dependent phases of consolidation. First, there is fast reorganisation at cell and synapse levels that occurs within seconds of learning. Second, there are changes to dispersed neural systems taking place over weeks, months or even years, which is 'systems-level consolidation' and involves the *same* memory trace being transferred to neocortical areas for more lengthy storage (Baddeley 2015; Winocur et al. 2010, p. 2340). These older traces, stored in neocortical regions, are therefore less vulnerable to retrograde amnesia occurring following damage to the medial temporal lobes.

One dissenting model is the 'multiple trace hypothesis' (Baddeley 2015, p. 447). This accepts the two-stage process of the other models, but also states that a trace is left of the remembered item in the hippocampus, and that the hippocampus is then involved in retrieval (Baddeley 2015). Retrograde amnesia, in this account, occurs when there is hippocampal damage, resulting in a loss of traces and making retrieval difficult (Baddeley 2015). This alternative hypothesis is discussed in more detail later.

Nadel and Moscovitch (1997, p. 271) describe what they call the 'standard model' of retrograde amnesia, which developed from the early research on Henry Molaison (Scoville and Milner 1957). In this account, they argue, it is supposed that the information to be remembered is primarily registered in neocortical areas. It is then consolidated by the hippocampus and other medial temporal lobe mechanisms in 'seconds' or at most 'tens of minutes' (Nadel and Moscovitch 1997, p. 217). It eventually becomes a memory trace that is deposited back in the neocortex, becoming independent of the hippocampus. They argue that this 'standard model' receives partial support from evidence that hippocampal lesions may leave distant memories intact, suggesting that the traces are deposited somewhere away from the hippocampal region (Nadel and Moscovitch 1997).

Nadel and Moscovitch (1997) maintain, however, that this standard model is unable to explain retrograde amnesia following extensive damage to the medial temporal lobes. Such amnesia can extend back 25–40 years, or even encompass the person's whole life, and they argue that, according to the standard model, this would mean that the medial temporal lobes were still engaged in consolidation for memories this old. However, this would not make sense, as such a lengthy process would have no 'adaptive basis' (Nadel and Moscovitch 1997, p. 218). They propose, rather, that the hippocampal region must be involved in the retrieval of even very distant memories, explaining the extensive retrograde amnesia seen in medial temporal lobe damage (Nadel and Moscovitch 1997).

Nadel and Moscovitch (1997) developed a multistage model to explain how the hippocampal region and the neocortex work together to form, maintain and retrieve episodic memories. First, the hippocampal region is *obliged* to encode any items that a person pays attention to or tries to consciously apprehend, after which the items are 'sparsely encoded' in the hippocampal complex (Nadel and Moscovitch 1997, p. 223). The encoding neurons then act as a pointer to the realms of the neocortex where the item is represented and this hippocampus–neocortex nexus functions as the memory trace for the item (Nadel and Moscovitch 1997).

An important point in this model is that each time the memory trace is activated, the neural and experiential settings are different, meaning that every new activation results in a fresh trace in the hippocampus (Nadel and Moscovitch 1997). In addition, because each fresh trace acts as a pointer to the arrangement of neurons in the neocortex that encodes the initial event, the trace itself will also contain information about that event (Nadel and Moscovitch 1997). The construction of manifold traces permits the extraction of facts about the world that are derived from the event trace, for example that Big Ben is in London, and these facts are subsequently stored separately to the trace for the event, as part of *semantic* memory (Nadel and Moscovitch 1997). Finally, these authors argue that the space and time contexts that make the trace an *episodic* item depend on ongoing engagement of the hippocampus for spatial aspects, and the frontal cortex for temporal components (Nadel and Moscovitch 1997).

This multiple traces of memory account is not based on the notion that items are transferred from the hippocampus to the neocortex, but that both regions continually work together (Nadel and Moscovitch 1997). This would explain the temporal gradient in retrograde amnesia, as recent traces, with fewer representations, would be more vulnerable to disruption than more established ones with manifold representations (Nadel and Moscovitch 1997). In addition, it would help explain the extent of retrograde amnesia, because the trace in the hippocampus is meagre and spread out, meaning that damage in the region could impair the acquiring, retaining or recovering of any memory (Nadel and Moscovitch 1997). In both cases, the gradient and the extent of retrograde amnesia would be functions of the scale of hippocampal damage (Nadel and Moscovitch 1997).

These ideas were subsequently developed in work by Winocur et al. (2010), who argued that the hippocampus is involved for as long as the memory maintains episodic elements. This episodic memory then facilitates the development of a 'schematic version' of the initial memory in the neocortex, which encompasses the key elements of the original event but lacks details about the setting (Winocur et al. 2010, p. 2344). In this sense, the hippocampus plays a role in the development of *semantic* memory, which is 'transformed' once stored in the neocortex, so that it is now independent of context (Winocur et al. 2010, p. 2344).

Key differences from SCT are that this transformed memory is *different* from the hippocampus-dependent memory, and that these two distinct traces can co-exist (Winocur et al. 2010). Winocur et al. (2010) maintain that their model provides a better explanation of retrograde amnesia for episodes just preceding hippocampal damage, as it implies that the ensuing disruption of memory transformation would result in situation-specific items being lost.

The model promulgated by Winocur et al. (2010) has implications for occupational therapy practice. These authors stress that the retrieval process is *dynamic* and is not a simple extraction of a pre-structured trace. Rather, the cues for retrieval and the information to-be-retrieved interact, so that the emergent memory is a *reconstruction*, an amalgam of the retrieved items, the cues and, crucially for occupational therapists, 'the demands of the particular task' (Winocur et al. 2010, p. 2353). The authors, here, draw on the theories of memory retrieval developed by Bartlett (1995) and Tulving (1985) that were encountered in Chapter 1.

In addition, it will be remembered that, in research on prospective memory, it has been shown that a retrieval cue that is closely associated with the action-to-be-remembered is more effective and makes successful retrieval more likely (Dismukes 2010). Similarly, Craik and Lockhart (1972) found that a cue to retrieve an item was more effective if it matched the initial coding, meaning that the original 'learning context' could be restored. Indeed, it has been shown that people with amnesia may benefit more from contextual cues in aiding retrieval than people without neurological impairment (Kopelman 2002). So, the cues and the context of retrieval make a difference to how memory emerges. This means, for example, that aspects of occupational performance underpinned by memory may appear impaired in an unfamiliar hospital kitchen or bathroom, when compared with the familiar facilities of the patient's usual place of residence. In addition, an occupational therapist supporting a memory-impaired child in the classroom, or an adult returning to work following TBI, should consider carefully the type of cues that will be most useful in supporting occupational performance.

Anterograde Amnesia

Anterograde amnesia implies impairment in the encoding, storage and retrieval of 'new information' about episodes that have happened at or after the occurrence of the illness or trauma, and would normally be available for future use (Baddeley 2015; Bradley and Kapur 2012; Eichenbaum 2012, p. 383). Short-term memory – that is, memory of one minute or less – may be intact, but the person has no ability to form new long-term memories (Dewar et al. 2009).

Henry Molaison, whose history was outlined in Chapter 1, has been described as 'a classic case of anterograde amnesia' (Baddeley 2015, p. 438). Molaison, for example, was found to have a normal digit span recall, while he was unable to form new long-term episodic or semantic memories (Milner et al. 1968).

Generally, the key impairment in anterograde amnesia is in episodic memory, and other areas, such as working and semantic memory, may be unaffected (Baddeley 2015). Kopelman (2002) points out differences between remembering and knowing: when we remember, we recreate the *feeling* of the experience, while 'knowing' information is less personal and does not imply a reliving of the past. While people with amnesia may be impaired in both areas, there is greater impairment in remembering (Kopelman 2002).

Kopelman (2002) cites the case of a man with damage in the left hippocampus, perirhinal and entorhinal cortices and parahippocampal gyrus, but with comparative sparing of the inferior lateral region of the temporal cortex (Kopelman 2002). This person performed very poorly on episodic memory tasks, but did have some semantic memory and was able to recognise personal life events and personally known individuals (Kopelman 2002). It seemed he was able to learn new semantic information despite the near absence of anterograde episodic memory. For example, he was not aware that his daughter had reached maturity but could identify former US president Ronald Reagan (Kopelman 2002). In keeping with these insights, Baddeley (2015) suggests that there is a consensus position among researchers that the main problem in amnesia is an inability to locate an episode in its temporal and spatial context.

Explaining Anterograde Amnesia

Early findings with densely amnesic patients showed that they were able to recall a three-digit number or word pair for several minutes, but would forget it as soon as their attention shifted to a new item (Scoville and Milner 1957). It was argued that the ongoing refocusing of attention required in everyday situations meant that these patients had seemingly total anterograde amnesia (Scoville and Milner 1957). Scoville and Milner (1957) reported, for example, that Henry Molaison had no memory of prior tests once his attention was diverted to a fresh task, and they noted similar findings for other patients, named as D.C. and M.B., who had also undergone surgery removing parts of the hippocampus and hippocampal gyrus bilaterally. Overall, then, the early view was that anterograde amnesia resulted from impaired attention.

These initial insights have been questioned. Dewar et al. (2009, p. 3), for example, suggest that amnesic forgetting may stem from a failure to consolidate new learning as result of 'retroactive interference', rather than shifting attention away from the learned items, as previously supposed. They argue that memories are initially vulnerable but become consolidated over time. However, this process can be disrupted if the person is required to devote additional cognitive resources to another task during the consolidation period.

Interesting evidence for this view is presented by Kopelman (2002), who cites a study in which concussed American football players were able to provide quite detailed accounts of their injury straight after the event but were later unable to remember anything, suggesting a failure of consolidation. In addition, Baddeley (2015) argues that it is widely accepted that anterograde, like retrograde, amnesia may be underpinned by failures of consolidation, which, as shown earlier, is thought to be a function of the hippocampal region.

Dewar et al. (2009) tested this hypothesis in an experiment in which they tested 12 amnesic individuals and 12 neurologically intact controls. The participants were given four trials learning lists of 15 words. Their immediate recall of the lists was assessed. There was then a nine-minute delay, after which their recall was once again tested (Dewar et al. 2009). However, there were three different conditions for the delay period that involved an interfering picture recognition task occurring at different intervals during the nine minutes. In the 'early' condition the interfering activity occurred in the first three minutes; in the 'mid' condition it occurred after three minutes; and in the 'late' condition it occurred in the final three minutes (Dewar et al. 2009, p. 13). Also, during the times where there was no interfering task being performed, the participants were directed to relax in a quiet, dimly lit room (Dewar et al. 2009).

It was found that the patients' delayed recall was significantly improved in the late condition, where there was an unfilled delay of six minutes, compared with the early condition, where there was an unfilled delay of three minutes (Dewar et al. 2009). This effect was not observed in the non-impaired control group (Dewar et al. 2009). In addition, each of the 12 patients increased their scores significantly in the late interference condition when compared with the early condition, including eight patients who had initially scored zero in the early condition (Dewar et al. 2009). The longer relaxation periods associated with the later conditions allowed more time for consolidation of learning, and the authors therefore maintain that amnesia occurs at least in part because of disruption of consolidation (Dewar et al. 2009).

Key Characteristics of Amnesia

Ryan et al. (2000) argued that there were two approaches to understanding amnesia. The first is the view that amnesia involves impairment in the declarative memory for the relations between items or events that normally allows the 'binding' of constituents (Kopelman 2002, p. 2158). The second is the approach that sees amnesia as a limitation in explicit, conscious memory for information (Ryan et al. 2000). These researchers tested these hypotheses in an experiment, described next.

Ryan et al. (2000) asked 12 neurologically intact people and 6 people with amnesia resulting from brain impairments to view a series of scenes. Some of these scenes were shown initially in a non-manipulated format and then with the relation of items from the scene manipulated in various ways (Ryan et al. 2000). The eye movements of the participants were recorded and two variables were measured, the 'number of fixations' and the 'number of regions sampled' (Ryan et al. 2000, p. 456).

It was found that the healthy participants showed a manipulation effect, whereby the manipulated segments of the scenes had a significantly higher number of fixations when compared with the novel or repeated images (Ryan et al. 2000). However, there was no effect of manipulating the images for the amnesic individuals (Ryan et al. 2000). The authors argue that this is confirmation of the hypothesis that amnesia is actually the impaired declarative memory for the *relations* between the key elements of items or events, the 'relational memory binding of all manner of relations' (Ryan et al. 2000, p. 460).

Alzheimer's Type Dementia

Prevalence

ATD is a neurodegenerative condition and is defined by progressive impairments in two or more domains of cognition or areas of behaviour (Chatzikostopoulos et al. 2022). It is the most common cause of dementia, affecting 11% of people over the age of 65 (Breijyeh and Karaman 2020; Snowden 2012; Tortora and Derrickson 2011). Internationally, there are about 24 million people with the condition and this is predicted to increase fourfold by 2050 (Breijyeh and Karaman 2020).

Manwell et al. (2022) argue the occupational patterns of millennials, who were born between 1980 and 1995, and generation Z, born between 1996 and 2012, mean that existing epidemiological projections may underestimate future levels of ATD and related dementias. These authors present evidence that 17–19-year-olds spend an average of six hours each day on 'mobile digital devices', while generation Z individuals spend three hours more on this occupation each day when compared with millennials (Manwell et al. 2022, p. 6). In addition, they show that large amounts of time looking at screens has been linked to learning and memory impairment, maintaining that this can be associated with evidence that excessive time on screen is linked to thinning of the hippocampus and temporal cortex, and reduced volume in the orbitofrontal cortex (Manwell et al. 2022). They suggest that, taking these factors into account, predictions of the prevalence of ATD and related dementias in the United States, for example, which currently suggest this will double by 2100, should be adjusted to an increase of between four and six times current levels (Manwell et al. 2022).

Aetiology

Key neuropathological features of ATD are the presence of accumulations of beta-amyloid protein (Aβ) outside of the neurons, which are known as plaques (Breijyeh and Karaman 2020). These plaques, which accumulate in the hippocampus, amygdala and neocortex, are key in disrupting neural processes and the neurons themselves (Breijyeh and Karaman 2020). In addition, neurofibrillary tangles, which are deposits of tau protein that has undergone hyperphosphorylation – that is, it has had phosphate groups added to the point of saturation – appear in the cell body, dendrites and axon of the neuron (Breijyeh and Karaman 2020).

These plaques and tangles contribute to the damage and loss of synapses, although the precise role of the abnormal protein accumulation in triggering the cerebral changes causing dementia has been debated (Breijyeh and Karaman 2020). Key areas of protein deposition and neural damage are in the medial temporal lobes and temporoparietal regions of the neocortex; in particular, there is marked atrophy in the hippocampus (Crossman and Neary 2020; Snowden 2012). The location of the disease sites helps explain the distinct pattern of amnesia in the disease, which is discussed further on.

In order to understand the role of genetics in ATD, it is first helpful to recall some basic information about the role of genes in development. A gene is a portion of a molecule of deoxyribonucleic acid (DNA) located in the nucleus of a cell. It is responsible for inherited characteristics and for synthesising proteins, and therefore for controlling most body activities (Tortora and Derrickson 2011). Genes are organised in chromosomes, which are lengthy DNA molecules, normally 46 pairs in human body cells, with 23 chromosomes from each parent (Tortora and Derrickson 2011); 22 of the pairs are homologous chromosomes, known as autosomes, which have the same structure and control the same physical characteristics, for example hair or eye colour (Martini 2018). The genome is the total complement of genes in an organism or cell (Tortora and Derrickson 2011).

Genes controlling the same characteristics are located on the equivalent position, or locus, on each homologous chromosome (Martini 2018). Despite this, the fact that genes originate with different parents means that they may have different forms, known as alleles (Martini 2018). These different alleles control the exact manner in which genes affect characteristics (Martini 2018). A mutation occurs due to variations in the sequence of subunits making up a gene (Martini 2018). Mutations may be linked to specific diseases.

Early-onset ATD, which occurs at or under the age of 65, is linked to mutations in genes including amyloid precursor protein (APP), presenilin 1, on chromosome 14, and presenilin 2, on chromosome 1 (Hillam 2004; Martini 2018; Breijyeh and Karaman 2020; Chatzikostopoulos et al. 2022). These mutations are linked to aggregations of Aβ, which has led to an 'amyloid cascade hypothesis' positing that Aβ deposits trigger malfunction of synapses, destruction of neurons and development of neurofibrillary tangles (Hascup and Hascup 2020, p. 2).

For late-onset ATD, occurring after age 65, the key genetic risk factor, second only to age, is the presence of an allele of the gene coding for apolipoprotein E (apoE), *apoE ε4* (Hascup and Hascup 2020; Gustavson et al. 2023; Snowden 2012). In addition to these genetic risk factors, there are over 40 genes or genome locations associated with ATD risk, and when combined they give a 'polygenic risk score' for ATD (Gustavson et al. 2023, p. 2).

In addition to the changes already described, another brain factor in ATD is reduced synthesis of the neurotransmitter acetylcholine (ACh; Breijyeh and Karaman 2020). ACh plays a key role in cognitive processes including learning, memory and attention (Breijyeh and Karaman 2020). Depletion of this neurotransmitter may therefore have an impact on these processes (Breijyeh and Karaman 2020).

There is a range of environmental risk factors for Alzheimer's disease (Breijyeh and Karaman 2020; Hascup and Hascup 2020). The first of these is ATD linked to TBI. TBI is defined as involving impact to the head resulting in brain injury, frequently in the temporal and frontal regions (Hascup and Hascup 2020). Primary developments following TBI include oedema, reduced blood flow, excitotoxicity and changes in glial cells that lead to the death of neurons (Hascup and Hascup 2020). This loss of neurons may be a factor in cognitive impairment in ATD, particularly if *apoE ε4* is also present (Hascup and Hascup 2020).

Chronic traumatic encephalopathy (CTE) occurs as a result of repeated impact affecting the brain over an extended period, and has become a prominent issue in sports such as rugby. Aβ deposits and neurofibrillary tangles have been found in CTE and have also been revealed in the brain in the years following TBI; the precise mechanisms of this remain unclear, however (Hascup and Hascup 2020). Ultimately, the evidence linking TBI and ATD is inconsistent, with some research showing the presence of dementia following trauma and some not, and methodological limitations and heterogeneity lead Hascup and Hascup (2020) to call for further investigation of this putative connection.

ATD can also be linked to blood–brain barrier (BBB) impairment (Hascup and Hascup 2020). The BBB normally functions to sustain the extracellular fluid in the central nervous system (CNS) and to block microbes and toxic substances from entering the CNS via the bloodstream (Hascup and Hascup 2020). As a person ages, there can be a reduction in blood flow to the cerebrum, alongside failure of the BBB in the association and limbic regions. The result is reduced supply of 'energy substrates' and impaired removal of damaging protein accumulation (Hascup and Hascup 2020, p. 4). Compromised vascular processes such as these may lead to the progression of ATD, and people with ATD do demonstrate reduced blood flow in the cerebrum as the condition progresses (Hascup and Hascup 2020).

Age-related damage in the BBB first occurs in the hippocampus and is more marked in those with cognitive impairments. This may lead to both reduced cerebral blood flow and increased permeability in blood vessels and may result in toxic substances entering the CNS and causing destruction of neurons (Hascup and Hascup 2020). In addition, impaired vascular function may lead to the build-up of Aβ deposits in the vessels.

Some researchers have developed a 'two-hit vascular hypothesis', which posits that factors such as diabetes, hypertension and obesity lead to impaired BBB and reduced blood flow, and compromised relations between the vascular system and the CNS. This results in neural damage, which then leads to Aβ build-up, progressing to ATD via increased Aβ and tau deposits and ultimately accelerating cognitive decline (Hascup and Hascup 2020).

Another factor is 'metabolic syndrome' (MetS), which encompasses conditions such as type 2 diabetes, hyperglycaemia and hypercholesterolaemia (Hascup and Hascup 2020, p. 4). Resistance to insulin, for example, is a risk factor for ATD and has been found to lead to damage in the dentate area of the hippocampus as a result of reduced blood glucose levels (Hascup and Hascup 2020). Insulin is produced within the brain and has been linked to a range of benefits, including glucose consumption, curbing effects of inflammation-causing cytokines, plasticity of synapses and enhanced cognition. Conversely, insulin impairment is associated with more rapid ageing and has been identified in the hippocampus in people with ATD (Hascup and Hascup 2020). Resistance to insulin is also linked to raised deposits of Aβ and hyperphosphorylation of tau, which may in turn lead to raised levels of inflammation-causing cytokines in glial cells that can cross the BBB. Overall, the effect is to increase changes associated with ATD and destruction of neurons (Hascup and Hascup 2020).

Another possible environmental factor is disturbed sleep, which has increased in recent times as a result of extensive working hours and time spent on screens (Hascup and Hascup 2020). Chronic sleep disruption has been implicated in impaired cognition and the onset of MetS (Hascup and Hascup 2020). It has also been linked to ATD, particularly when involving breathing disturbance or insomnia, and deprivation of sleep has been linked to Aβ aggregation and disruption of apoE transport to the brain, which may have an impact on myelination, plasticity in synapses and cognitive function (Hascup and Hascup 2020). Overall, however, Hascup and Hascup (2020) stress that more research is required on the role of sleep disturbance.

Further environmental factors include air pollution and diet. Exposure to air contamination has been linked to inflammation in the brain, degeneration of neurons and also increased presence of tau and Aβ (Breijyeh and Karaman 2020). Regarding diet, consumption of antioxidants, which protect against the damaging effects of food being exposed to oxygen, and vitamins and fish, for example, has been found to be protective. Conversely, a high-calorie diet rich in saturated fatty acids as well as malnutrition have been identified as risk factors (Breijyeh and Karaman 2020). These dietary factors may be linked to obesity, which is linked to cardiovascular disease and type 2 diabetes, which are risk factors for Alzheimer's disease (Breijyeh and Karaman 2020).

The environmental factors outlined provide support for occupational therapy conceptual practice models that stress the role of environment and occupation in occupational performance. For example, patterns of occupation are shifting for many towards increased screen time. In addition, the exposure of some populations to contaminated environments reveals the impact of socioeconomic injustice. These issues are discussed further in Chapter 4.

Treatment

At present there are only two categories of pharmacological treatment for ATD. The first category is drugs that inhibit the enzyme cholinesterase, which normally breaks down ACh (Breijyeh and Karaman 2020; Hascup and Hascup 2020; Tortora and Derrickson 2011). The inhibition of this enzyme increases the availability of ACh at the synapse (Breijyeh and Karaman 2020; Hascup and Hascup 2020; Tortora and Derrickson 2011). Examples of these drugs, known as acetylcholinesterase inhibitors, are donepezil, galantamine and rivastigmine (Breijyeh and Karaman 2020).

The other category is drugs that inhibit NMDA receptors. These receptors can become overactive, leading to a damaging influx of calcium ions into the neuron, so inhibition helps to restore normal function (Breijyeh and Karaman 2020). The only approved medication of this type is memantine (Breijyeh and Karaman 2020).

Neither of these drug classes treats the underlying disease, only the symptoms (Breijyeh and Karaman 2020; Hascup and Hascup 2020). There are ongoing attempts to reverse the underlying disease process, which involve the presence of Aβ plaques and neurofibrillary tangles (Hascup and Hascup 2020). One widely reported recent trial of a new treatment that does target the disease process itself is discussed next.

Lecanemab is an antibody that binds soluble Aβ in people with early-stage ATD. A phase three randomised controlled trial was conducted with participants between 50 and 90 years old who had a diagnosis of mild cognitive impairment (MCI) or mild ATD (van Dyck et al. 2023). All had episodic memory impairments (van Dyck et al. 2023).

The participants were randomised to a group given intravenous lecanemab, with 729 eventually completing the trial, and a group given a placebo, where 757 completed (van Dyck et al. 2023). The primary outcome measure was the 'Clinical Dementia Rating – Sum of Boxes' (CDR-SB; van Dyck, et al. 2023, p. 3). The CDR-SB is based on a semi-structured interview conducted with patients and their carers. The interviewer uses their judgement to score from 0 to 3 on each of six domains: 'memory, orientation, judgement and problem solving, community affairs, home and hobbies, and personal care' (Morris 1993, p. 2412; van Dyck et al. 2023). Each score is associated with a descriptor, for example in the memory domain a score of zero matches to the statement 'no memory loss or slight inconstant forgetfulness', while three is matched with 'severe memory loss; only fragments remain' (Morris 1993, p. 2413). A *higher* score in the CDR-SB indicates a greater level of impairment (van Dyck et al. 2023). A main secondary outcome measure was the difference in amyloid load, which is measured in centiloids, following treatment, measured using positron emission tomography (PET; van Dyck et al. 2023).

All measurements were taken at baseline and then again at 18 months. The mean baseline score on CDR-SB was 3.2 for both the lecanemab and placebo groups, while at 18 months the mean score for the lecanemab group was 1.21 and for the placebo group 1.66, a statistically significant difference indicating lower impairment levels for the lecanemab (van Dyck et al. 2023).

The amyloid load was evaluated in a subgroup of 698 individuals. At baseline there were 77.92 centiloids in the lecanemab group and 75.03 centiloids in the placebo group; at 18 months there were −55.48 centiloids in the lecanemab group, which took this group below the threshold for elevated amyloid load in the brain, and 3.64 centiloids in the placebo group (van Dyck et al. 2023). Overall, then, there were lower levels for the lecanemab group and these differences were statistically significant (van Dyck et al. 2023). In addition, the lecanemab group showed lower levels of impairment on a clinician-rated outcome measure of cognitive function.

Memory in Alzheimer's Type Dementia

Hascup and Hascup (2020) show that cerebral atrophy and anterograde amnesia are key features of ATD. In keeping with this, ATD is characterised by impaired episodic memory, working memory and executive function (Chatzikostopoulos et al. 2022; Gustavson et al. 2023; López-Pérez et al. 2023).

López-Pérez et al. (2023) point out that episodic memory is underpinned by medial temporal lobe mechanisms, particularly those involving the hippocampus and the surrounding entorhinal, perirhinal and parahippocampal cortices, and pathways between anterior and posterior cortical areas. As pointed out already, these are the key regions affected in ATD. Furthermore, 'associative memory', which these authors suggest is a component of episodic memory and involves temporal, spatial and other components of experience being bound together into an individual episode by medial temporal lobe mechanisms, has been found to be impaired in people with MCI with a likelihood of developing Alzheimer's disease (Chatzikostopoulos et al. 2022, p. 2; López-Pérez et al. 2023, p. 9).

Gustavson et al. (2023) tested a hypothesis that the polygenic risk score, as discussed earlier, would be associated with changes in episodic memory and executive function. In their study, 1168 male twins were recruited from a cohort who had all served in the US military between 1965 and 1975, all of whom were cognitively unimpaired when the first of three assessments, conducted at an average of 56, 62 and 68 years, was undertaken (Gustavson et al. 2023). Genetic data was used to compile polygenic risk scores along with genotyping of apoE (Gustavson et al. 2023). For apoE, weighted scores were given for different alleles, with the highest score for *apoE ε4* (Gustavson et al. 2023).

It was found that higher polygenic risk scores were significantly associated with a greater drop in episodic memory and executive function scores (Gustavson et al. 2023). In addition, when apoE variants were taken out of the polygenic risk scores, the association was generally non-significant, although in one statistical analysis the relationship with episodic memory scores remained significant, while those for executive function, including working memory, remained non-significant. The authors argue that these latter results indicate that episodic memory impairment, although being driven predominantly by the *apoE ε4* allele, may involve other genetic risk factors, while executive function impairments resulted mainly from *apoE ε4* (Gustavson et al. 2023). This research provides interesting evidence linking the aetiology of ATD with the memory impairments experienced in the condition.

Chatzikostopoulos et al. (2022) discuss the diagnostic value of episodic memory in ATD. Especially useful for occupational therapists is their point that episodic memory impairment is the 'best predictor' of shopping skills in ATD (Chatzikostopoulos et al. 2022, p. 3).

Furthermore, they describe 'amnesic mild cognitive impairment' (aMCI; Chatzikostopoulos et al. 2022, p. 1), which is a subtype of MCI involving memory deficits. It has been found that changes in episodic memory performance can be used as an index to chart different phases of aMCI and the period between onset of ATD and development of more marked symptoms (Chatzikostopoulos et al. 2022). So, knowledge of episodic memory status can help therapists assess levels of impairment in Alzheimer's disease, including in performance of activities of daily living.

Chatzikostopoulos et al. (2022) used scores on the Doors and People test battery, which deploys four subtests for evaluating episodic memory in a manner considered to have ecological validity, in order to track changes in episodic memory in people with aMCI and ATD. People with early aMCI, late aMCI and

ATD, with an average age of 76, were tested with Doors and People (Chatzikostopoulos et al. 2022).

The aMCI patients were divided into early- and late-stage groups based on the results of a range of neuropsychological tests (Chatzikostopoulos et al. 2022). It was found that there were statistically different results on all of the Doors and People subtests for the early aMCI and late aMCI groups, indicating that episodic memory performance could be used to distinguish these categories (Chatzikostopoulos et al. 2022). In addition, it was found that the results of the 'people' component of the test, which involves the person recalling the occupation and name of individuals presented in pictures, could be used to distinguish between early aMCI and mild ATD (Chatzikostopoulos et al. 2022). Overall, the conclusion was that a neuropsychological test of episodic memory could be used to distinguish early and late aMCI and mild ATD. The authors propose that the differing performance in the groups might be linked to progressive pathology in the hippocampus (Chatzikostopoulos et al. 2022). Again, the results point to the important roles of this brain region and episodic memory in understanding ATD.

As well as ATD, there is a range of other cause of dementia, which are discussed in Box 3.1.

BOX 3.1   SUBTYPES OF DEMENTIA

There are four main subtypes of dementia: Alzheimer's type (ATD), vascular, Lewy body (LBD) and front-temporal dementia (FTD). Warchol (2006) notes that ATD accounts for around 60% of dementia cases. Estimates for the prevalence of vascular dementia range from 15% to 20% of dementia cases (O'Brien and Thomas 2015; Warchol 2006). LBD accounts for 20% of cases (Warchol 2006). FTD may account for between 3% and 26% of dementia cases (Bang et al. 2015). People with vascular dementia, LBD and FTD are all likely to be encountered by occupational therapists. These subtypes are therefore discussed in more detail in this box.

Vascular Dementia

As has been discussed, vascular dementia is the most frequent cause of dementia after Alzheimer's disease (O'Brien and Thomas 2015). Vascular disease affecting subcortical regions is the main cause (O'Brien and Thomas 2015). There is a range of subtypes of vascular dementia and three are described here. The first is multi-infarct dementia, which involves extensive infarcts in the cortex; the second is small vessel dementia, also known as subcortical vascular dementia, which involves lesions in white matter regions; and the third is ATD with cardiovascular disease, which involves a combination of vascular impairments, medial temporal lobe damage, atrophy and a mix of tau and amyloid pathology with vascular disease (O'Brien and Thomas 2015, p. 1699).

Aetiology

Risk factors for developing vascular dementia include age, with the risk doubling every 5.3 years, and stroke, with 15–30% of stroke survivors developing the condition within three months following the event (O'Brien and Thomas 2015). The risk of developing post-stroke vascular dementia is increased by being female, having low education levels, and the presence of atrophy in the medial temporal lobe and other brain regions (O'Brien and Thomas 2015). General risk factors include late-life depression, also noted as a risk for Alzheimer's disease (O'Brien and Thomas 2015). In addition, impairments affecting vascular function, such as hypertension, ischaemic heart disease, atrial fibrillation and obesity, are risk factors for both Alzheimer's disease and vascular dementia (O'Brien and Thomas 2015).

Memory, Other Cognitive Impairments and Mortality

While memory is a key impairment in ATD, which also has a well-defined pattern of progression, vascular dementia has a more varied presentation. Clinically, the presentation depends on the brain regions affected by vascular disease (O'Brien and Thomas 2015; Skilbeck 2012). Vascular disease in subcortical regions is often present and has impacts on fronto-striatal neural circuitry, leading to impaired executive function, attention and information processing (O'Brien and Thomas 2015). The impact on language, praxis and memory is more varied. However, apathy and depression are frequent and mortality levels are higher than for Alzheimer's disease, normally three to five years following onset, mainly due to the presence of vascular disease (O'Brien and Thomas 2015).

One distinguishing feature between Alzheimer's disease and vascular dementia is that people with Alzheimer's often have little insight into their condition from quite early on in the disease. However, people with vascular dementia may maintain insight, unless there is marked frontal lobe involvement (Skilbeck 2012).

Treatment

Treatment of vascular dementia involves blood pressure reduction, although O'Brien and Thomas (2015) report methodological problems in research in this area. It is possible that medication controlling hypertension is effective in preventing vascular dementia as it may reduce the risk of stroke (O'Brien and Thomas 2015). Positive findings have also come from treatment programmes that combine vascular treatment, cognitive work, exercise and instruction on nutrition (O'Brien and Thomas 2015). Skilbeck (2012) suggests that activities such as dancing and playing games may benefit the person, possibly via increasing blood supply to the brain.

Fronto-temporal Dementia

Prevalence

FTD is the third most widespread type of dementia across all age groups, behind ATD and LBD (Bang et al. 2015). In the United Kingdom, the prevalence of FTD is 3–26 per 100 000 in people aged from 45 to 65 years. It usually occurs in people in their 50s and 60s and affects females and males to the same extent. The disease process cannot be treated, although medication may be used to modify behaviour (Bang et al. 2015). It has also been known as Pick's disease, although, as shown further on, this term is now applied to a subtype of FTD (Bang et al. 2015).

Subtypes of Fronto-temporal Dementia

Like the other types of dementia discussed here, FTD is a neurodegenerative condition (Bang et al. 2015). The key features are atrophy in the frontal or temporal lobes, and of the fronto-insular area in particular (Bang et al. 2015). Snowden (2012, p. 567) points out that the circumscribed anatomy of these dementias leads to them being labelled 'focal dementias', despite the fact that atrophy can be more far-reaching than in ATD and the weight of the brain at death is usually lighter than in ATD.

There are three subtypes of FTD. The first is the behavioural variant, with a presentation involving executive impairments and changes in behaviour; the second is non-fluent primary progressive aphasia, which involves progressive impairments in word production and grammar; and the third is 'semantic variant primary progressive aphasia', which entails progressive deficiencies in semantic knowledge and names (Bang et al. 2015, p. 1672).

These subtypes may blend in with each other as the disease spreads throughout the frontal and temporal lobes. The results may be cognitive impairments of a global nature, parkinsonism and, in about 12.5% of behavioural variant cases, motor neurone disease, although mild motor neurone disease symptoms occur in around 40% of FTD cases overall (Bang et al. 2015).

The final point of the disease may entail difficulty in eating and swallowing and movement problems, and death usually occurs about eight years after disease onset, often from infections such as pneumonia (Bang et al. 2015). Snowden (2012) points out that some people may live for 10–15 years with the condition, but that those who develop motor neurone disease may die within 2–3 years.

Snowden (2012, p. 567) offers a slightly different classification of these dementias. This author gives an umbrella label of 'fronto-temporal lobar degeneration' that covers FTD, 'progressive non-fluent aphasia', and 'semantic dementia' (Snowden 2012 p. 567). In this account, FTD is linked to atrophy in right and left anterior temporal and frontal lobes. Progressive non-fluent aphasia, meanwhile, results from atrophy in the left perisylvian region, the area around the lateral fissure of the cerebrum that encompasses Broca's and Wernicke's areas. Finally, semantic dementia occurs following bilateral degeneration in middle and inferior temporal regions (Snowden 2012). Notwithstanding this classification, the remainder of this section will use the taxonomy described by Bang et al. (2015).

The three subtypes require more detailed description. In the behavioural variant, initial features may include changes in personality, uncharacteristic disinhibited actions and crimes such as theft, sexual approaches, public urination or involvement in 'hit-and-run' traffic accidents (Bang et al. 2015, p. 1673). People may exhibit reduced impulse control and lack of concern for the consequences of their actions. There may also be apathy; reduced empathy for family and others; neglect of personal care; excessive consumption of sweets, biscuits and chocolates, alcohol or cigarettes; walking around unclothed; and lack of insight into their condition (Bang et al. 2015; Snowden 2012). Leocadi et al. (2023) state that such behaviour may be labelled sociopathic, in that the person knows they are acting in an improper manner, but does not care about this.

Impaired executive function in behavioural variant FTD, in line with frontal lobe pathology, may involve perseveration, problems with switching attention, planning and organisation; the person may also be distractible and unconcerned about their performance on tests (Snowden 2012). In addition, repetitive motor behaviour can occur, which could range from rubbing the hands and tapping the feet to more complex patterns, such as following a particular route or performing the same task daily at the same time (Snowden 2012). These repeated patterns can be triggered by environmental cues, such as signs in the street (Snowden 2012).

Primary progressive aphasia involves reduced linguistic ability, without behavioural challenges, for the initial two years following onset, characterised by impairments in naming, comprehending and syntax (Bang et al. 2015). The person may become very frustrated at failure to retrieve a word from their vocabulary (Snowden 2012).

Semantic variant primary progressive aphasia is described as 'perhaps the most homogeneous of all neurodegenerative disorders' (Bang et al. 2015; Snowden 2012, p. 572). It results from anterior temporal lobe and amygdala degeneration. There is aphasia for semantic items and impaired conceptual understanding affecting multiple modalities (Bang et al. 2015; Snowden 2012). For example, the person may fail to recognise tactile, olfactory or gustatory stimuli (Snowden 2012). There may also be associative agnosia, where the person has problems identifying the use of objects. In all these cases, they may perceive the stimulus correctly but are unable to assign meaning to it (Bang et al. 2015; Kartsounis 2012; Snowden 2012). They may also have difficulty with names of people, objects and places and reduced comprehension (Bang et al. 2015).

Aetiology

A familial occurrence of dementia is reported in 40% of FTD cases, though only 10% of cases are explained by autosomal dominance; that is, inherited directly from a parent (Bang et al. 2015; Snowden 2012; Martini 2018).

Memory

The key features of FTD are altered behaviour, executive function and language impairments (Bang et al. 2015). The presence of memory problems *early on* in primary progressive aphasia, for example, suggests that ATD may be the cause rather than FTD, although the two conditions can occur together (Bang et al. 2015).

In semantic dementia, verbal and non-verbal semantic information are affected, while episodic items are relatively intact (Kopelman 2002). This pattern fits with evidence from magnetic resonance imaging (MRI) that shows atrophy of the lateral and inferior temporal regions with comparative sparing of the medial temporal area (Kopelman 2002). In addition, the right temporal region is usually less affected, although if it is involved, this is linked to impaired visual semantic information (Kopelman 2002). Furthermore, it has been found that 'superordinate' category words, for example 'animal', are more affected than 'subordinate' category words, such as 'horse' (Kopelman 2002, p. 2164).

People with semantic dementia may be more impaired recalling names, places and factual items that are part of general knowledge, and less disadvantaged on names, places and other items with a personal connection (Kopelman 2002). Memory problems in semantic variant primary progressive aphasia are specific to semantic items, for example names of people or things, while daily episodic memory and awareness of time are preserved, unlike in 'classical amnesia', as seen in ATD, and the person is able to maintain a level of independence in activities of daily living (Snowden 2012, p. 571).

Memory impairments in FTD also fit with a pattern of frontal lobe atrophy, so that the person has difficulties with general recall tasks but performs better when the task is more constrained, such as in multiple choice or when cues are provided (Snowden 2012). The person can retain items following a 30-minute period and this suggests that memory problems stem from registration, rather than preservation, of information (Snowden 2012). Topographical information appears to be retained, unlike in ATD, as seen when the person repetitively traces the same path (Snowden 2012). Snowden (2012) suggests that poor performance in memory tests might be linked to distractibility, impulsiveness when responding, tendency to perseverate or failure to stick to the goal of the task.

Pick's Disease

Pick's disease is a variant of FTD that involves 'knife-edge atrophy', a marked thinning affecting the temporal, frontal and cingulate gyri (Bang et al. 2015, p. 1677). In addition, there are protein deposits known as 'Pick bodies' present (Bang et al. 2015, p. 1677). There may also be swollen neurons, known as 'Pick cells' (Snowden 2012, p. 567). Snowden (2012, p. 568) states that the disease is now referred to as 'tau-positive' or 'Pick-type' dementia.

Lewy Body Dementias

LBD is an umbrella term for a range of conditions (Walker et al. 2015). A key feature of LBD is the presence of α-synuclein deposits within neurons, known as 'Lewy bodies' when occurring in the cell body and 'Lewy neurites' when located in neuronal processes (Walker et al. 2015, p. 1684). The Lewy bodies may spread progressively from the brainstem to the limbic system and then the neocortex (Walker et al. 2015).

Subtypes of Lewy Body Dementia

The key subtypes of LBD are first, dementia with Lewy bodies, which can appear alongside parkinsonism or within 12 months of the initiation of motor symptoms, and may include 10% of all dementia cases. The second is Parkinson's disease dementia, which has an onset at or after 12 months of

Parkinson's disease onset. The third is MCI in Parkinson's disease and the fourth, is Lewy body disease, which indicates the presence of Lewy body pathologies (Walker et al. 2015). In addition, a more recent term has been put forward, 'major and mild neurocognitive disorder with Lewy bodies or due to Parkinson's disease', which corresponds to dementia with Lewy bodies and Parkinson's disease dementia, respectively (Walker et al. 2015, p. 1684).

Prevalence

LBD is the second most frequent neurodegenerative dementia type in people over 65 years (Walker et al. 2015). Around 80% of people with Parkinson's disease eventually develop dementia and, although dementia with Lewy bodies is a distinct clinical syndrome, the two conditions become quite similar, hence the use of an umbrella term (Walker et al. 2015).

Aetiology

LBD generally has a sporadic occurrence, but there have been unusual cases of parent–child inheritance (Walker et al. 2015). There is evidence of the increased presence of *apoE ε4* in sporadic cases, although this presence is lower than in ATD (Walker et al. 2015). For dementia with Lewy bodies there is some evidence of familial clusters (Walker et al. 2015).

Signs and Symptoms

Key symptoms of dementia with Lewy bodies include executive, attentional and visuospatial impairments (Walker et al. 2015). In addition, a patient may have a history of falls and transient loss of conscious that is unexplained (Walker et al. 2015). The person may also experience visual hallucinations, frequently of animals, people or children, that may be very vivid and that the person can describe in some detail. The hallucinations are not usually perceived of as presenting a threat and frequently make no noise (Snowden 2012; Walker et al. 2015).

There is often a presentation of fluctuating cognitive impairments (Walker et al. 2015). Indeed, people close to the patient may report that sometimes they seem lucid but then confused again over the course of a day (Snowden 2012). In MCI in Parkinson's disease there may be impaired working memory and in Lewy body disease there is evidence of problems with memory retrieval (Walker et al. 2015).

Another distinct feature of dementia with Lewy bodies is 'rapid eye movement sleep behaviour disorder' (RBD; Walker et al. 2015, p. 1683). RBD may lead a person to dream they are being attacked, causing them to lash out with arms and legs and scream while sleeping, and environmental adaptations may be needed to reduce risk of injury (Walker et al. 2015).

Radiographs reveal a pattern of global atrophy affecting grey matter in dementia with Lewy bodies, although with less atrophy in the medial temporal lobe than would be seen in ATD. This can act as a diagnostic criterion for dementia with Lewy bodies (Walker et al. 2015).

Treatment

Again, there are no pharmacological options for treating the disease. Acetyl-cholinesterase inhibitors such as rivastigmine have, however, been linked to moderate improvements in cognitive status and performance of daily living tasks in people with Parkinson's disease dementia, and drugs of this class are therefore recommended by Walker et al. (2015) for treating LBD in general.

Post-traumatic Stress Disorder

PTSD can happen following violent offences, head injuries, traffic accidents or large-scale disasters (Kopelman 2002). The condition has also been observed in Holocaust survivors, victims of floods, war and concentration camps, explosions, earthquakes, torture and kidnapping (Kopelman 2002).

It is characterised by unwelcome memories or 'flashbacks' of the traumatic event (Kopelman 2002, p. 2172). PTSD has been reported even when the person has total amnesia for the event and people with the condition have displayed evidence of anterograde amnesia even years following the trauma (Kopelman 2002). The amnesia in PTSD is of psychological origin, rather than resulting from organic brain impairment as in dementia (Kopelman 2002).

Amnesia in PTSD may be 'situation specific', involving loss of memory for a particular event (Kopelman 2002, p. 2171). This may occur when someone has committed, or been the victim of, a violent act, in episodes of childhood sexual abuse, or for the incidents that result in PTSD (Kopelman 2002). For example, between 25% and 45% of perpetrators of homicide aver that they have amnesia for the event (Kopelman 2002). There may be isolated oases of memory within the amnesia, and semantic and procedural memory are often unaffected (Kopelman 2002).

Montag (2021) points out that retrograde amnesia in PTSD may occur either as the loss or removal of memories, or on account of a failure to retrieve existing memories. In addition, this author points out that PTSD is associated particularly with associative memories that build on information from a variety of domains, such as sensory and emotional (Montag 2021).

'Dual Representation' Approach to Memory in Post-traumatic Stress Disorder

Brewin (2001) argued that intensely stressful events may affect hippocampal and non-hippocampal–based memory in different ways and that these differences may explain the phenomenon of PTSD. He suggested that memory in PTSD is fragmentary, making construction of a clear account challenging, but that this is accompanied by unpredictable 'flashbacks' in which the person relives the event, while maintaining a feeling of 'unreality' in relation to the episode (Brewin 2001, p. 374). The flashbacks are generally triggered by an external signal and are difficult to control and, in addition, contain vivid perceptual elements that are absent from standard painful memories (Brewin 2001).

Furthermore, there is an altered feeling of personal time, meaning that the episode is experienced as happening *now* (Brewin 2001).

Brewin (2001) suggests that there are two categories of trauma memory. First, there is VAM, which can be retrieved and examined, set in a personal timeline and deposited in a long-term memory store. Second, there is the SAM that underpins the flashbacks and disturbing dreams typical of PTSD (Brewin 2001). SAM contains basic perceptual information and somatic responses related to the event, meaning that flashbacks are more vivid and affective than VAM. It may also be difficult to describe SAM in words, making communication and inclusion in one's personal narrative challenging (Brewin 2001).

SAM is difficult to control because it is initiated by environmental triggers that lead the person to relive the 'fear, helplessness and horror' of the initial event (Brewin 2001, p. 375). Brewin (2001) suggests that these traumatic memories are untypical of hippocampal-based memories, which are bound into a coherent episode, contextualised and located in personal time. Rather, they bypass the hippocampus and activate the amygdala following environmental triggers, making them unavailable for conscious retrieval and judgement (Brewin 2001). In addition, SAM cannot be manipulated and reconstructed like hippocampal-dependent VAM, explaining the repetitive images and 'perceptual representation' associated with flashbacks in PTSD (Brewin 2001, p. 379).

Environmental triggers may lead to the SAM being reactivated repeatedly. Reliving the experience means that even innocuous situations may appear to the person as threatening and uncertain, while they may view themselves as unworthy or incapable of coping, a condition described by Brewin (2001, p. 384) as 'catastrophic interference'. Brewin (2001) suggests that psychological therapy should focus on attending to the events and internal shifts associated with the traumatic episode, ultimately allowing the creation of a VAM, based on hippocampal activation, that is located in time, and also allowing cortical inhibition of the amygdala.

Massazza et al. (2021) provided evidence in support of Brewin's view that there are two ways of representing traumatic memories. They researched the differences between the intrusive traumatic memories characteristic of PTSD and non-intrusive memories for the same events.

Their sample consisted of 104 survivors of earthquakes that affected central Italy in 2016–2017. First, they identified a number of features associated with traumatic experience, such as 'mental defeat, somatoform dissociation, cognitive overload, immobility and distress' (Massazza et al. 2021, p. 8). The participants were then asked to rate the extent to which they experienced a range of reactions during the event and also to indicate the negative emotions experienced during intrusive and non-intrusive recall of the episode (Massazza et al. 2021).

First, 49% of their sample reported intrusive memories of the events linked to the earthquakes. The researchers found that intrusive memories were characterised by significantly higher levels of dissociation, immobility, distress and cognitive overload, both for memories reported by an individual and for memories compared between different members of the sample (Massazza et al. 2021). In addition, the emotions experienced at recall for intrusive compared to non-intrusive memories showed significantly higher instances of 'anxiety, fear and helplessness' when compared for one person, and significantly higher fear and anxiety when compared between participants (Massazza et al. 2021, p. 14).

Massazza et al. (2021) argue that their results are evidence of the centrality of encoding at the time of the events. This is because intrusive memories were more characterised by a reliving of the emotions occurring during the event. In addition, they suggest that the results support Brewin's dual representation hypothesis, in that intrusive memories appear to be supported by different mechanisms than other autobiographical items. Finally, they maintain that the traumatic episode is best conceived of as a sequence of 'micro-events', rather than a single event (Massazza et al. 2021).

Brewin (2016) highlights some controversies in PTSD research. These focus, first, on whether a traumatic episode can be fully forgotten (Brewin 2016). Brewin (2016) comments that clinical research indicates that recovery of traumatic memory *is* possible. A debate linked to this centres on whether memories in PTSD are fragmented – that is, they do not flow, meaning they are marked by repetition, filtered speech and unfinished thoughts; and disorganised – that is, they are confused and not joined up (Brewin 2016).

Furthermore, there has been discussion about whether memories in PTSD can be fitted into the person's life narrative, with some authors arguing that such recollections become centrally integrated as reference points for subsequent events and projections into the future (Brewin 2016). Brewin (2016) maintains, however, that this does not necessarily contradict his own position, which is that the traumatic memory creates a rupture with earlier views of the self and subsequent ones.

Brewin (2016) suggests that a resolution to some of these disagreements may be a refreshed view of PTSD that recognises that, at a broad level, well-rehearsed painful memories may be as coherent as non-traumatic items. However, at the granular level there is fragmentation, marked by greater use of the present tense, incomplete thoughts and less evidence of reflection (Brewin 2016).

Conclusion

This chapter has involved an overview of various causes of amnesia. There was also a detailed discussion of the concept of PTA. Furthermore, there was discussion of contemporary debates about the precise relationship between the medial temporal lobes and representation in the neocortex in the formation of memory.

It was shown that the 'multiple trace hypothesis' proposes that memory retrieval involves context-dependent reactivation of memory traces, which are actually slightly different according to the context. This may help in occupational therapy task analysis. For example, if the therapist asks a person with memory impairment to perform a familiar task in an unfamiliar environment, the change in context may affect memory retrieval.

There was also extensive discussion of ATD. This is justified by the frequency with which occupational therapists are likely to encounter people with this condition in clinical practice. It was shown that a key early feature of ATD is impaired episodic memory. This was explained by the involvement of the medial temporal lobes, and the hippocampus in particular, in the condition. This is in keeping with evidence that was outlined in Chapters 1 and 2 on the centrality of this region for memory performance.

The pharmacological options for treatment for Alzheimer's disease were outlined. It was stressed that these did not, in general, affect the underlying disease process. A recent trial of lecanemab was discussed. This drug does target the underlying disease process and also may have some beneficial effect on the rate of cognitive decline in people with the condition. It should be stressed, though, that this latter finding was based on a clinician-rated outcome measure and that the precise relationship between changes in the underlying pathology and memory function remains unclear. Overall, these limitations underline the importance of non-pharmacological treatments for ATD, such as occupational therapy. These are discussed further in Chapter 7.

Vascular dementia, FTD and LBD were also described. Although the primary clinical presentation in these dementias is not necessarily memory, as it often is in ATD, memory impairments may be involved at some stage. In addition, these are relatively common causes of dementia and occupational therapists may well encounter people with these conditions.

Finally, the character of memory impairments in PTSD was discussed. It was shown that these memories are characterised by flashbacks. Brewin's hypothesis that these flashbacks are examples of 'situationally accessible' memories that bypass the medial temporal lobes was outlined.

In addition, flashbacks can be triggered by unanticipated environmental cues. Again, this underlines the importance for the occupational therapist of an awareness of the environment when working with this population. This is a key feature of some of the conceptual practice models developed within occupational therapy, which are discussed in more depth in Chapter 4.

Points for Discussion

Case Study Vignette

Faiza was involved in a road traffic accident six weeks ago. Initially she could not remember any personal information for about five months prior to the accident. However, she has now fairly clear recall for events that occurred about two weeks before the crash. Despite this memory impairment, Faiza is now able to prepare one of her preferred meals from before the crash without any problems.

1. Name the subtype of amnesia that Faiza is experiencing.
2. Using knowledge from this and the previous chapters, explain why Faiza has memory impairment for personal information but can still perform instrumental activities of daily living independently.

Activities

Activity 1

Seren is an occupational therapist working with Faiza. Seren has been using a meal preparation task as a means of assessing and treating working memory impairments. As cues, Seren writes down the location of items in the kitchen, for example:

- Onions are in the cupboard over the sink.
- Pans are in the cupboard to the left of the sink.
- Knives are in the drawer nearest the door.

However, Faiza consistently fails to identify the location of these items without further visual and verbal cues from Seren.

1. How could Seren change the cues she is giving to Faiza so as to improve performance?
2. Make a list of possible cues.

Activity 2

Matilda is a 13-year-old school student with working memory impairments. Lloyd, her occupational therapist, notices that the class teacher tends to provide lengthy verbal explanations to the class about where to place different items once a task is completed. Matilda consistently forgets where things are supposed to go.

1. How could Lloyd advise the teacher to change the cues he is providing to the class in order to help Matilda?
2. Make a list of possible cues.

Activity 3

Jo is an occupational therapy team leader on a stroke rehabilitation unit and has been training her team on the muscles of the upper limb. She usually does this by using a PowerPoint® slide presentation. However, she is frustrated that, when supervising team members during 'upper limb treatment sessions' with stroke survivors, they seem to have remembered very little.

1. How could Jo support learning and memory of this information by adjusting her approach to delivery?
2. What cues might be useful for her team to support memorisation of this information?

References

Amaral, D.G. and Strick, P.L. (2013). The organisation of the central nervous system. In: *Principles of Neural Science*, 5e (ed. E.R. Kandel, J.H. Schwartz, T.M. Jessell, et al.), 337–369. New York: McGraw Hill Education.

Baddeley, A. (2015). When memory systems fail. In: *Memory* (ed. A. Baddeley, M.W. Eysenck, and M.C. Anderson), 435–466. London: Psychology Press.

Bang, J.M.D., Spina, S.M.D., and Miller, B.L.P. (2015). Frontotemporal dementia. *Lancet* 386 (10004): 1672–1682.

Bartlett, F.C. (1995). *Remembering: A Study in Experimental and Social Psychology*. Cambridge: Cambridge University Press.

Bear, M.F., Connors, B.W., and Paradiso, M.A. (2016). *Neuroscience: Exploring the Brain*, 4e. Philadelphia, PA: Wolters Kluwer.

Bradley, V. and Kapur, N. (2012). Neuropsychological assessment of memory disorders. In: *The Handbook of Clinical Psychology* (ed. J.M. Gurd, U. Kischka, and J.C. Marshall), 159–183. Oxford: Oxford University Press.

Breijyeh, Z. and Karaman, R. (2020). Comprehensive review on Alzheimer's disease: causes and treatment. *Molecules* 25 (24): 5789.

Brewin, C.R. (2001). A cognitive neuroscience account of posttraumatic stress disorder and its treatment. *Behaviour Research and Therapy* 39 (4): 373–393.

Brewin, C.R. (2016). Coherence, disorganization, and fragmentation in traumatic memory reconsidered: a response to Rubin et al. (2016). *Journal of Abnormal Psychology* 125 (7): 1011–1017.

Chatzikostopoulos, A., Moraitou, D., Tsolaki, M. et al. (2022). Episodic memory in amnestic mild cognitive impairment (aMCI) and Alzheimer's disease dementia (ADD): using the 'Doors and People' tool to differentiate between early aMCI–late aMCI–mild ADD diagnostic groups. *Diagnostics* 12 (7): 1768.

Craik, F.I.M. and Lockhart, R.S. (1972). Levels of processing: a framework for memory research. *Journal of Verbal Learning and Verbal Behavior* 11 (6): 671–684.

Crossman, A.R., Neary, D., and Crossman, B. (2020). *Neuroanatomy: An Illustrated Colour Text*, 6e. Amsterdam: Elsevier.

Dewar, M., Garcia, Y.F., Cowan, N., and Della Sala, S. (2009). Delaying interference enhances memory consolidation in amnesic patients. *Neuropsychology* 23 (5): 627–634.

Dismukes, R.K. (2010). Remembrance of things future: prospective memory in laboratory, workplace, and everyday settings. *Reviews of Human Factors and Ergonomics* 6 (1): 79–122.

van Dyck, C.H., Swanson, C.J., Aisen, P. et al. (2023). Lecanemab in early Alzheimer's disease. *New England Journal of Medicine* 388 (1): 9–21.

Eichenbaum, H. (2012). *The Cognitive Neuroscience of Memory: An Introduction*, 2e. Oxford: Oxford University Press.

Gazzaniga, M.S., Ivry, R.B., and Mangun, G.R. (2009). *Cognitive Neuroscience: The Biology of the Mind*, 3e. New York: Norton.

Gustavson, D.E., Reynolds, C.A., Hohman, T.J. et al. (2023). Alzheimer's disease polygenic scores predict changes in episodic memory and executive function across 12 years in late middle age. *Journal of the International Neuropsychological Society* 29 (2): 136–147.

Hascup, E.R. and Hascup, K.N. (2020). Toward refining Alzheimer's disease into overlapping subgroups. *Alzheimer's and Dementia: Translational Research and Clinical Interventions* 6 (1): e12070.

Hillam, J. (2004). *Dementia: Your Questions Answered*. Orlando, FL: Elsevier Health Sciences.

Kartsounis, L.D. (2012). Assessment of perceptual disorders. In: *The Handbook of Clinical Psychology* (ed. J.M. Gurd, U. Kischka, and J.C. Marshall), 120–138. Oxford: Oxford University Press.

Kopelman, M.D. (2002). Disorders of memory. *Brain* 125 (10): 2152–2190.

Kosch, Y., Browne, S., King, C. et al. (2010). Post-traumatic amnesia and its relationship to the functional outcome of people with severe traumatic brain injury. *Brain Injury* 24 (3): 479–485.

Leocadi, M., Canu, E., Paldino, A. et al. (2023). Awareness impairment in Alzheimer's disease and frontotemporal dementia: a systematic MRI review. *Journal of Neurology* 270 (4): 1880–1907.

López-Pérez, J., García-Herranz, S., and Díaz-Mardomingo, M.D.C. (2023). Acquisition and consolidation of verbal learning and episodic memory as predictors of the conversion from mild cognitive impairment to probable Alzheimer's disease. *Aging, Neuropsychology, and Cognition* 30 (4): 638–653.

Manwell, L.A., Tadros, M., Ciccarelli, T.M., and Eikelboom, R. (2022). Digital dementia in the internet generation: excessive screen time during brain development will increase the risk of Alzheimer's disease and related dementias in adulthood. *Journal of Integrative Neuroscience* 21 (1): 28.

Martini, F. (2018). *Fundamentals of Anatomy & Physiology*, 11e. Harlow: Pearson.

Massazza, A., Joffe, H., and Brewin, C.R. (2021). Intrusive memories following disaster: relationship with peritraumatic responses and later affect. *Journal of Abnormal Psychology* 130 (7): 727.

Milner, B., Corkin, S., and Teuber, H.-L. (1968). Further analysis of the hippocampal amnesic syndrome: 14-year follow-up study of H.M. *Neuropsychologia* 6 (3): 215–234.

Montag, D. (2021). Retrograde amnesia – a question of disturbed calcium levels? *Frontiers in Cellular Neuroscience* 15: 746198.

Morris, J.C. (1993). The Clinical Dementia Rating (CDR): current version and scoring rules. *Neurology* 43 (11): 2412–2414.

Nadel, L. and Moscovitch, M. (1997). Memory consolidation, retrograde amnesia and the hippocampal complex. *Current Opinion in Neurobiology* 7 (2): 217–227.

O'Brien, J.T.P. and Thomas, A.P. (2015). Vascular dementia. *Lancet* 386 (10004): 1698–1706.

Reed, J.M. and Squire, L.R. (1998). Retrograde amnesia for facts and events: findings from four new cases. *Journal of Neuroscience* 18 (10): 3943–3954.

Ribot, T. (1882). *Diseases of Memory*. New York: D. Appleton.

Russell, W.R. and Nathan, P.W. (1946). Traumatic amnesia. *Brain* 69 (4): 280–300.

Ryan, J.D., Althoff, R.R., Whitlow, S., and Cohen, N.J. (2000). Amnesia is a deficit in relational memory. *Psychological Science* 11 (6): 454–461.

Scoville, W.B. and Milner, B. (1957). Loss of recent memory after bilateral hippocampal lesions. *Journal of Neurology, Neurosurgery, and Psychiatry* 20 (1): 11.

Skilbeck, C. (2012). The neuropsychology of vascular disorders. In: *The Handbook of Clinical Psychology* (ed. J.M. Gurd, U. Kischka, and J.C. Marshall), 521–540. Oxford: Oxford University Press.

Snowden, J. (2012). The neuropsychological presentation of Alzheimer's disease and other neurodegenerative disorders. In: *The Handbook of Clinical Psychology* (ed. J.M. Gurd, U. Kischka, and J.C. Marshall), 561–584. Oxford: Oxford University Press.

Squire, L.R., Clark, R.E., and Knowlton, B.J. (2001). Retrograde amnesia. *Hippocampus* 11 (1): 50–55.

Tortora, G.J. and Derrickson, B. (2011). *Principles of Anatomy and Physiology*, 13e. Hoboken, NJ: Wiley.

Trevena-Peters, J., McKay, A., Spitz, G. et al. (2018). Efficacy of activities of daily living retraining during posttraumatic amnesia: a randomized controlled trial. *Archives of Physical Medicine and Rehabilitation* 99 (2): 329–337.

Tulving, E. (1985). Memory and consciousness. *Canadian Psychology* 26 (1): 1.

Walker, Z.D., Possin, K.L., Boeve, B.F. et al. (2015). Lewy body dementias. *Lancet* 386 (10004): 1683–1697.

Warchol, K. (2006). Facilitating functional and quality-of-life potential: strength-based assessment and treatment for all stages of dementia. *Topics in Geriatric Rehabilitation* 22 (3): 213–227.

Warrington, E.K. and Shallice, T. (1984). Category specific semantic impairments. *Brain* 107 (3): 829–853.

Wilson, B.A. (2012). The natural recovery and treatment of learning and memory disorders. In: *The Handbook of Clinical Psychology* (ed. J.M. Gurd, U. Kischka, and J.C. Marshall), 184–201. Oxford: Oxford University Press.

Winocur, G., Moscovitch, M., and Bontempi, B. (2010). Memory formation and long-term retention in humans and animals: convergence towards a transformation account of hippocampal–neocortical interactions. *Neuropsychologia* 48 (8): 2339–2356.

Woolsey, T.A., Hanaway, J., and Gado, M.H. (2003). *The Brain Atlas: A Visual Guide to the Human Central Nervous System*, 2e. Hoboken, NJ: Wiley.

Worthington, A.D. (2012). The natural recovery and treatment of executive disorders. In: *The Handbook of Clinical Psychology* (ed. J.M. Gurd, U. Kischka, and J.C. Marshall), 369–386. Oxford: Oxford University Press.

4 Occupational Therapy Assessment, Goal Setting and Action Planning with the Person with Memory Impairment

In this chapter the concept of 'occupation' as used by occupational therapists is defined and Yerxa's concept of 'homo occupacio' is discussed. Features of occupational therapy interventions, modelled as the 'occupational therapy process', are also described.

Conceptual practice models are defined and discussed. Prominent conceptual practice models include the Model of Human Occupation (MOHO), the ecological systems model, the Person-Environment-Occupation (PEO) model, the Canadian Model of Occupational Performance (CMOP) and the Canadian Model of Occupational Performance and Engagement (CMOP-E).

A key feature of all these models is that they show that the person performs occupations in specific environmental contexts. The Kawa model, which is based on a critique of these models as over-individualistic in their focus, is also explained.

There is a detailed explanation of the functional information processing model (FIPM), which explicitly addresses cognitive functions such as memory and attention. It is shown that this represents a detailed and systematic approach to cognitive assessment for occupational therapists. In addition, there is a range of standardised assessment tools linked to this model. Some of these appear to meet the requirement of assessing cognitive function in a valid way that is not biased by aspects such as culture and language.

The concept of 'frames of references' in occupational therapy is described. It is shown that these provide sources of evidence from outside the profession that can underpin clinical practice. Nonetheless, it is suggested that none of

Memory Impairment and Occupation: A Guide to Evaluation and Treatment, First Edition.
Jonathon O'Brien.
© 2024 John Wiley & Sons Ltd. Published 2024 by John Wiley & Sons Ltd.

the established frames of reference fits neatly with the ideas discussed in this book. A tentative proposal is made that occupational therapists should recognise a new 'cognitive neuroscience' frame of reference.

The chapter includes a critical discussion of a number of standardised assessments used to assess cognitive status by occupational therapists. In addition, there is a description of the continued efforts made to develop evaluations that are standardised, ecologically valid and true to occupational therapy principles.

The Assessment of Motor and Process Skills (AMPS), the Kettle Test and the Kitchen Task Assessment are presented as occupational therapy–specific assessments. One limiting factor is that all these tests assess memory along with other cognitive components. This is likely to be because, in practice, memory processes are not deployed in isolation but are embedded within the wider task performance.

Remedial and functional approaches to treatment of the person with memory impairment are contrasted. The use of the memory checklist is introduced. This was developed by the present author and presents a method for applying evidence from learning and memory theory in task analysis.

The importance of goal setting in therapy is explained. In particular, the principle of SMART goals is described, along with some practical suggestions about achieving these.

The use of the Canadian Occupational Performance Measure (COPM) is discussed. In addition, the goal attainment scaling (GAS) approach to goal setting is explained, as well as the ABCDE approach to SMART goal setting. Goal-oriented cognitive rehabilitation, which embeds goal setting in the rehabilitation process, is described. Finally the Mental Capacity Act (2005) is covered; this guides occupational therapists' work with people with cognitive impairment in England and Wales.

Assessment of Memory Impairment and the Philosophy of Occupational Therapy

Occupational therapy aims at preserving, or improving, the fit between a person's capacities, the requirements of their occupations and environmental demands (Creek 2003). Occupational therapy intervention is also based on the concept that what a person *does* can be harnessed in order to enhance this fit (Pentland et al. 2018).

'Occupation' has been defined in various ways (Molineux 2017). A broad definition encompasses both physical and cognitive purposeful activities that humans 'need, want, or are obliged to do' and that require capacities such as attention, memory and other skills (Molineux 2017; Wilcock 2006, p. 343). In addition, occupation has meaning for the person and may also have cultural relevance (Molineux 2017). In this sense, occupation is not limited to what can be observed, but also entails 'being, becoming and belonging' (Wilcock 2006, p. 3).

Yerxa (2000b) stressed the importance of personal agency in occupation, involving the person in self-initiated actions to achieve congruence with an environment that presents challenges as well as 'affordances' (Yerxa 2000b, p. 94, 2000a). In addition, different cultures categorise occupations in various ways, and occupational therapists have often used the categories of 'self-maintenance, productivity and leisure' (Creek 2003, p. 33; Yerxa 2000a).

Yerxa (2000a, p. 91) coined the term 'homo occupacio' in order to highlight an inherent human drive to engage in occupation in order to 'take possession' of our world. Homo occupacio is conceived of as an open system, interacting with the environment and operating at multiple levels (Yerxa 2000b). For example, at the level of the nervous system, synaptic plasticity underpins the learning and memory of new skills and declarative knowledge (Rose 1992; Deacon 1998).

The person develops a 'repertoire of skills' throughout the life course that are built into energy-conserving 'habits' and 'routines' (Yerxa 2000a, p. 93, 2000b, p. 197). Occupations are performed in specific environments, although Pentland et al. (2018, p. 13) prefer the term 'context' as it expresses the way in which the environment, personal factors and the actor's history are woven together.

Some occupational therapy authors have identified the succession of actions that constitute an occupational therapy intervention as the 'occupational therapy process' (Creek 2003, p. 15). This includes steps such as referral, information gathering, initial assessment, identification of requirements and goal setting. In addition, this account includes planning actions, implementing the plan, assessment of progress and revising the plan where needed, measuring outcomes, discharging the person and reviewing the intervention (Creek 2003). The process may not be followed in a linear manner, and the therapist may repeat elements or work on others simultaneously (Creek 2003; Duncan 2011a). Other models of the process present a cyclical rather than linear pattern (Hagedorn 2001).

Conceptual Practice Models

Occupational therapy theorists have developed conceptual practice models to support clinical work and research. Again, these have been defined in various ways. For Creek (2003), a model is a simplification of complex reality that describes relationships and explains data. In Pentland et al.'s (2018) account, conceptual practice models help the therapist understand the person at certain points of the life course. Duncan (2011b) defines models as theoretical schemes that facilitate the description of occupational therapy process and interventions. For Molineux (2017), they give direction to practice and research and may have specific associated assessment tools. There are a number of prominent conceptual practice models, which are discussed in this section.

Model of Human Occupation

MOHO builds on 'dynamical systems theory' (Kielhofner 1995, p. 10). This proposes that the constituent parts of a system interact with unpredictable outcomes. 'Occupational behaviour', for instance, is seen as something novel that emerges from the interaction of biological and psychological processes with a social, cultural and physical context (Kielhofner 1995, p. 21).

MOHO views the human as constituted of three complementary, rather than hierarchical, subsystems. First, a 'volitional subsystem' involves the inclinations and knowledge of self that attract a person towards specific occupational behaviour (Kielhofner 1995, pp. 28, 30). Second, a 'habituation subsystem' governs repeated forms of behaviour, for example a daily self-care or work routine, allowing the person to allocate attention to other areas (Kielhofner 1995, p. 30). Third, the 'mind-brain-body performance subsystem' indicates the neurological, musculoskeletal, cognitive, perceptual and other body functions that underpin the 'capacity for occupational performance' (Kielhofner 1995, p. 33).

Learning and memory mechanisms would be included in this latter subsystem and the procedural memory for specific skills would support the habituation subsystem. Volition, meanwhile, could require procedural knowledge of certain skills, but would also draw on semantic and episodic memory.

MOHO stresses the dialectical relationship between people and their environments, meaning that, as humans change their environments, the environment also shapes their performance and destiny (Kielhofner 1995). The environment 'affords' opportunities for occupational behaviour. Alternately, when the environment, which could, for example, include the physical arrangement of items or the expectations of others, provides a *requirement* for a specific behaviour, this is described as 'press' (Kielhofner 1995, pp. 92–93). Press can be negative because an environment that demands too much from a person may provoke anxiety and helplessness, while one that demands too little may lead to boredom and withdrawal (Kielhofner 1995). Occupational therapy researchers have applied the concept of environmental press in order to understand and improve the experience of people with memory impairment and dementia, and also to carer–person with dementia dyads (Gitlin et al. 2003, 2012). This work is discussed in more detail in Chapter 7.

The physical environment may be natural or built, and contains objects such as plants and animals, or made items (Kielhofner 1995). Alternatively, the social environment consists of enduring groups of people, joining together with different levels of formality, and providing varying amounts of press towards commitment to the group (Kielhofner 1995). The social environment also involves 'occupational forms', which are culturally acknowledged and named purposeful actions, guided by culturally sanctioned rules regarding the correct manner of executing them (Kielhofner 1995, p. 101). These occupational forms could include hunting, making conversation, cooking or many other action sequences (Kielhofner 1995). Kielhofner (1995, p. 105) provides a 'taxonomy' of locations in which occupational behaviour may occur. These may include the home, the neighbourhood, the school or workplace and public locations, such as libraries or restaurants (Kielhofner 1995).

Ecological Systems Model

Howe and Briggs (1982, p. 322) described an 'ecological systems model' that shares MOHO's concept of the person as an 'open system', shaping, and being shaped by, their environments. The individual, placed at the centre of the model, is the product of all the influences in their 'ecosystem' (Howe and Briggs 1982, p. 323). During individual development, their style of information processing becomes more specific to that person, constituting an 'inner life space' (Howe and Briggs 1982, p. 323).

Howe and Briggs (1982) conceived of the person as existing within various 'environmental layers', which may be facilitatory or may present barriers

(Howe and Briggs 1982, p. 323). The initial layer encompasses home, family or neighbourhood and those people who are encountered regularly (Howe and Briggs 1982). The second layer consists of 'social networks' such as schools, transportation or health services, while the final 'ideological layer' refers to social and cultural values (Howe and Briggs 1982, pp. 323–324).

The occupational therapist aims for 'operational harmony' between the individual and these layers of the environment (Howe and Briggs 1982, p. 324). Environmental layers constitute an 'extended life space', in which the person must perform tasks and roles, using 'life skills' (Howe and Briggs 1982, p. 324). The model also places importance on the goal-directed nature of performance, both for basic survival and for achieving self-actualisation (Howe and Briggs 1982, p. 325).

Person-Environment-Occupation Model

Law et al. (1996, p. 9), in their PEO model stressed that the person and their environment were interdependent. This 'transactional approach' maintains that behaviour is inseparable from context, time and the person's psychological and physical factors (Law et al. 1996, p. 9). As with some of the other models described, the environment encompasses a range of factors, including physical, social, cultural, political, legal and economic, and may influence behaviour at the personal level, or at the level of home or neighbourhood, community or country (Law et al. 1996).

The PEO model is represented graphically by three interlocking circles, indicating the person, the environment and the occupation, while the central area of overlap represents 'occupational performance' (Law et al. 1996, p. 13). Occupational performance is ameliorated when the 'fit' of the components, represented by the overlapping area of the three circles, is improved, for example by adapting the environment to better suit the person (Law et al. 1996).

It is worthwhile describing the 'person' and 'occupation' components of PEO in more detail. First, the person is conceived of as a spiritual, physical and mental whole, who performs roles throughout their life that last varying times and have differing levels of importance (Law et al. 1996). The person has different 'performance components' that support occupational performance, which could include personality or cultural formation, and they possess 'personal competencies' that might encompass sensory and motor capabilities, or cognitive factors such as memory (Law et al. 1996, p. 16).

The concept of 'occupation' in PEO is broken down into activities, tasks and occupations (Law et al. 1996, p. 16). At the most basic level, an activity could involve, for example, typing on a computer keyboard, underpinned by procedural and working memory. A task then consists of a number of grouped activities, for example those involved in preparing a university or workplace presentation, which may also involve semantic memory. Activities and tasks are then grouped together in the performance of occupation, which takes place as part of a role in particular environments, for example that of lecturer, occupational therapist, or student (Law et al. 1996). It will be noted that 'activity' here is the equivalent of the term 'task', and task is equivalent to activity as used by writers on occupational therapy in the United Kingdom, such as Creek (2003). Creek's (2003) taxonomy is more commonly used and is the one employed throughout this book.

Canadian Model of Occupational Performance

CMOP was launched in 1997 (Sumsion et al. 2011). Similar to PEO, CMOP conceptualised occupational performance as emerging from the interaction of the person, the environment and the occupation (Sumsion et al. 2011). The person is analysed as having physical, affective and cognitive performance components, while 'spirituality' is placed at the centre of the model, albeit the authors acknowledge that this concept is not clearly defined (Sumsion et al. 2011).

The environment is defined in a similar manner as in PEO (Law et al. 1996). This model has subsequently developed into CMOP-E, which has added an extra component designed to show that the core concern of the therapist is occupation (Sumsion et al. 2011).

Kawa Model

Iwama et al. (2009) state that most conceptual practice models originate from the West and their underlying principles reflect a particular world view. They maintain, for example, that MOHO and CMOP both centre on the individual, who is seen as separated from their environment and the natural world (Iwama et al. 2009). In these models, they argue, well-being correlates with successful control of the person's situation within the environment (Iwama et al. 2009).

In opposition to these views, Iwama et al. (2009) state that in an 'Asian and Aboriginal worldview', and in societies influenced by Buddhist or Confucian philosophies, the individual is part of an 'inseparable whole' that sees life happenings as determined by factors in and outside the body (Iwama 2006; Iwama et al. 2009, p. 1127). Furthermore, they suggest that the Western perspective emphasises individual agency in shaping one's destiny, while a Japanese person, for example, may focus more on their future as being determined by a 'collective will' (Iwama 2006, p. 26; Iwama et al. 2009). Overall, they suggest that Western conceptual practice models may exclude those from outside the Western cultural sphere (Iwama 2006).

Based on this critique, Iwama et al. (2009) have developed a fresh conceptual practice model, the Kawa (river) model. This is constructed on a metaphor of the life course as a river, which they propose contrasts with the 'mechanical' and 'system' approaches of the Western models they criticise (Iwama et al. 2009, p. 1128). In this metaphor, the sides and floor of the river, or Kawa Zoko, represent the physical and social contexts of the person, while rocks stand for barriers such as disease. Driftwood represents 'personal attributes or resources', which could include, for example, personality traits, family support or financial wealth (Iwama et al. 2009, p. 1132). The spaces between these items represent the locations where the person's 'life energy' flows, offering the hope of recovery or healing, because of either intrinsic or environmental factors (Iwama 2006, p. 151; Iwama et al. 2009). Facilitation of 'life flow' via analysis of all the factors influencing that flow is the aim of occupational therapy (Iwama 2006, p. 141).

Functional Information Processing Model

FIPM is based on the earlier Cognitive Disabilities Model, developed by Claudia Allen and described as one of the main approaches used by occupational therapists in the treatment of elderly populations (Bar-Yosef et al. 2000; Pool 2011, p. 105). It is based on Allen's cognitive levels, which describe levels of cognitive function, relating these to the person's occupational engagement and relations with others (Pool 2011, p. 106).

In FIPM, cognition is defined as the capacity that specifies which objects the person attends to. It also determines their motor response and verbal capability, guiding how the person engages in occupation and with their environment (Pool 2011, p. 106). Cognition can be assessed, therefore, via analysis of the person's performance of tasks and activities (Pool 2011).

In FIPM, cognition progresses along two tracks, verbal and motor. These are bridged by attention, which is defined as noticing and using information and is assessable via motor or verbal performance (Pool 2011). Allen defined a number of mental 'structures' that underpin learning and thinking and the structures are chosen in a given context that is a function of the person's purpose (Pool 2011, p. 107). The first structure, 'observations', refers to attending to, and understanding, cues and stimuli. The second, 'speed', involves the pace of information processing. Third are 'visual spatial' mechanisms, viewed as part of working memory, which include sensing, perceiving and imagining. Fourth, 'verbal propositional' structures, also part of working memory, allow understanding of verbal and non-verbal communication, conceptual abstraction, awareness of time and social norms. Finally, memory processes are grouped into explicit/declarative plans to learn and implicit/non-declarative learning that occurs without awareness of storage or retrieval of items (Pool 2011, p. 107).

Allen's Cognitive Levels

As stated earlier, FIPM is based on Allen's cognitive levels. Level zero is when the person is completely unconscious, alive but unresponsive to stimuli. At level one, the individual can provide general responses, such as an altered heart rate, to stimuli, as well as specific responses to other stimuli. At level two, the person can transfer to sitting and standing, do simple exercises, and supportive equipment may be needed. A person at level three can reach and grasp items, although they do not assess the effect of this, meaning that supervision is needed at all times. At level four, the person can perform normal activities of daily living (ADL) independently, although they may require support in the event of any changes to the environment or if there are any hazards. At level five, the person can learn new skills through performing them, although supervision is still needed as the person may fail to recognise hazards. At level six, the person is able to foresee the results of their actions and takes pleasure in creativity and finding out new things (Pool 2011). In addition, for each stage there are five 'modes of performance' that permit a more detailed description of the person's level (Pool 2011, p. 108).

Functional Information Processing Model Assessment Tools

FIPM also has a number of linked assessment tools. These include the Allen Cognitive Levels Screen (ACLS), which has been found to be valid and reliable

(Pool 2011). Also, the Routine Task Inventory (RTI), intended for patients being discharged to relatively unchanging or familiar environments, facilitates assessment of procedural memory via performance of ADL (Pool 2011). Cognitive Performance Tests focus on the assessment of working memory for patients who will be discharged to changing, unpredictable environments (Pool 2011). The focus here is also on performance of activities, such as dressing, travelling or washing hands (Pool 2011).

In addition, the Allen Diagnostic Module (ADM) projects use a range of standardised craft activities in order to assess working memory (Pool 2011). Furthermore, Sensory-Motor Stimulation Kits are available for assessment of people with marked cognitive impairment, for example following traumatic brain injury or late-stage Alzheimer's type dementia (ATD; Pool 2011). An emphasis is also placed on environmental adjustment to allow improved function (Pool 2011).

Henry et al. (1998) tested the earlier ACLS in a group of 62 female and 38 male patients following admission to an acute psychiatric unit. Data was gathered retrospectively on pre-admission living status, diagnosis, roles, discharge destination and scores on ACLS (Henry et al. 1998). The authors found that there was a significant difference between ACLS scores for patients discharged to independent living and those discharged to supported living, with independent living patients scoring higher. It was also found that, after pre-admission living status, the ACLS score was the next best predictor of supported or independent living on discharge (Henry et al. 1998).The authors comment that the cognitive levels provided a useful tool to communicate the occupational therapists' findings to the multidisciplinary team (Henry et al. 1998).

Velligan et al. (1998) stress that cognition is multifaceted, and regard executive functions as the main influences on ACLS scores. In their view, executive functions include the capacity for behaviours aimed at goal accomplishment, sequencing of thoughts and behaviours, and maintenance of goal direction, while resisting distraction and inhibiting inappropriate behaviour.

Velligan et al. (1998) tested the validity of ACLS with a group of 110 people with schizophrenia. All were assessed with ACLS on discharge from hospital, while subgroups of 64 were also assessed using the Functional Needs Assessment (FNA), which assesses performance of ADL, and 40 were assessed using a battery of neuropsychological tests (Velligan et al. 1998). It was found that there was a positive correlation between the ACLS and FNA scores and that ACLS predicted community functioning such as levels of work obtained (Velligan et al. 1998). Overall, the authors argue that ACLS has good validity in determining current functional levels and predicting future function (Velligan et al. 1998).

The Large Allen Cognitive Levels (LACL) test is a development of ACL that is designed to factor in visual and motor impairments encountered in normal ageing (Roitman and Katz 1997). Roitman and Katz (1997) evaluated the test–retest reliability and concurrent and predictive validity of LACL. It was found that LACL had moderate to high test–retest reliability in a subgroup of the sample who were recruited from an elderly living apartment complex, but low reliability in another subgroup recruited from day centres (Roitman and Katz 1997). Roitman and Katz (1997) also found that there was moderate to high inter-rater reliability for ADM and that there was moderate and statistically significant predictive validity for LACL, based on correlation with ADM scores.

Language Issues and the Functional Information Processing Model

Velligan et al. (1995) point out that cognitive assessments can be biased based on beliefs, language and value systems, but that ACLS, based on non-verbal responses in an assessment, may have a lower threat of bias. Velligan et al. (1995) were interested in assessing the concurrent validity of ACLS against FNA, which was described earlier. Specifically, they wished to assess this across a range of ethnic groups in people with schizophrenia or schizoaffective disorder (Velligan et al. 1995). The sample consisted of non-Hispanic white people, Mexican Americans and African Americans (Velligan et al. 1995). In addition, levels of acculturation were assessed for the Mexican Americans using a scale that measured areas such as language use, cultural activities of preference and country of origin (Velligan et al. 1995).

Velligan et al. (1995) found that the FNA and ACLS scores were significantly positively correlated and that there were no significant differences between these correlations (Velligan et al. 1995). In addition, there were no effects of ethnicity or sex on the ACLS scores. Furthermore, there was no significant correlation between levels of acculturation and ACLS scores for the Mexican Americans (Velligan et al. 1995). They conclude that ACLS assesses the person's cognitive function in a non-biased manner. On the basis of the results reported, it may be the case that, by implication, LACL, which is based on ACLS, is also an appropriate test for assessing cognitive function in a valid manner.

Bar-Yosef et al. (2000) translated the Cognitive Performance Test, used in FIPM, into Hebrew, and adjusted some aspects of the test to make it more culturally appropriate for an elderly Israeli population. They were able to demonstrate that the test is reliable and valid for this population, whether dementia was present or not.

Frames of Reference

Occupational therapists also use frames of reference. These are sets of concepts that are derived from other knowledge domains, but that occupational therapists apply to their own practice (Duncan 2011b; Molineux 2017). An example might be an occupational therapist working within the area of wheelchair provision and drawing on evidence from a 'biomechanical frame of reference' (McMillan 2011, p. 179).

It is interesting to note that most of the evidence discussed in this book would not fit neatly into any of the frames of reference identified by Duncan (2011b). Indeed, Feaver and Ezekiel (2011, p. 201) address the issue of cognitive rehabilitation following stroke and comment that the various approaches used do not align with a 'cohesive frame of reference'. It is possible that ideas discussed in Chapter 5 of this book would be relevant for occupational therapists applying concepts from a 'psychodynamic frame of reference' that draws on psychoanalysis, psychotherapy and other areas (Daniel and Blair 2011, p. 165). It is perhaps useful to recall the earlier work by Hagedorn (1992, p. 27), who described a 'cognitive frame of reference' that encompassed the processes of learning and memory. Also, as Hagedorn (1992) points out, in practice an occupational therapist is unlikely to confine themselves to one frame of reference and will move between these, depending on the developing needs of their patient.

Tentatively, it could be the case that occupational therapists should recognise a new 'cognitive neuroscience' frame of reference. As shown in Chapter 1, cognitive science emerged in the 1970s as an interdisciplinary approach to understanding cognitive processes (Miller 2003). Cognitive neuroscience was a development of this. It uses neuroscientific evidence to explain mental function, while applying concepts from psychology in order to deepen understanding of the brain (Gazzaniga et al. 2009). This is the broad approach taken in this book, which also seeks to apply these concepts to occupational therapy.

General Principles of Memory Assessment

Informant-Based Measures

Taylor-Rowan et al. (2023, p. 580) suggest that commonly used cognitive screening tests only give a 'snapshot' of the person's cognitive level at the time of testing and do not measure the *change* in status that is inherent in dementia. For this reason, 'informant'-rated measures, where a carer or other person close to the patient is asked to evaluate the change in performance, may be useful (Taylor-Rowan et al. 2023).

An example of an informant-rated measure is the Informant Questionnaire on Cognitive Decline in the Elderly (IQCODE), which is based on answers to 39 questions that the informant is asked to rate on a five-point scale. It includes questions on aspects of memory such as acquiring new items and retrieving information (Jorm 2004). It has been found to have moderate correlation with tests of episodic memory and has good reliability (Jorm 2004).

Taylor-Rowan et al. (2023) conducted an analysis of systematic reviews in order to evaluate the accuracy of various informant-based assessments for cognitive screening. They found that IQCODE was sufficiently sensitive and specific in identifying dementia. Another measure, the Eight-Item Informant Interview to Differentiate Aging and Dementia (AD8®), also showed sensitivity and specificity (Taylor-Rowan et al. 2023, p. 580). A further tool, the General Practitioner Assessment of Cognition (GPCOG), has both patient- and informant-rated components; however, when only the informant aspect was evaluated it was found to have poor specificity for detection of dementia (Taylor-Rowan et al. 2023, p. 580). Overall, the authors argue that AD8 and IQCODE can be compared with clinician-rated cognitive screens such as the Montreal Cognitive Assessment (MoCA) and the Mini-Mental State Examination (MMSE) and are best used alongside other assessments, or in the event that the person refuses assessment by another route (Taylor-Rowan et al. 2023).

Carer Burden

It was noted earlier that occupational therapy conceptual practice models emphasise the 'person-in-context' (Pentland et al. 2018, p. 14). In this sense, it is important that occupational therapists consider the person with memory impairment not in isolation, but in relation to their social and physical environments. Babulal et al. (2023) comment, for example, that cognitive screening and treatment planning should be bespoke to the needs of the person and that this should involve patient and carer self-reports that incorporate patient and caregiver accounts in a tailored manner (Babulal et al. 2023). This is discussed further in this section.

Amato et al. (2021) point out that family members may provide up to 40 hours/week assisting with daily tasks for people with dementia. This may create 'caregiver burden', which they define as the varied financial, physical, emotional, psychological and social reactions to the carer role, and which may be greater for dementia than for other illnesses (Amato et al. 2021, p. 237). These stresses can lead to deterioration in the relationship between the carer and the person with dementia (Amato et al. 2021).

Amato et al. (2021) surveyed 62 carers living with people with dementia. About one-third of those with dementia had ATD, and it can therefore be assumed that memory impairment was a key issue. The survey examined the level of assistance provided for different activities and the level of difficulty experienced by the carer (Amato et al. 2021). They also measured caregiver burden using the standardised Zarit Burden Inventory (ZBI; Amato et al. 2021).

It was found that the bulk of assistance was needed for ADL, particularly getting showered and dressed, tasks that required moderate to maximal assistance (Amato et al. 2021). The burden of caregiving was also correlated significantly with assistance in getting dressed and using the shower and toileting, and with assistance provided for instrumental activities of daily living (IADL), for example shopping and cooking, although the burden did not correlate significantly with the amount of assistance needed (Amato et al. 2021). There was also a significant correlation between perceived burden and IADL, including social situations and controlling fall risks (Amato et al. 2021). The authors suggest that the findings underline the importance of taking carers' perspectives into account when designing treatment programmes for those with dementia.

There is a range of standardised cognitive screening tests available to support clinical practice. Some of these are explored in Box 4.1.

BOX 4.1   STANDARDISED COGNITIVE SCREENING TESTS

This box discusses some standardised cognitive screening tests often used by occupational therapists in the clinical setting. A key point here is that two of the tests described, Mini-Mental State Examination (MMSE) and Montreal Cognitive Assessment (MoCA), are designed by medical doctors for the use of medical doctors. They may therefore be of limited relevance to occupational therapy practice. Other tests discussed, such as the Oxford Cognitive Screen (OCS) and the Rivermead Behavioural Memory Test (RBMT), may be more useful but were still not designed exclusively for occupational therapy. Finally, three occupational therapy–specific tests are described: Assessment of Motor and Process Skills (AMPS), the Kettle Test and the Kitchen Task Assessment.

Carnero-Pardo (2014) explains that cognitive screening tests are generally designed to allow medical doctors to quickly evaluate cognitive status in order to support diagnosis. This author lists a number of desiderata for such screens. First, and most crucially, they should be quick to use. Second, they should be applicable to all relevant populations, so the results should not be affected by variables such as social class background, culture, personality style, educational status and so on, minimising bias in the results (Carnero-Pardo 2014). Third, the cognitive screen should demonstrate inter- and intra-rater reliability and should also show validity, part of which means that it should be able to discriminate between those with and without impairment (Carnero-Pardo 2014). The test should also encompass a range of cognitive domains, including episodic memory and executive function as a minimum (Carnero-Pardo 2014). Two commonly used cognitive screening tests are discussed next.

Mini-Mental State Examination

MMSE has been used as a screening test of cognitive status in clinical practice and in research trials since its introduction in 1975 (Folstein et al. 1975; Bukhbinder et al. 2023). The test covers a range of domains, including orientation, attention, recall, repetition, reading and writing, and comprehension (Carnero-Pardo 2014). MMSE has been very influential, as these areas, with some variation, have been included in subsequent tests (Folstein 1989).

It is perhaps important to note that there was no clear scientific justification for testing these domains and, in a light-hearted account of the 'birth' of MMSE, the main author comments that he 'included those items that had been clinically useful to me and that could be scored with little interpretation' and that 'the weighting of the scores was completely intuitive' (Folstein 1989, p. 18). He also suggested that a reason for the widespread use of the test was that, up until that time, it was free to use (Folstein 1989).

The validity of MMSE has been questioned. Bukhbinder et al. (2023), for example, were interested in revealing the factors influencing MMSE scores in a cohort of 3404 Mexican Americans. They found that the variable most linked to MMSE score was years spent in education, with more years associated with higher scores (Bukhbinder et al. 2023). In addition, age and the presence of anxiety were influential variables (Bukhbinder et al. 2023). The authors point out that their results may mean that MMSE requires adjustment for educational levels and question whether it is appropriate to use it as a screening tool in research (Bukhbinder et al. 2023). Household income was also found to be a variable affecting scores (Bukhbinder et al. 2023).

Considerations such as those have caused some researchers to question the use of MMSE. Carnero-Pardo (2014), for example, argues that while MMSE was ground breaking when launched, it is no longer fit for purpose. First, it was originally developed for use with psychiatric patients and this is reflected in the comparatively small space devoted to memory testing, with only 3 of the 30 available test points relating to memory (Carnero-Pardo 2014). In addition, the test cannot be used with people who cannot read or write, since some components require a written response or reading of a command. Furthermore, as highlighted by Bukhbinder et al. (2023), MMSE is 'systematically' affected by the respondent's educational level, leading to bias in the results (Carnero-Pardo 2014, p. 477). Also, the test has poor diagnostic accuracy for dementia, which may be explained in part by the findings that people with higher education consistently perform better (Carnero-Pardo 2014). At a financial level, MMSE was purchased by a corporation in 2001, meaning that use of the test without payment is now fraudulent (Carnero-Pardo 2014).

Montreal Cognitive Assessment

MoCA was originally intended for medical doctors to detect the presence of mild cognitive impairment (MCI; Nasreddine et al. 2005). MoCA evaluates areas including short-term and working memory, executive function, attention, orientation to place and time, and language (Nasreddine et al. 2005).

Nasreddine et al. (2005) compared MMSE and MoCA in detection of MCI and found that MMSE had poor sensitivity, identifying only 18% of those with MCI, while MoCA showed high sensitivity, detecting 90% of those with the condition (Nasreddine et al. 2005). In addition, MMSE detected 78% of cases of people with a likely diagnosis of Alzheimer's type dementia (ATD), which is considered poor, while MoCA detected 100% (Nasreddine et al. 2005).

The authors suggest that this greater sensitivity is because MoCA uses more words in its memory tests, as well as giving a longer delay for recall tests and fewer practice trials (Nasreddine et al. 2005). The authors acknowledged the bias in results caused by the educational levels of participants by the addition of one point to any score less than 30 for participants with 12 or fewer years of education (Nasreddine et al. 2005).

The main author of MoCA made a number of assumptions in the design of the assessment based on, in their own words, 'clinical intuition' about the cognitive domains assessed (Nasreddine et al. 2005, p. 696). These issues are picked up in research by Coen et al. (2016), who point out that some subtest titles in MoCA do not fit the putative domain being assessed, with, for example, visuospatial and executive components being grouped under the same title (Coen et al. 2016). The authors conclude that, while MoCA is a useful medical screening tool, more granular neuropsychological assessment is required to provide detailed information on specific cognitive impairments (Coen et al. 2016).

Oxford Cognitive Screen

OCS was designed specifically for evaluating cognitive function in stroke (Demeyere et al. 2015). It assesses cognitive domains including language, calculation, memory, praxis and attention and executive function (Demeyere et al. 2015). The test is considered inclusive, in that it can be adapted for respondents with aphasia or spatial neglect (Demeyere et al. 2015). Another advantage of OCS is that it explicitly distinguishes between memory systems, encompassing orientation, episodic, recognition and recall memory (Demeyere et al. 2015).

OCS consists of 10 tasks and the authors estimate that it can be administered in around 15 minutes (Demeyere et al. 2015). The presentation of the test results, which involves a visual graphic that can be shaded in and presented to facilitate discussion in multidisciplinary team meetings, was designed with input from occupational therapists working on acute stroke units (Demeyere et al. 2015). Furthermore, the assessment is free to access and comes with extensive support materials, including training videos.

OCS has been found to have test–retest reliability for assessment of stroke survivors (Demeyere et al. 2015). The subtests were also found to be valid when compared with components of other assessments testing the same domains, and the specificity and sensitivity of each subtest were generally found to be high (Demeyere et al. 2015). Although OCS has been designed for use with stroke survivors, the authors state that they are optimistic that it will be useful for screening cognition in other neurological populations, such as in people with Parkinson's disease (Demeyere et al. 2015).

Some authors have questioned the relevance of many neuropsychological tests to the everyday life of the person with cognitive impairment. Wilson et al. (1989), for example, somewhat sardonically describe the reaction of a spouse observing their significant other labouring over the Rey–Osterrieth figure and wondering aloud what relevance it has. Occupational therapy researchers have also questioned the relevance of such 'table-top' assessments in predicting levels of real-world function (Hartman-Maeir et al. 2009; Harper et al. 2019, p. 219). Efforts have therefore been therefore, to design assessments with ecological validity. Some of these are discussed next.

Rivermead Behavioural Memory Test

Wilson et al. (1989) describe the development of RBMT, which is intended as a 'bridge' between 'laboratory-based measures of memory' and assessment based on observation (Wilson et al. 1989, p. 856). RBMT has 12 subtests, including short- and long-term memory, prospective memory, visuospatial memory, recognition and delayed recall (Wilson et al. 1989; Bolló-Gasol et al. 2014). Prospective memory, for example, involves the respondent remembering to ask for the location of some hidden items when a specific sentence is uttered (Bolló-Gasol et al. 2014). Like the other tests described, the domains covered in the subtests were decided partly based on clinical observations of memory problems that patients encountered (Wilson et al. 1989).

Wilson et al. (1989) tested RBMT on 176 individuals with brain injuries caused by strokes, multiple sclerosis and other causes, such as carbon monoxide poisoning (Wilson et al. 1989). Inter-rater reliability was tested on a subset of 40 participants and found to be high (Wilson et al. 1989). In addition, 'parallel-form validity' was tested by administering two versions of the test with 118 of the participants (Wilson et al. 1989, p. 858). RBMT's claim to ecological validity was tested by comparing results with checklists completed by occupational therapists and physiotherapists working with patients that listed the categories of memory difficulties that the patients actually encountered (Wilson et al. 1989). RBMT was found to have high levels of inter-rater reliability, parallel-form validity and ecological validity (Wilson et al. 1989).

Bolló-Gasol et al. (2014) tested RBMT on people with MCI, those with ATD and neurologically healthy controls. RBMT was administered at baseline and again after 12 months. It was found that the healthy group scored significantly higher than the MCI group, and that those with MCI scored significantly higher than those with ATD, indicating that the test successfully discriminated between these groups (Bolló-Gasol et al. 2014). In addition, it was found that those who transitioned from MCI to ATD after 12 months scored significantly lower in the overall RBMT score and in the majority of the subtest scores at baseline, compared to those with stable MCI (Bolló-Gasol et al. 2014). Overall, the authors conclude that RBMT is able to distinguish between groups and between those with MCI who will progress to ATD and those who will not (Bolló-Gasol et al. 2014).

Assessment of Motor and Process Skills

Occupational therapy researchers have developed tests of memory and other aspects of cognition that focus on task and activity performance. AMPS is based on observation of activities of daily living (ADL) and assesses across the domains of 16 motor and 20 process skills (Linden et al. 2005; Fabricius et al. 2023). Motor skills encompass goal-directed actions, while process skills are defined as those actions that can be observed and that allow sequencing of activities, choice of tools and other items, and adaptation of behaviour when problems arise (Linden et al. 2005).

The assessor chooses two tasks from a manual (Linden et al. 2005) and assesses performance on a four-point scale. A score of four indicates competence, three indicates that performance is 'questionable', two that performance is 'ineffective' and one indicates the presence of a 'deficit' (Fabricius et al. 2023, p. 180). Scoring involves conversion of raw values into 'logits' using computer software (Fabricius et al. 2023, p. 180).

Linden et al. (2005) assessed 16 adults with severe brain injuries using AMPS and a neuropsychological test battery that included tests of learning and memory, on admission to a treatment centre and again at 3, 6 and 12 months following admission (Linden et al. 2005). They found out that there was progress throughout the period on neuropsychological variables, including logical memory and forwards and backwards digit span, although verbal memory scores did not return to normal values within the 12 months (Linden et al. 2005).

Despite these overall improvements, there were not similar gains in AMPS scores: 6 of the participants were still below the process skills cut-off for independent living at 12 months and 13 patients actually deteriorated in process skills following discharge (Linden et al. 2005). The authors suggest that the variance in scores between the tests may show that AMPS is actually better at assessing capacity for living independently and gives a clearer picture of people with brain injuries' vulnerability to their environment (Linden et al. 2005).

Fabricius et al. (2023) compared AMPS with a multidisciplinary outcome measure, the Functional Independence Measure (FIM), in predicting the length of stay of people with brain injuries in a rehabilitation setting. They administered AMPS to 647 patients in a rehabilitation centre over a 10-year period; the patients had also been assessed using FIM. Length of stay was defined as the number of days in the setting after AMPS assessment was conducted (Fabricius et al. 2023).

Fabricius et al. (2023) found that independence in process abilities, measured by AMPS, was associated with a 31% shorter stay, which was a statistically significant difference to patients who were not assessed as independent. Independence, as measured by FIM cognition scores, was associated with a 38% shorter stay, which was also a significant difference to those who were not independent (Fabricius et al. 2023). The authors conclude that AMPS is, at a minimum, as effective as FIM as a predictor of length of stay, and may provide a more fine-grained analysis of ADL performance (Fabricius et al. 2023).

Kettle Test

While AMPS represents a validated test of memory performance that is grounded in occupational therapy concepts, it has been pointed out that it necessitates costly and extensive training (Hartman-Maeir et al. 2009; Fabricius et al. 2023). The Kettle Test, therefore, was developed as an attempt to provide an occupation-focused, ecologically valid assessment of cognition that uses resources available to most occupational therapists (Hartman-Maeir et al. 2009).

The Kettle Test is based on the activity of preparing a hot drink, which is deconstructed into 13 stages that are scored by the examiner, who indicates the level of cues needed for each task (Harper et al. 2019). There are 13 indices covering tasks such as putting the kettle together, switching the tap on and filling the kettle. Scores depend on the cues and support required to complete the tasks and range from 0 to 52, with 0 indicating total independence Harper et al. (2019, p. 219). The Kettle Test takes around 20 minutes to complete (Harper et al. 2019).

The Kettle Test also challenges higher cognitive functions; for example, the person is asked to prepare a drink both for themselves and for the therapist, and the therapist's drink has some extra requirements, placing a burden on working memory (Hartman-Maeir et al. 2009). In addition, the electric kettle is initially not fully assembled, increasing the need for problem solving and safety awareness, while additional items are placed in the workspace, making demands on attentional mechanisms (Hartman-Maeir et al. 2009).

Hartman-Maeir et al. (2009) assessed the inter-rater reliability of the Kettle Test with 21 stroke survivors on a rehabilitation unit and it was found to be high. Construct validity was tested by comparing the Kettle Test scores with scores on other outcome measures, including MMSE and the cognitive component of FIM (Hartman-Maeir et al. 2009). Moderate but statistically significant correlations were found between the Kettle Test and the other measures, indicating construct validity.

In addition, ecological validity was measured by comparing the Kettle Test results with the motor component of FIM, measurements of instrumental ADL performance and measures of safety. Again, significant correlations were found, indicating that the Kettle Test has ecological validity (Hartman-Maeir et al. 2009). Furthermore, the authors report that the Kettle Test results were not affected by the educational status of the participants, indicating that the results were not biased in the ways researchers have found for MMSE (Hartman-Maeir et al. 2009).

Harper et al. (2019) compared the Kettle Test with the MMSE and the cognitive component of FIM (cFIM). In addition, they tested how well the three measures predicted functional independence by comparing the results of the tests when administered at admission to results for the same patients on the motor component of FIM (mFIM) once discharged (Harper et al. 2019). They explain that cFIM assesses five cognitive domains, including memory and problem solving, and rates these on a seven-point scale, with a score of one indicating complete dependence and a score of seven meaning complete independence (Harper et al. 2019).

They found that the scores on the Kettle Test were moderately but significantly correlated with MMSE and cFIM (Harper et al. 2019). In addition, they found that, while the Kettle Test and cFIM taken at admission correlated significantly with the mFIM on discharge, the strongest correlation was with the Kettle Test, which accounted for 21.5% of the variance in mFIM scores (Harper et al. 2019). The authors concluded that the Kettle Test is a valid test of cognitive function and can also be used to predict the person's function on discharge (Harper et al. 2019).

Harper et al. (2019) subsequently evaluated the correlation between scores on MMSE, cFIM and the Kettle Test in 97 people on admission and discharge from a geriatric rehabilitation centre. They found significant correlations between all three tests at both time points (Harper et al. 2019). They also found that the Kettle Test and cFIM significantly predicted scores on mFIM on discharge, with the Kettle Test explaining 21.5% of the variance in mFIM (Harper et al. 2019). The authors conclude that the Kettle Test is a useful assessment of cognitive status as part of an occupation-based approach and could, for example, be used in the context of conceptual practice models such as the Person-Environment-Occupation model (Harper et al. 2019).

Kitchen Task Assessment

Another kitchen activities–based assessment is the Kitchen Task Assessment (Baum and Edwards 1993). This uses the activity of preparing a pudding from a packet mix and, the authors state, can be carried out in a clinical or home setting (Baum and Edwards 1993). A range of specified tasks are scored: 'initiation', 'organisation', performing all stages, 'sequencing', safety and judgement, and task 'completion' (Baum and Edwards 1993, p. 432). Each is scored on a four-point scale as follows: zero indicates 'independent', one indicates that 'verbal cues' were needed, two that 'physical assistance' was required and three that they were incapable of performing the task (Baum and Edwards 1993, p. 433).

The authors state that a main aim of the assessment is to provide a measure of the type of support strategies that a carer can employ to assist the person with dementia. The authors tested the assessment on 106 people with ATD and assessed construct validity by comparing the results with those of standard neuropsychological tests (Baum and Edwards 1993). They found that the Kitchen Task Assessment had good inter-rater reliability and that the correlations of scores with those of other tests were highly significant (Baum and Edwards 1993).

Cognitive Rehabilitation in Occupational Therapy

Katz (1994) defines cognition as the ability to acquire and utilise information in order to adapt to environmental requirements. Cognitive rehabilitation is then defined as a therapeutic process aimed at enhancing the person's capacity to use information (Katz 1994). According to Katz (1994), cognitive rehabilitation in occupational therapy uses two approaches.

First, the remedial approach focuses on the person's areas of impairment. The assumptions here are that there is scope for recovery, that the therapist can treat the impairments and, in addition, that therapy will facilitate recovery in the brain. Furthermore, it is assumed that there will be generalisation to other areas of function, although this does not take place spontaneously and needs to be explicitly tackled in treatment (Katz 1994). The remedial approach also assumes that the person must adapt themselves to the requirements of the environment (Katz 1994).

Second, the functional approach is based on the supposition that the person has limited scope for recovery, that there will be no spontaneous transfer of trained skills to other areas and that explicit skill training is needed (Katz 1994). In this approach, treatment will include adapting the task and/or environment to fit the capacity of the person (Katz 1994).

Katz (1994) points out that both remedial and functional approaches may be used together or in sequence. In the early stages of treatment, for example, a remedial approach may be taken and a functional approach used when it is felt that further recovery is not possible and a stable level has been reached. The key unifying factor is the deployment of purposeful activities tailored to the person (Katz 1994).

Memory Checklist: An Occupation-Focused Approach to Assessment of Memory Impairment

One approach to assessing the attentional and memory components of task and activity performance, developed by the author in his own clinical practice, is the use of the memory checklist shown in Table 4.1.

The memory checklist is based on the author's clinical experience. It will be recalled that well-known cognitive assessments originate from their creators' subjective clinical analyses, for example MMSE, whose author reported that the domains covered in the assessment were 'conceived in one night' (Folstein 1989, p. 18), MoCA (Nasreddine et al. 2005) and RBMT (Wilson et al. 1989). The memory checklist has the advantage of addressing those memory domains discussed in other parts of this book, which have been developed from research in the fields of neuropsychology and cognitive neuroscience. In addition, it incorporates attention domains. It is not yet standardised, but is offered here as a useful guide for observing attention and memory processes during occupation-based assessment.

The first part of the checklist covers attention. This is divided into three domains. First, selective attention allows the person to ignore irrelevant stimuli and focus on what is needed (Grieve and Gnanasekaran 2008). Second, sustained attention is the ability to maintain focus on a stimulus or task over an extended period (Grieve and Gnanasekaran 2008). Third, divided attention refers to the ability to attend simultaneously to different activities and allows 'multitasking' in occupational performance (Grieve and Gnanasekaran 2008, p. 130).

The process is based on the occupational therapy core skill of task analysis. First, the therapist explains the task to the person, demonstrating the location and use of all necessary items; the author usually does this twice to facilitate

Table 4.1 The memory checklist.

Attention
Selective
Sustained
Divided
Memory
Procedural
Semantic
Episodic
Prospective
Working memory
Visuospatial
Phonological

Source: © Jonathon O'Brien.

Table 4.2 Rough notes made by the occupational therapist during assessment.

Assessment: making a cup of tea with beans on toast.

Needed verbal prompt to locate teabags.

Needed verbal prompt to initiate use of toaster.

Allowed beans to start burning while watching toast preparing.

Failed to stir beans as soon as toast popped up, as specified during instructions.

Forgot to pour beans on top of toast, as specified in spoken instructions.

Needed prompt to fill kettle.

Forgot to turn off tap after filling kettle.

During conversation did not seem to remember personal care practice from this morning.

Tried to put teabags in kettle, thinking it was a teapot.

Became distracted by noise outside assessment kitchen, began to make irrelevant conversation and needed verbal prompt to return to the task.

Source: © Jonathon O'Brien.

learning. Then, the occupational therapist observes the person performing the task. During observation, the therapist makes concurrent rough notes on everything they observe the person doing during task performance. An example of this can be seen in Table 4.2. Finally, the therapist organises their observations under the headings of the memory checklist and uses this to produce a report and recommendations. An example of a completed memory checklist is shown in Table 4.3.

The author has found that kitchen tasks work particularly well, as the task and the environment can be easily adjusted by the therapist according to the capacities of the person. Kitchen tasks may also be modified so as to provide a challenge in order to probe particular memory domains.

The memory checklist can be used to establish priority areas for memory impairment treatment. Goals should be decided in collaboration with the person, their carer if appropriate and the multidisciplinary team. A structured approach to goal setting is recommended, for example using the GAS approach, explained further on in the chapter. An example of two GAS goals for the patient just described is in Table 4.4.

Goal Setting for the Person with Memory Impairment

Bovend'Eerdt et al. (2009) stress that rehabilitation is a complex intervention but that goal setting can support cohesion and clarity in a multidisciplinary team. They comment that 'goal setting is an essential part, and indeed the central part of the interdisciplinary rehabilitation process' (Bovend'Eerdt et al. 2009, p. 353). Other authors emphasise that communication with other staff members is vital and can be facilitated by writing goals into the person's care plan, or having them displayed above their bed (Jogie et al. 2021).

Turner-Stokes (2009), Pentland et al. (2018) and Jogie et al. (2021) state that collaborative goal setting with the patient or service user is of great importance. Turner-Stokes (2009) maintains that this approach allows the person to

Table 4.3 Completed memory checklist.

Attention
Selective
Appears to be intact, as patient was able to focus on tasks at the start of the assessment.
Sustained
There may be impairments, as patient's attention wandered at some points and he needed verbal prompts to return the task.
Divided
Evidence of impairment. When the patient's attention was focused on the toaster, he did not attend to the beans, which almost burned.
Memory
Procedural
Appears intact as the patient was able to complete the tasks needed for the activity, although he required prompts.
Semantic
Evidence of impairment. Patient thought that the kettle was a teapot.
Episodic
Evidence of impairment. Patient did not appear to remember that the occupational therapist had already seem him the same morning for personal care practice.
Prospective
Impaired, as patient did not remember to stir the beans once toast popped up from the toaster, which had been specified during the original instructions.
Working memory
Visuospatial
Impaired, as patient forgot the location of teabags, which had been indicated visually twice during the instructions.
Phonological
Impaired, as patient failed to pour beans on top of the toast, which had been explained verbally twice during the instructions.

Source: © Jonathon O'Brien.

formulate their own desired outcome; fosters decision making, involvement and communication; and also allows multidisciplinary co-working (Turner-Stokes 2009).

Engagement of family or carers has been found to support effective goal development too (Jogie et al. 2021). Furthermore, conversation about the person's previous occupations and interests helps in goal setting, as does breaking down activities and only setting a limited number of goals (Jogie et al. 2021).

Goals should be specific to the person. This means that the same goal could mean entirely different things to different people. For example, 'able to identify location of items for meal preparation with visual prompts' could indicate a successful treatment outcome for one person and failure for another (Rockwood et al. 1997). Rockwood et al. (1997) also make the important point that goals should be written as an observable outcome, and that the treatment plan and

Table 4.4 Goal attainment scaling example.

Scores	−2	−1	0	1	2
Goal one	After two weeks, patient makes cup of tea and beans on toast with maximal verbal and visual prompts to locate items	After two weeks, patient makes cup of tea and beans on toast with repeated verbal and visual prompts to locate items	After two weeks, patient makes cup of tea and beans on toast with occasional verbal and visual prompts to locate items	After two weeks, patient makes cup of tea and beans on toast with occasional visual prompts only to locate items	After two weeks, patient makes cup of tea and beans on toast independently
Goal two	After two weeks, patient does not remember to stir beans when toast pops up	After two weeks, patient remembers to stir beans when toast pops up with an explicit verbal cue only	After two weeks, patient remembers to stir beans when toast pops up with a general verbal cue only	After two weeks, patient remembers to stir beans when toast pops up with a visual cue only	After two weeks, patient remembers to stir beans when toast pops up independently

the goal should not be confused. (In the author's clinical and teaching experience these are frequent errors made in goal setting by occupational therapists and occupational therapy students.)

Bovend'Eerdt et al. (2009) state that goals are an effective way to promote change in rehabilitation, provided they are relevant to the person and they are realistic and specific. They call for goals to be 'specific, measurable, achievable, realistic/relevant and timed (SMART)' (Bovend'Eerdt et al. 2009, p. 353). This fits with a general principle that should underpin occupational therapy activities, in that the focus should be on areas that are meaningful and valuable to the person (Pentland et al. 2018). Bovend'Eerdt et al. (2009) propose a four-step process for SMART goal setting.

First, the goal target should be defined as explicitly as possible. This should be focused on a specific desired behaviour and will often be at the level of participation or activity, rather than focused on isolated skills (Bovend'Eerdt et al. 2009) Second, the level of support needed to accomplish the goal should be described. This could include support from another person, in the form of prompts or cues, or from items in the environment, for example a timer to support memory or provision of a list (Bovend'Eerdt et al. 2009).

The third step involves defining the quantitative, measurable aspects of the performance needed to achieve the goal. Bovend'Eerdt et al. (2009) describe three aspects to quantification. First, it is possible to state the time that will be needed for a particular part of the activity, such as the time needed to assemble the items needed for a kitchen task. Second is the amount of 'continuous activity' that will be executed in a specified time, for example the occupational therapist might specify the maximum time needed to prepare the hot drink component of a meal preparation activity for a patient prone to distraction due to attention impairments (Bovend'Eerdt et al. 2009, p. 356). Third, the 'frequency' of a delimited activity can be indicated, which could include an increase in something wanted, such as the number of kitchen items found without prompts, or conversely a *decrease* in something negative, such as the number of cues needed to locate the items (Bovend'Eerdt et al. 2009, p. 356).

The fourth step is the specification of the time by which the goal should be achieved; the authors recommend a minimum period of four weeks for this (Bovend'Eerdt et al. 2009), although it should be borne in mind that in settings such as stroke units in the United Kingdom, the target length of stay is normally around three weeks.

Jogie et al. (2021) conducted a scoping review examining approaches to goal setting for people with MCI or dementia. They found that facilitators of goal setting included a systematic approach, for which a range of tools are available. The first, COPM, is based on a semi-structured interview with the patient or service user that explores limitations they are experiencing in the areas of leisure, productivity and self-care (Law et al. 1990). Once problem areas are identified, the person is asked to weight the importance of these on a scale of 1–10, allowing prioritisation of five areas to work on in therapy (Law et al. 1990). The person then rates their performance in these areas and their levels of satisfaction with each, also on scale of 1–10. These latter ratings allow baseline scores to be calculated that can then be measured again at the end of a specified period and following treatment (Law et al. 1990).

The Bangor Goal Setting Interview has similarities to COPM. It is also based on a semi-structured interview that allows goal identification for people with cognitive impairment (Jogie et al. 2021).

Goal Attainment Scaling

Another structured method is GAS, an approach in which 'each patient has their own outcome measure' (Turner-Stokes 2009, p. 363). It also allows grading of goals, avoiding a simple pass/fail dichotomy (Turner-Stokes 2009). GAS has been found to encourage patients in goal achievement and, in that sense, has therapeutic value in itself (Turner-Stokes 2009). In one study, GAS was compared with seven other standardised outcome measures and was found to be the most responsive to changes of clinical importance and, in addition, was found to have high inter-rater reliability (Rockwood et al. 1997).

There are a number of stages in the GAS process (Turner-Stokes 2009). First, the criteria defining successful accomplishment of the goal are agreed between therapist, patient and carers. Second, a value of zero is given to a goal based on these criteria. A four-stage gradation is then developed. A value of +1 indicates that the goal achievement is 'somewhat more' than expected and +2 indicates that the level of accomplishment is 'much more' than expected. Conversely, −1 means that attainment was 'somewhat less' than predicted and −2 means that it was 'much less' than anticipated (Turner-Stokes 2009, p. 364). An example of GAS is shown in Table 4.1.

Weighting of goals is optional and can reflect the importance the person places on the goal, and/or the difficulty that the treatment team foresees in attaining the goal (Turner-Stokes 2009). For example, if memory were a key problem it may be weighted as 'two', indicating that memory impairments were 'twice as clinically important' as other areas of impairment identified (Rockwood et al. 1997, p. 582).

The final stage is the calculation of an aggregate 'T score' that constitutes GAS, at an agreed follow-up date. Turner-Stokes (2009) reports that a spreadsheet formula is available free of charge to facilitate this if needed.

Turner-Stokes (2009, p. 365) also states that goals formulated via the GAS process should be SMART, defined here as 'specific, measurable, attainable, realistic and timely'. The author also recommends developing a time-saving 'menu' of pre-written goals that occur commonly in clinical practice, to save time (Turner-Stokes 2009, p. 367).

ABCDE Approach

Another approach to SMART goal setting, the 'ABCDE' approach, is outlined by Shumway-Cook and Woollacott (2012, p. 145). ABDCE is an initialism that describes the stages required to construct an effective goal. First the 'Actor', the person who will perform the activity specified in the goal, is defined. This is followed by specification of the desired Behaviour. Then comes 'Condition', the circumstances in which performance will take place. 'Degree' quantifies task performance, for example stating how many and what type of prompts the person will need to achieve the goal. Last, the 'Expected time' needed to accomplish the goal is stated (Shumway-Cook and Woollacott 2012, p. 145). An example is shown in Table 4.5 for two patients with memory impairment, Sean and Shola.

Dutzi et al. (2019) conducted research that compared a semi-structured and a structured approach to goal setting with people with mild–moderate dementia. This was a cohort study of 101 people with dementia attending a rehabilitation centre. First, in the semi-structured interview participants were asked to state goals that had personal relevance to them; the style of questioning was adjusted if the person did not appear to understand what was being requested (Dutzi et al. 2019). A structured interview was then conducted with the same participants. Here, 19 areas were selected from the core set and the person was asked to score the relevance of each area from 0 to 2 and their abilities in each area from 0 to 5 (Dutzi et al. 2019).

The researchers reported that the semi-structured interview was less effective in enabling goal setting. For example, 18 participants, who did not differ in cognitive status from the rest of the cohort, failed to provide any goals (Dutzi et al. 2019). The structured interview, however, provided a clearer picture of the person's self-perceived needs. For instance, around 70% reported improving mobility and about 50% reported cognitive issues, including attention and memory, as priorities (Dutzi et al. 2019). In addition, significant correlations were found between goals and clinical assessments of function, indicating that the participants remained insightful into their impairments (Dutzi et al. 2019). The authors conclude that goal setting in collaboration with individuals with

Table 4.5 Examples of SMART goals written using the ABCDE checklist.

Actor	Behaviour	Condition	Degree	Expected time
Sean	Will pick children up from school	On foot	Using his phone calendar only as a cue	Within four weeks
Shola	Will complete staff development plans	In a quiet room in her workplace	Within three hours	In eight weeks' time

dementia is feasible and that this is supported by a structured rather than semi-structured approach (Dutzi et al. 2019).

Efforts have been made to develop treatment approaches that embed goal setting into rehabilitation for people with cognitive impairments. Although not developed exclusively by occupational therapists, they fit well with the profession's principles. One of these is discussed next.

Clare et al. (2019) argue that standard approaches to cognitive rehabilitation with ATD, which use training on pre-specified tasks addressing particular areas of cognitive function, have shown limited success. They suggest that where results have been positive, there is no evidence to support the clinical significance of any improvements or generalisability to other areas (Clare et al. 2010). These authors describe their own approach of 'goal-oriented cognitive rehabilitation' (Clare et al. 2010, p. 928). They explain that cognitive rehabilitation is person centred, guided by goals and based on problem solving (Clare et al. 2019). The therapist works collaboratively with the person, their carers and others providing support (Clare et al. 2019). They need to evaluate the person's capacity and current abilities and assess the necessities of the task or activities involved in the goal, identifying any disparity between current abilities and goal requirements (Clare et al. 2019). The therapist must then use evidence-based approaches to rehabilitation as they aim to overcome these disparities (Clare et al. 2019). Techniques could include adapting the environment, prompting, using memory aids or compensatory schemes, or learning specific skills (Clare et al. 2019). Cognitive rehabilitation is carried out in the person's home and is evaluated using participant or carer rating (Clare et al. 2019).

Clare et al. (2010, p. 928) reported on the results of a randomised controlled trial of goal-oriented cognitive rehabilitation for people with early-stage Alzheimer's disease. In their study, COPM was used to identify up to five goals for each participant (Clare et al. 2010). The person rated their current performance of and level of satisfaction with these targeted areas (Clare et al. 2010). They were then randomly allocated to one of three groups. There was a goal-oriented cognitive rehabilitation group, one control group that underwent guided relaxation and one that received no treatment (Clare et al. 2010). Measurements with COPM were taken at baseline and then again after the eight-week period of the intervention (Clare et al. 2010). The goal-oriented cognitive rehabilitation group experienced bespoke treatment based around one or two of their COPM goals (Clare et al. 2010).

At the end of the intervention, the goal-oriented cognitive rehabilitation group showed higher performance and satisfaction scores in COPM, when compared with baseline, while the two control groups did not show any change. When the scores for the groups were compared, the higher scores for the goal-oriented cognitive rehabilitation group were statistically significant (Clare et al. 2010). In addition, although COPM was not used at a six-month post-intervention follow-up, another cognitive screening tool showed that the cognitive rehabilitation group showed a significantly higher level of satisfaction with memory performance when compared with controls (Clare et al. 2010).

Clare et al. (2019) reported on the results of a multicentre randomised controlled trial of goal-oriented cognitive rehabilitation. The participants had mild–moderate cognitive impairment, resulting from ATD, vascular dementia and mixed dementia (Clare et al. 2019). The Bangor Goal-Setting Interview

(BGSI) tool was used to set three personal goals in collaboration with each participant (Clare et al. 2019, p. 711). Once the goals were set, the person was asked to use BGSI to score their level of attainment for each goal at baseline. They were then randomised to one of two groups: a usual treatment plus goal-oriented cognitive rehabilitation group; and a usual treatment group (Clare et al. 2019). The goal-oriented cognitive rehabilitation group had 10 one-hour treatment sessions each week over three months, with 4 follow-up maintenance sessions in the six months following treatment. The goal-oriented cognitive rehabilitation sessions were facilitated by nine occupational therapists and one nurse (Clare et al. 2019).

The key outcome measure was the participant-rated scores for attainment of their BGSI goals at baseline and at the three-month endpoint (Clare et al. 2019). In addition, they were asked to rate their satisfaction levels with their goal attainment at three months and then at nine months, while carers and supporters, labelled the 'study partner', were asked to rate goal attainment at three and nine months (Clare et al. 2019, p. 710). It was found that participant rating of attainment, satisfaction and study partner–rated attainment were all significantly different for the goal-oriented cognitive rehabilitation group, which had higher scores, at three and nine months. This figure is for all goals, not necessarily only the average of two that were targeted in therapy. However, when only the goals worked on during goal-oriented cognitive rehabilitation treatment were analysed, it was found that improvements in scores met predefined criteria for clinical significance (Clare et al. 2019). There were no significant differences identified on secondary measures of cognitive status, suggesting that improvements in function had occurred without any remedial changes to cognition (Clare et al. 2019).

Occupational therapists treating people with memory impairment must have regard for the legal framework guiding aspects of this work. The Mental Capacity Act 2005 is a key piece of legislation affecting England and Wales. It is discussed in Box 4.2.

BOX 4.2   MENTAL CAPACITY ACT 2005

The legal concept of mental capacity refers to a person's ability to make decisions in areas affecting them, such as social care and healthcare, welfare and also matters of finance and property (Johnston and Liddle 2007; Nicholson et al. 2008). The Mental Capacity Act became law in England and Wales when Royal Assent was given in April 2005, and was implemented in 2007 (Johnston and Liddle 2007).

The Act applies to people over the age of 16 who lack mental capacity. Lack of capacity to make a decision at a particular time is defined as inability to comprehend information that is relevant; inability to retain this information; and incapacity to use or assess this information when making decisions (Johnston and Liddle 2007). Clearly, these impairments touch on areas of learning and memory.

It is important to stress that capacity only applies to the decision in question and in that sense has been described as a 'functional approach' to assessment, rather than a 'status approach', where the person would be evaluated according to a standard benchmark (Nicholson et al. 2008, p. 324). The Act also stresses that just because a decision may appear unwise, for example to an occupational therapist or other healthcare professional, the person should not be judged to want capacity (Johnston and Liddle 2007).

The Act is intended to support the person in making the maximum possible number of decisions for themselves (Johnston and Liddle 2007). Importantly, it makes a 'presumption of capacity' that means that the person should not be judged not to have capacity, for example on the basis of their behaviour, age or appearance, and also states that the person should receive all possible support in making decisions (Johnston and Liddle 2007, p. 94). The present author has direct of experience of this through his work with stroke survivors with aphasia. Here, joint treatment sessions with a speech and language therapist, who was able to provide the person with alternative, non-verbal communication strategies, were essential in establishing mental capacity.

If a person cannot make decisions for themselves, then those making decisions for them must act in their 'best interests' (Johnston and Liddle 2007, p. 94). This latter concept does not just include questions of healthcare, but also consideration of their earlier wishes, beliefs and feelings (Johnston and Liddle 2007; Nicholson et al. 2008). In addition, best interest decisions about treatment should evaluate the possible benefits or disadvantages the treatment may bring for the person (Johnston and Liddle 2007).

Other people such as carers, a person with 'lasting power of attorney' or a court-appointed deputy, such as a family member or senior figure from social services, may make decisions in what is considered the person's best interests (Johnston and Liddle 2007, p. 95; Nicholson et al. 2008). Lasting power of attorney may be granted by a person at or above 18 years old enabling another, a 'proxy', to make decisions for them in their best interests (Johnston and Liddle 2007, p. 95). In cases where there is disagreement with the person with lasting power of attorney, then these may be referred to a 'court of protection', whose scope was extended by the Act to include health and welfare matters, for a decision to be made (Johnston and Liddle 2007, p. 95; Nicholson et al. 2008).

In addition, the Act established the role of the 'independent mental capacity advocate' who can support the person if they have no one close to them to provide support, and whose views must be taken into account when planning treatment for the person (Johnston and Liddle 2007, p. 97; Nicholson et al. 2008, p. 322). The present author believes that this role would be well suited to occupational therapists.

Conclusion

Occupation is the central concern of occupational therapy. Occupational therapy theorists have also attempted to model the stages of professional reasoning and intervention as the 'occupational therapy process'.

Numerous efforts have been undertaken to develop conceptual practice models that can guide professional reasoning and problem solving. Despite the variety of these models, at their heart they focus on the person performing occupations in specific environments. Prominent models include MOHO, PEO and CMOP-E. The Kawa model is based on a critique of these others, which its authors have described as biased towards a Western approach to occupation.

In addition, occupational therapists draw on evidence from other fields. These fields of knowledge are described as different 'frames of reference'. It was argued that there is not, currently, a single frame of reference that fits the approach taken to memory impairment and assessment described in this book. The author tentatively proposes that a new 'cognitive neuroscience' frame of reference might be recognised that could fulfil this function.

The chapter also considered the role of standardised cognitive screening tests. It was shown that MMSE is, in some ways, the 'grandparent' of many of these screens. MMSE influenced the domains assessed in more contemporary assessments, such as MoCA. This is despite the fact, as MMSE's main author openly acknowledged, that the assessment was put together very quickly and was based purely on the authors' professional subjective judgements.

A number of occupational therapy–specific assessments were discussed. These do not focus on memory per se. Rather, they assess aspects of cognition as embedded in task and activity performance. They range from the extensive, and costly, AMPS to quicker assessments based on readily available materials, such as the Kettle Test.

The chapter also described the memory checklist, developed by the present author to support his own clinical occupational therapy practice with stroke survivors. The checklist is based on categories of attention and memory derived from neuropsychology and cognitive neuroscience that are described in other chapters. It is currently non-standardised.

The importance of goal setting with the person with memory impairment was a concern of this chapter. It was shown that various authors have stressed the importance of this as guiding effective therapy and also facilitating multi-disciplinary working. A number of structured and easy-to-use approaches to producing and grading SMART goals were described. In addition, an ambitious programme of goal-centred rehabilitation for people with cognitive impairments was described. In the author's clinical experience, effective goal setting for people with memory impairments is sometimes a challenge for occupational therapists working clinically. It is hoped that the evidence discussed in this chapter will be useful in guiding training in both clinical and academic contexts.

Finally, the Mental Capacity Act 2005 was discussed. It was shown that this important Act provides a framework for decision making for people with cognitive impairments in England and Wales. In particular, it guarantees them certain rights to make decisions about treatment, even where professionals may consider these decisions unwise. It was also suggested that the role of independent mental capacity advocate would be a fitting one for occupational therapists.

Activities

Case Study Vignette 1

Angela has a diagnosis of ATD. She has been admitted to hospital following a fall, but she is eager to return to home.

Angela lives alone and is normally fairly independent in ADL. How could you use the memory checklist to:

1. Assess her memory performance when performing cooking activities?
2. Assess her memory performance during personal care tasks?

Case Study Vignette 2

Andriy has left his own country as a result of war. He has post-traumatic stress disorder characterised by unanticipated flashback memories. He is a chef and would like to work in this area in Wales, where he now lives. He is concerned that a kitchen environment might trigger flashbacks.

1. How could a cognitive neuroscience frame of reference support your professional reasoning when working with Andriy?
2. What would be an appropriate conceptual practice model for this case?
3. Describe how COPM could be used to identify treatment goals for Andriy.
4. Use the ABCDE approach to establish two SMART goals for Andriy.
5. Grade these SMART goals using the GAS approach.
6. How would the Mental Capacity Act 2005 be relevant in this case?

Case Study Vignette 3

Alan has Huntington's disease. He has been admitted to hospital following a fall. He has recently developed memory impairments in addition to motor control problems.

You have been asked to facilitate Alan's discharge from hospital. You conduct an assessment of Alan's home environment.

He lives in a flat at the top of a building of several storeys. It is accessible only via a long stairway constructed from stone. The flat is almost derelict.

In your professional opinion, Alan would be at severe risk of falls, injury or even death if he returned there. However, Alan is insistent that he will accept being discharged only to this property and has even threatened to kill himself if he is discharged elsewhere.

Alan has been found to have mental capacity to make the decision regarding his discharge destination.

1. How would the Mental Capacity Act 2005 inform your professional reasoning and intervention planning in this case?

References

Amato, C., Burridge, G., Basic, D. et al. (2021). Assistance provided in daily tasks and difficulty experienced by caregivers for people living with dementia. *Australian Occupational Therapy Journal* 68 (3): 236–245.

Babulal, G.M., Zhu, Y., and Trani, J.-F. (2023). Racial and ethnic differences in neuropsychiatric symptoms and progression to incident cognitive impairment among community-dwelling participants. *Alzheimer's and Dementia* 19 (8): 3635–3643.

Bar-Yosef, C., Weinblatt, N., and Katz, N. (2000). Reliability and validity of the cognitive performance test (CPT) in an elderly population in Israel. *Physical & Occupational Therapy in Geriatrics* 17 (1): 65–79.

Baum, C. and Edwards, D.F. (1993). Cognitive performance in senile dementia of the Alzheimer's type: the Kitchen Task assessment. *American Journal of Occupational Therapy* 47 (5): 431–436.

Bolló-Gasol, S., Piñol-Ripoll, G., Cejudo-Bolivar, J.C. et al. (2014). Ecological assessment of mild cognitive impairment and Alzheimer disease using the Rivermead Behavioural Memory Test. *Neurología* 29 (6): 339–345.

Bovend'Eerdt, T.J.H., Botell, R.E., and Wade, D.T. (2009). Writing SMART rehabilitation goals and achieving goal attainment scaling: a practical guide. *Clinical Rehabilitation* 23 (4): 352–361.

Bukhbinder, A.S., Hinojosa, M., Harris, K. et al. (2023). Population-based Mini-Mental State Examination norms in adults of Mexican heritage in the Cameron County Hispanic Cohort. *Journal of Alzheimer's Disease* 92 (4): 1323–1339.

Carnero-Pardo, C. (2014). Should the Mini-Mental State Examination be retired? *Neurología* 29 (8): 473–481.

Clare, L.P.D., Linden, D.E.J., Woods, R.T. et al. (2010). Goal-oriented cognitive rehabilitation for people with early-stage Alzheimer disease: a single-blind randomized controlled trial of clinical efficacy. *American Journal of Geriatric Psychiatry* 18 (10): 928–939.

Clare, L., Kudlicka, A., Oyebode, J.R. et al. (2019). Individual goal-oriented cognitive rehabilitation to improve everyday functioning for people with early-stage dementia: a multicentre randomised controlled trial (the GREAT trial). *International Journal of Geriatric Psychiatry* 34 (5): 709–721.

Coen, R.F., Robertson, D.A., Kenny, R.A. et al. (2016). Strengths and limitations of the MoCA for assessing cognitive functioning: findings from a large representative sample of Irish older adults. *Journal of Geriatric Psychiatry and Neurology* 29 (1): 18–24.

Creek, J. (2003). *Occupational Therapy Defined as a Complex Intervention*. London: College of Occupational Therapists.

Daniel, M.A. and Blair, S.E.E. (2011). An introduction to the psychodynamic frame of reference. In: *Foundations for Practice in Occupational Therapy* (ed. E.A.S. Duncan), 165–178. London: Churchill Livingstone.

Deacon, T.W. (1998). *The Symbolic Species: The Co-evolution of Language and the Human Brain*. London: Penguin.

Demeyere, N., Riddoch, M.J., Slavkova, E.D. et al. (2015). The Oxford Cognitive Screen (OCS): validation of a stroke-specific short cognitive screening tool. *Psychological Assessment* 27 (3): 883–894.

Duncan, E.A.S. (2011a). Skills and processes in occupational therapy. In: *Foundations for Practice in Occupational Therapy* (ed. E.A.S. Duncan), 33–42. London: Churchill Livingstone.

Duncan, E.A.S. (2011b). An introduction to conceptual models of practice and frames of reference. In: *Foundations for Practice in Occupational Therapy* (ed. E.A.S. Duncan), 43–48. London: Churchill Livingstone.

Dutzi, I., Schwenk, M., Kirchner, M. et al. (2019). 'What would you like to achieve?' Goal-setting in patients with dementia in geriatric rehabilitation. *BMC Geriatrics* 19 (1): 280–280.

Fabricius, J., Huynh, M.N.M., Pedersen, A.R., and Pilegaard, M.S. (2023). Predicting length of stay with assessment of motor and process skills in subjects with acquired brain injury. *Brain Injury* 37 (3): 179–184.

Feaver, S. and Ezekiel, L. (2011). Theoretical approaches to motor control and cognitive-perceptual function. In: *Foundations for Practice in Occupational Therapy* (ed. E.A.S. Duncan), 195–205. London: Churchill Livingstone.

Folstein, M.F. (1989). The birth of the MMS. *American Journal Occupational Therapy* 43: 391–397.

Folstein, M.F., Folstein, S.E., and McHugh, P.R. (1975). 'Mini-mental state': a practical method for grading the cognitive state of patients for the clinician. *Journal of Psychiatric Research* 12 (3): 189–198.

Gazzaniga, M.S., Ivry, R.B., and Mangun, G.R. (2009). *Cognitive Neuroscience: The Biology of the Mind*, 3e. New York: Norton.

Gitlin, L.N., Winter, L., Corcoran, M. et al. (2003). Effects of the home environmental skill-building program on the caregiver–care recipient dyad: 6-month outcomes from the Philadelphia REACH initiative. *Gerontologist* 43 (4): 532–546.

Gitlin, L.N., Kales, H.C., and Lyketsos, C.G. (2012). Nonpharmacologic management of behavioral symptoms in dementia. *JAMA* 308 (19): 2020–2029.

Grieve, J.I. and Gnanasekaran, L. (2008). *Neuropsychology for Occupational Therapists: Cognition in Occupational Performance*, 3e. Oxford: Blackwell Publishing.

Hagedorn, R. (1992). *Occupational Therapy: Foundations for Practice: Models, Frames of Reference and Core Skills*. Edinburgh: Churchill Livingstone.

Hagedorn, R. (2001). *Foundations for Practice in Occupational Therapy*, 3e. Edinburgh: Churchill Livingstone.

Harper, K.J., Llewellyn, K., Jacques, A. et al. (2019). Kettle test efficacy in predicting cognitive and functional outcomes in geriatric rehabilitation. *Australian Occupational Therapy Journal* 66 (2): 219–226.

Hartman-Maeir, A., Harel, H., and Katz, N. (2009). Kettle test—a brief measure of cognitive functional performance: reliability and validity in stroke rehabilitation. *American Journal of Occupational Therapy* 63 (5): 592–599.

Henry, A.D., Moore, K., Quinlivan, M., and Triggs, M. (1998). The relationship of the Allen Cognitive Level Test to demographics, diagnosis, and disposition among psychiatric inpatients. *American Journal of Occupational Therapy* 52 (8): 638–643.

Howe, M.C. and Briggs, A.K. (1982). Ecological systems model for occupational therapy. *American Journal of Occupational Therapy* 36 (5): 322–327.

Iwama, M.K. (2006). *The Kawa Model: Culturally Relevant Occupational Therapy*. Edinburgh: Churchill Livingstone/Elsevier.

Iwama, M.K., Thomson, N.A., and Macdonald, R.M. (2009). The Kawa model: the power of culturally responsive occupational therapy. *Disability and Rehabilitation* 31 (14): 1125–1135.

Jogie, P., Rahja, M., van den Berg, M. et al. (2021). Goal setting for people with mild cognitive impairment or dementia in rehabilitation: a scoping review. *Australian Occupational Therapy Journal* 68 (6): 563–592.

Johnston, C. and Liddle, J. (2007). The Mental Capacity Act 2005: a new framework for healthcare decision making. *Journal of Medical Ethics* 33 (2): 94–97.

Jorm, A.F. (2004). The informant questionnaire on cognitive decline in the elderly (IQCODE): a review. *International Psychogeriatrics* 16 (3): 275–293.

Katz, N. (1994). Cognitive rehabilitation: models for intervention and research on cognition in occupational therapy. *Occupational Therapy International* 1 (1): 49–63.

Kielhofner, G. (1995). *A Model of Human Occupation: Theory and Application*, 2e. Baltimore, MD: Williams & Wilkins.

Law, M., Baptiste, S., McColl, M. et al. (1990). The Canadian occupational performance measure: an outcome measure for occupational therapy. *Canadian Journal of Occupational Therapy* 57 (2): 82–87.

Law, M., Cooper, B., Strong, S. et al. (1996). The person-environment-occupation model: a transactive approach to occupational performance. *Canadian Journal of Occupational Therapy* 63 (1): 9–23.

Linden, A., Boschian, K., Eker, C. et al. (2005). Assessment of motor and process skills reflects brain-injured patients' ability to resume independent living better than neuropsychological tests. *Acta Neurologica Scandinavica* 111 (1): 48–53.

McMillan, I.R. (2011). The biomechanical frame of reference in occupational therapy. In: *Foundations for Practice in Occupational Therapy* (ed. E.A.S. Duncan), 179–193. London: Churchill Livingstone.

Miller, G.A. (2003). The cognitive revolution: a historical perspective. *Trends in Cognitive Sciences* 7 (3): 141–144.

Molineux, M. (2017). *A Dictionary of Occupational Science and Occupational Therapy*. Oxford: Oxford University Press.

Nasreddine, Z.S., Phillips, N.A., Bédirian, V. et al. (2005). The Montreal Cognitive Assessment, MoCA: a brief screening tool for mild cognitive impairment. *Journal of the American Geriatrics Society* 53 (4): 695–699.

Nicholson, T.R.J., Cutter, W., and Hotopf, M. (2008). Assessing mental capacity: the Mental Capacity Act. *British Medical Journal* 336 (7639): 322–325.

Pentland, D., Kantartzis, S., Clausen, M.G., and Witemyre, K. (2018). *Occupational Therapy and Complexity: Defining and Describing Practice*. London: Royal College of Occupational Therapists.

Pool, J. (2011). The functional information-processing model. In: *Foundations for Practice in Occupational Therapy* (ed. E.A.S. Duncan), 105–115. London: Churchill Livingstone.

Rockwood, K., Joyce, B., and Stolee, P. (1997). Use of goal attainment scaling in measuring clinically important change in cognitive rehabilitation patients. *Journal of Clinical Epidemiology* 50 (5): 581–588.

Roitman, D.M. and Katz, N. (1997). Predictive validity of the Large Allen Cognitive Levels Test (LACL) using the Allen Diagnostic Module (ADM) in an aged, non-disabled population. *Physical & Occupational Therapy in Geriatrics* 14 (4): 43–59.

Rose, S.P.R. (1992). *The Making of Memory*. London: Bantam.

Shumway-Cook, A. and Woollacott, M.H. (2012). *Motor Control: Translating Research into Clinical Practice*, 4e. Baltimore, MD: Lippincott Williams & Wilkins.

Sumsion, T., Tischler-Draper, L., and Heinicke, S. (2011). Applying the Canadian model of occupational performance. In: *Foundations for Practice in Occupational Therapy* (ed. E.A.S. Duncan), 81–91. London: Churchill Livingstone.

Taylor-Rowan, M., Nafisi, S., Owen, R. et al. (2023). Informant-based screening tools for dementia: an overview of systematic reviews. *Psychological Medicine* 53 (2): 580–589.

Turner-Stokes, L. (2009). Goal attainment scaling (GAS) in rehabilitation: a practical guide. *Clinical Rehabilitation* 23 (4): 362–370.

Velligan, D.I., True, J.E., Lefton, R.S. et al. (1995). Validity of the Allen Cognitive Levels Assessment: a tri-ethnic comparison. *Psychiatry Research* 56 (2): 101–109.

Velligan, D.I., Bow-Thomas, C.C., Mahurin, R. et al. (1998). Concurrent and predictive validity of the Allen Cognitive Levels Assessment. *Psychiatry Research* 80 (3): 287–298.

Wilcock, A.A. (2006). *An Occupational Perspective of Health*, 2e. Thorofare, NJ: Slack.

Wilson, B., Cockburn, J., Baddeley, A., and Hiorns, R. (1989). The development and validation of a test battery for detecting and monitoring everyday memory problems. *Journal of Clinical and Experimental Neuropsychology* 11 (6): 855–870.

Yerxa, E.J. (2000a). Confessions of an occupational therapist who became a detective. *British Journal of Occupational Therapy* 63 (5): 192–199.

Yerxa, E.J. (2000b). Occupational science: a renaissance of service to humankind through knowledge. *Occupational Therapy International* 7 (2): 87–98.

5 Occupational Therapy Action Planning and Treatment Implementation for Children and Adolescents with Memory Impairment

The phonological loop component of the multicomponent working memory model may underpin language acquisition in children. Conversely, this chapter also shows evidence that impairments in this area may impede language development. The importance of this in the UK context is underscored by the fact that early reading and writing skills are taught using 'synthetic phonics'.

Performance on tests based on the multicomponent working memory model can also predict performance on national curriculum tests. This is particularly the case for the central executive and visual spatial aspects of the multicomponent model. Furthermore, it is shown that impairments in verbal working memory may help explain specific language impairments (SLIs) for some children.

It is argued that the occupational therapists supporting children in classroom settings should apply knowledge of the multicomponent working memory model during task analysis. In particular, an understanding of the 'episodic buffer' can help the occupational therapist when guiding the teacher or classroom assistant to facilitate 'bridging' between new items and items from long-term memory. Examples of 'chunking' in order to support learning are also described.

The role of conceptual practice models in guiding occupational therapy interventions with children in the classroom is outlined. It is shown that insights from learning and memory theory can help the occupational therapist guide the

Memory Impairment and Occupation: A Guide to Evaluation and Treatment, First Edition.
Jonathon O'Brien.
© 2024 John Wiley & Sons Ltd. Published 2024 by John Wiley & Sons Ltd.

teacher as part of environmental or task analysis. Working memory, and visuospatial skills in particular, may also help explain mathematical performance in the classroom.

Children with attention deficit/hyperactivity disorder (ADHD) may have working memory difficulties. In addition, children with behavioural problems linked to oppositional defiant disorder (ODD) may have working memory impairments. Furthermore, there is evidence that children with anxiety may experience working memory difficulties.

The psychodynamic and cognitive behavioural frames of reference are described briefly in this chapter. These are linked to the concept of overgeneral autobiographical memory (OAM). Rather like the age of offset of infantile amnesia, discussed in Chapter 3, this concept provides an experimental paradigm through which to analyse environmental factors influencing memory in children and adolescents.

The CaR-FA-X model, which attempts to account for problems with memory retrieval in people with anxiety and depression, is described. It is shown how this relates to the multicomponent working memory model and also understanding of executive function. Evidence from neuroimaging is presented that suggests that mental health conditions such as major depressive disorder (MDD) could have an impact on hippocampal development and, by implication, the development of memory.

Working Memory Impairments in the Classroom

Researchers have investigated the extent to which performance in the multicomponent working memory model domains might explain language learning and impaired linguistic development in children. They have also explored the relationship between working memory ability and attainment in standardised education tests. Further work has examined the impact of working memory on mathematics performance and also on specific learning impairments in mathematics. This work has relevance to occupational therapists supporting children and teachers in the classroom and is described in more detail later in the chapter.

Gathercole and Baddeley (1989) investigated the relationship between language acquisition and the phonological loop component of working memory. They tested 104 children on entrance to primary school at age 4–5 and again one year later. They assessed children's phonological skills by asking them to repeat groups of non-words of different levels of complexity. The assumption was that learning new words must involve assimilating initially unfamiliar spoken word sounds with the aid of articulatory rehearsal within phonological memory, and that the non-word repetition test could be taken as a model of this process (Gathercole and Baddeley 1989).

The test scores were analysed in relation to the children's scores on a vocabulary test, the short form of the British Picture Vocabulary Scale (BPVS; Gathercole and Baddeley 1989). The authors found what they describe as a high level of correlation between non-word repetition and BPVS scores at age 4–5 and one year later (Gathercole and Baddeley 1989). They also found that most of the variance noted in the BPVS scores was explained by performance on the non-word recognition task.

When the children were tested a year later, it was found that chronological age did not explain any of the variance in BPVS scores, while the non-word repetition test accounted for 24% of performance (Gathercole and Baddeley 1989). Overall, the authors suggest that phonological working memory capacity predicts vocabulary acquisition during a child's first school year, although they are clear that the relationship they identified is one of correlation, rather than causation (Gathercole and Baddeley 1989).

In a subsequent study, Gathercole and Baddeley (1990) investigated whether children with delayed language development also had impaired phonological memory. They compared a group of six children with language impairments and six children with normal development on performance of the non-word repetition task. They found that children with language impairments performed less well on the task, and that the differences in scores were statistically significant (Gathercole and Baddeley 1990).

In a second experiment, Gathercole and Baddeley (1990) found that children with impairments had lower non-word repetition scores, although they only noted significant differences for three- and four-syllable non-words, while one- and two-syllable non-words did not show the same pattern. Using the data from this experiment, Gathercole and Baddeley (1990) were able to show that children with impaired language were performing non-word repetition at a rate around four years behind their chronological age. The authors concluded that the phonological memory skills involved in non-word recognition may underpin language development, and suggested that phonological memory is important at the point where children are learning to relate groups of letters to sounds (Gathercole and Baddeley 1990).

These findings are especially important for occupational therapists working in education settings. In the United Kingdom, the government-mandated approach to teaching reading and writing in early years and Key Stages 1 and 2 is 'synthetic phonics' (Wallace 2015). This is based on speech sounds and the ways these sounds are combined to build up words (Wallace 2015). The evidence provided by Gathercole and Baddeley (1989, 1990) suggests that children with impairments in the phonological loop aspect of working memory may be disadvantaged when using this approach. Occupational therapists may therefore support reading and writing progress by suggesting classroom strategies beneficial to children with working memory difficulties.

Gathercole and Pickering (2000) used a test battery to evaluate the working memory of children undertaking standard assessment tests of their performance on the English national curriculum. They tested 83 children between 6 and 7 years old and found that children who performed poorly on national curriculum assessments also performed poorly on central executive and visual-spatial tasks (Gathercole and Pickering 2000). They discovered that scores on the working memory test successfully predicted the membership of 83.1% of the children in the normally performing group and 82.6% of the children in the poorly performing group (Gathercole and Pickering 2000). They point out that a range of working memory component scores predicted group membership, and therefore speculate that performance on the national curriculum tests reflected general working memory (Gathercole and Pickering 2000). They found that performance on the central executive components and on visuospatial memory were particularly strong predictors of national curriculum test scores.

Gathercole and Pickering (2000) suggest that the central executive is heavily involved in higher cognitive ability and may underpin literacy and numeracy skills by functioning as a 'mental workspace' where the outcomes of ongoing procedures are cached and merged with simultaneous complex cognitive tasks (Gathercole and Pickering 2000, p. 189). They list some typical classroom activities that might depend on the central executive: working out a word while also keeping in mind words from a text that has been previously decoded; writing while also thinking about what to write next; and mental arithmetic (Gathercole and Pickering 2000). They point out that all of these tasks involve holding information while also integrating it with items in working memory or information drawn from long-term memory, all of which should engage the central executive (Gathercole and Pickering 2000).

Some children fail to progress as expected in the national curriculum and may be eligible for special educational needs (SEN) support. Gathercole and Pickering (2001) were interested in a possible link between working memory impairment and SEN. They tested 57 children between 7 and 8 years old using a battery of working memory tests. They found that children's SEN status had a significant impact on some of the test battery scores at age 7. They discovered, for example, a significant effect of SEN status for scores on one of the central executive function tests and for some of the phonological loop tests (Gathercole and Pickering 2001).

When 54 of the children were retested one year later at age 8, the differences were more marked: significant differences were noted for two of the central executive tests and two of the visuospatial tests for the SEN group, although no differences were found for the phonological loop (Gathercole and Pickering 2001). At age 7, it was found that membership of the SEN or non-SEN group was predicted by working memory test scores for 91% of the children and at age 8 for 81% of the children (Gathercole and Pickering 2001). This evidence points to a strong association between working memory limitations and SEN.

Archibald and Gathercole (2006) tested 15 children with SLI, a condition leading to difficulties in using and understanding language, on tests of visuospatial working memory and visuospatial short-term memory. The children had an average age of 9 years and 8 months. They had also been tested previously by the researchers and found to have deficits in verbal working memory and verbal short-term memory (Archibald and Gathercole 2006). There were two control groups: 15 age-matched children and 15 children matched for language ability, with an average age of 6.

Archibald and Gathercole (2006) found no significant differences between the SLI group and the age-matched controls on the visuospatial working memory and visuospatial short-term memory tests. They argue that the results point to a specific impairment of verbal working and short-term memory in SLI, as opposed to a more general impairment also affecting visuospatial memory. In addition, they suggest that this offers further support to the multicomponent model of working memory (Archibald and Gathercole 2006). Again, these results show the importance of paediatric occupational therapists working in educational settings understanding working memory impairments.

Gathercole et al. (2004) tested two groups of children on subtests from the Working Memory Test Battery for Children (WMTB-C). One group consisted of 7–8-year-olds who had just completed national Key Stage 1 attainment tests, and the second consisted of 14–15-year-olds who had completed Key Stage 3 attainment tests (Gathercole et al. 2004). The authors found that at Key Stage 1, performance in English and maths was significantly correlated with performance on the WMTB-C subtests of digit recall and listening recall. This latter test involves the child judging the truth of a sequence of sentences and then recalling the final word of each sentence, therefore testing storage and processing ability simultaneously (Gathercole et al. 2004).

In the Key Stage 3 group, strong correlations were noted between maths and science scores and WMTB-C tests involving word list matching, backwards digit recall and listening recall. In word list matching, the child is presented with a sequence of words and the sequence is then presented again with the possibility that the position of some of the words has changed; the child has to state whether the sequence is the same or not, meaning that they must store and process information simultaneously (Gathercole et al. 2004). There was, however, a weaker correlation between these tests and their English scores (Gathercole et al. 2004).

The results of Gathercole et al.'s (2004) research were used to divide the children into low-, medium- and high-ability groups for various curriculum subjects. It was found that for the Key Stage 1 children, the effect of English ability group membership on non-word recognition, digit recall and listening recall scores was significant (Gathercole et al. 2004). The authors also found that for Key Stage 1 children, the effect of maths ability group on digit recall and listening recall was significant (Gathercole et al. 2004). For the Key Stage 3 students, it was found that the effect of maths group membership on listening recall and backward digits, considered to be tests of central executive function, was significant. In addition, the effect of science ability group on listening recall and word list matching was significant (Gathercole et al. 2004).

Gathercole et al. (2004) conclude, on the basis of the results described, that basic literacy learning may be underpinned by central executive function at Key Stage 1. However, at Key Stage 3 the relationship between English ability and central executive scores was weaker. The authors suggest that this may be because different areas were being assessed at the different stages: basic literacy for Key Stage 1 and higher-level reading, writing and comprehension skills for Key Stage 3 (Gathercole et al. 2004). They also argue that the strong connection between central executive tests and maths ability throughout the key stages may reflect a more general problem with the central executive, as opposed to a specific issue with number, as these children also showed impaired language recall, in addition to deficits in mathematical ability (Gathercole et al. 2004). These results seem to support the applicability of the multicomponent working memory model to educational attainment in English and maths.

In line with the evidence just presented, Alloway and Alloway (2015) argue that children with dyslexia have impairments in working memory. In relation to phonics, for example, the child with working memory problems may not have the 'internal look-up table' that mainstream students develop when memorising phonemes (Alloway and Alloway 2015, p. 29). This means that they must deploy working memory when decoding novel words, to such an extent that this memory system is not available to support them in understanding the broader text (Alloway and Alloway 2015). With regard to general classroom organisation, the child with working memory impairments may have difficulty remembering a list of tasks given by the teacher verbally, because they cannot internally rehearse all of these items using the phonological loop component of working memory.

The occupational therapist involved in supporting children with working memory impairments affecting reading and writing should apply an understanding of the multicomponent working memory model as part of their task analysis. For example, it was shown earlier that children with SLI did not necessarily have difficulties with *visuospatial* working memory (Archibald and Gathercole 2006). So, the occupational therapist might analyse the style of information processing required in a task, ensuring that the child is tapping their strengths. A topic such as the life cycle of the butterfly could, for example, be supported by visual representation of the egg, caterpillar, pupa and butterfly, rather than a solely written description. Also, a history timeline may be better presented vertically, rather than horizontally (Alloway and Alloway 2015).

The occupational therapist may recommend that the teacher should reduce the size or complexity of a text, meaning that the child will not need to deploy as much working memory simply to decode the words when reading, freeing capacity in order to understand the broader meaning (Alloway and Alloway 2015). In addition, the application of assistive technology has been defined as a 'context-dependent practice skill' for occupational therapists (College of Occupational Therapists 2016, p. 5). The occupational therapist could apply these skills, for example, by assessing for recording devices that allow the child to record what they wish to say prior to writing, which may support working memory (Alloway and Alloway 2015).

Alloway and Alloway (2015) also suggest that when presenting new information, the student with working memory impairments will benefit from connecting these novel items with pre-existing memories. This echoes the findings of Bartlett (1995), Craik and Lockhart (1972) and Craik and Tulving (1975), already discussed in Chapter 1. The use of mnemonic devices, such as 'Richard Of York Gave Battle In Vain' to remember the colours of the rainbow, is one example. At a higher level of abstraction, when introducing a new text the teacher or classroom assistant could demonstrate that the narrative structure of the story is the same as other stories the child has read. For instance, in the 'Three Little Pigs' the pigs are challenged by the wolf three times and then trick him, while in *The Gruffalo* (Donaldson and Scheffler 2014) the mouse encounters three different animals who want to eat it and tricks them in order to escape.

Alloway and Alloway (2015, p. 131) describe this process of linking new items with memory in the long-term store as creating a 'bridge' between the two. Bridging may be thought of as an application of the concept of the 'episodic buffer', which was added to the multicomponent working memory model by Baddeley (2000), p. 421, 2003 and was discussed in Chapter 1. It will be recalled that the episodic buffer was conceived as a 'workspace' in which, for example, freshly perceived visual or verbal items could be integrated with items from long-term memory in order to support task completion (Baddeley 2015, p. 82).

Baddeley (2000, p. 418, 2003, p. 835) has also suggested that 'visual semantics', which allows recognition of visually presented items, and language are part of 'crystallised knowledge', embedded in long-term memory.

With regard to the example of narrative structure, the child would be working within the episodic buffer when 'bridging' between their crystallised knowledge of the structure of the 'Three Little Pigs', stored in long-term memory, and learning to read *The Gruffalo*. This would enable them to grasp the overall pattern of the new text, freeing up working memory capacity to support, for example, analysis of the phonetic structures of novel words. Similarly, when using visual imagery to support learning, as in the example of the butterfly life cycle, the child would be bridging between crystallised visual semantic knowledge, for instance knowledge of what a caterpillar looks like, and new learning, such as the location of the caterpillar in the life cycle time line. In both examples, according to the multicomponent model, bridging would be facilitated by the episodic buffer.

Identifying the shared narrative structure of stories is also an application of Miller's (1956) concept of 'chunking', discussed in Chapter 1. Table 5.1 shows how the narratives of the 'Three Little Pigs' and *The Gruffalo* could be chunked.

Chunking narratives in the way suggested in Table 5.1 may support the child in grasping overall structure, releasing working memory capacity for decoding the language content of the stories. Baddeley et al. (2009) have also argued that the episodic buffer is involved in chunking words in order to facilitate sentence interpretation. They suggest that such chunking is a relatively automatic process, taking place in long-term memory, and that the central executive then manipulates the chunks within the episodic buffer (Baddeley et al. 2009).

The therapist should apply knowledge of memory theory when assisting the child or teacher with strategies to support occupational performance. For example, it will be recalled that, according to the multicomponent model, the length of time for which items are maintained in phonological memory can be increased by rehearsing them vocally or mentally (Baddeley 2012; Gathercole and Hitch 1993). The child with working memory impairments may therefore benefit from reading a word list out loud before reading it silently (Alloway and Alloway 2015).

Table 5.1 Chunking narratives.

Chunks	Examples from the 'Three Little Pigs'	Examples from *The Gruffalo*
Challenges	Wolf at the straw house	Fox
	Wolf at the stick house	Owl
	Wolf at the brick house	Snake
Tricks	Pigs trick the wolf	Mouse tricks the animals
Turns	Wolf comes down the chimney	Mouse meets the Gruffalo
Resolutions	Wolf runs away	Gruffalo runs away
Conclusions	Pigs live in peace	Mouse eats the nut

In Chapter 4, it was shown that occupational therapy theorists have developed conceptual practice models that suggest ways in which the environment could affect memory performance (Howe and Briggs 1982; Kielhofner 1995; Law et al. 1996). In Howe and Briggs's (1982, p. 323) ecological systems model, for example, the person's cognitive style of information processing is viewed as part of an 'inner life space' that is shaped by interaction with the environment. These insights, along with appreciation of memory theory, can support occupational therapy task analysis when working with a child with working memory impairments in order to support language-based learning.

The social environment should be analysed. This may include, for example, the style and context in which the educator presents language-based information. In Chapter 1, it was shown that retrieval cues work best if the retrieval situation matches the initial learning context (Craik and Lockhart 1972). The child with working memory impairments may thus benefit if the cues given to retrieve information match the environment in which it was initially presented. For instance, if a word was presented initially on coloured paper at a certain time in a particular part of the classroom, then it may be helpful to present the cue, for example part of the word, on the same coloured paper in the same part of the room at a similar time of day.

Occupational therapy conceptual practice models also emphasise the ways in which the physical environment shapes occupational performance (Howe and Briggs 1982; Kielhofner 1995; Law et al. 1996). Using these insights, the therapist should include the classroom surroundings in their task analysis. For example, is there excessive noise or clutter that is likely to place more demands on the central executive attentional component of working memory? Andersson (2008) describes four functions of the central executive: coordinating the execution of two individual tasks; alternating between different tasks; attention to specific items and inhibition of others; and activation and retrieval of items from long-term memory. If the child is moved to a quieter and less distracting environment, the central executive is then released to allocate attention to the phonological components of the reading or writing task (Alloway and Alloway 2015).

The treatment approaches suggested apply to the child with working memory impairments. However, techniques such as bridging, chunking, use of mnemonics and visual images, and adapting the social and physical environment may benefit all learners. Arguably, thinkers and educators have had an intuitive grasp of these techniques since ancient times. For example, the Jesuit missionary Cantova reported in 1721 that people in the Southern Pacific Caroline Islands included knowledge of star constellations in their children's education (Hogben et al. 1938). This can be seen as an example of chunking, grouping otherwise disparate stars into meaningfully named chunks to support memorisation. Similarly, early anatomists related parts of the body to pre-existing visual semantics, for example the hippocampus of the medial temporal lobe is named because of its resemblance to a seahorse, which supports recognition. Furthermore, if one views contemporary television programmes designed for a pre-school audience, which, at their best, have a strong educational content, one will see that the structure of each episode is usually identical, as are the set design and the presenter's costume; again, this releases attentional resources for processing the novel information presented in each episode.

Working Memory in Mathematics Performance

Working memory has been linked to performance in maths. Andersson (2008), for example, studied the role of different central executive components and the two working memory subsystems in maths skills with 141 children in years four and five. The children undertook tests of arithmetic performance alongside working memory tests. Andersson (2008) found that working memory performance accounted for 72% of the written maths outcomes. Performance on digit span, trail making, counting span and verbal fluency were all significant predictors of arithmetic abilities (Andersson 2008). Three central executive tasks, counting span, verbal fluency and trail making, and one phonological loop task, digit span, explained 59% of the variance in written maths performance (Andersson 2008).

Allen et al. (2020) explored the relationship between working memory and maths performance in 6–10-year-olds. The authors were interested in examining the relationship between working memory tasks of different complexity and maths skills. They point out that working memory tasks can be based on span, such as remembering lists or positions of visual stimuli in the order presented, which may be equivalent to basic short-term memory tasks (Allen et al. 2020). Alternatively, they may be complex dual tasks that require both storage and manipulation of presented items, for example remembering a list of words in order of presentation (Allen et al. 2020). They suggest, in addition, that working memory tasks may be placed on a 'horizontal continuum' from verbal to visuospatial, or on a 'vertical continuum' based on the amount of attentional control required (Allen et al. 2020, p. 850).

Allen et al. (2020) tested children's verbal working memory using forwards or backwards span tasks and a dual task, where children had to listen to four words and press a bar when they heard an animal mentioned. They then had to remember the last word in the list and, finally, give all of the last list words in order (Allen et al. 2020). To test visuospatial working memory, the children had to view a series of grids that contained different sequences of black squares; the task was to recall the position of the squares forwards or backwards (Allen et al. 2020). For the dual element, children needed to view grids with grey squares; the grids also displayed sequences of black dots and the participants had to indicate when they saw a black dot in a grey square and also state the position of the last dot viewed. They then needed to recall the sequence of the final dots seen in each viewing in order (Allen et al. 2020).

Allen et al. (2020) found that, for the various year groups, the strongest correlations with maths performance were with different working memory tests. In year two the dominant correlation was with backwards verbal span, while in year three it was with backwards verbal span and backwards matrices. For year four the strongest correlation was with backwards verbal span and forward matrices, and in year five it was with backwards matrices and the dual visuospatial test (Allen et al. 2020). The authors suggest that one explanation could be that the backwards tasks necessitate greater attention (Allen et al. 2020). Overall, the strongest correlation was with the backwards matrices and backwards word span tasks, pointing to a role for visuospatial and verbal working memory in mathematics performance

(Allen et al. 2020). In addition, the strength of correlation with two visuospatial tasks at year five led the authors to conclude that there may be greater reliance on visuospatial processes in this age group (Allen et al. 2020).

Attout and Majerus (2015) investigated the relationship between retention of serial order and developmental dyscalculia, a condition involving impaired learning of maths and number skills. They tested 16 children with developmental dyscalculia and 16 normally developing children from 8 to 12 years old. The participants were asked to perform two key tasks: an 'item' memory task and a serial order task (Attout and Majerus 2015, p. 436). For the item task, children had to repeat 30 monosyllabic words, with each word presentation being followed by a three-second delay in which they were asked to repeat an irrelevant non-word sound (Attout and Majerus 2015). For the serial order task, children were given lists of between two and seven animal names in different orders; they then had to place pictures of the animals in the correct order.

The authors found that the developmental dyscalculia group performed with significantly less accuracy on the serial order task, while there were no significant differences on performance of the item task sound (Attout and Majerus 2015). The authors therefore posit a relationship between impaired memory for serial order and developmental dyscalculia (Attout and Majerus 2015).

Metcalfe et al. (2013) conducted functional magnetic resonance imaging (fMRI) scans on children aged 7–9 performing mathematical tasks. The children were assessed for working memory ability using tests of central executive, visuospatial and phonological skills. The aim was to explore the neural mechanisms underpinning the visuospatial, phonological and central executive aspects of working memory during mathematics performance (Metcalfe et al. 2013).

Overlapping activation for visuospatial, phonological and central executive tasks was noted in the posterior parietal cortex, suggesting that this region may play a role in integrating the information required to perform mathematics (Metcalfe et al. 2013). This 'multimodal' association function of the posterior parietal cortex had been noted by Luria, who also remarked on the role of the parietal region in 'mathematical operations' (Luria 1973, pp. 73, 154). Metcalfe et al. (2013) note that the highest correlation was between the scores for the working memory test of visuospatial skill and ability to execute 'numerical operations', which are maths operations without any language requirements (Metcalfe et al. 2013, p. 164). The second highest correlation was between visuospatial scores and scores for 'mathematical reasoning', which describes maths problems with a language component (Metcalfe et al. 2013, p. 164). The authors conclude that visuospatial working memory is central to maths performance in this age group (Metcalfe et al. 2013).

Luria provided an explanation for the role of visuospatial function in mathematics. He noted that place value and tables, for example, depend on 'internal spatial schemes . . . with a similar structure to external spatial operations' (Luria 1973, p. 154). Luria also identified a role here for 'operative memory', a concept that appears similar to that of working memory as discussed throughout this book (Luria 1973, p. 154).

Bathelt et al. (2018) explored the relationship between changes in white and grey matter and working memory performance in children from 6 to 16 years of age. Participants were tested using digit recall, backwards digit span, dot matrix tests and 'Mr. X'. In the dot matrix test, the child had to recall the location of a dot that appeared in different segments of a sequence of matrices. For 'Mr. X', the child needed to state whether, in a series of simple human figures, the character was grasping a ball in identical or different hands, and then recall the ball's position at the end of each trial (Bathelt et al. 2018). These tests were from the Automated Working Memory Assessment (AWMA), which is discussed later in this chapter (Bathelt et al. 2018, p. 4). Some of the children were then assessed using T1-weighted MRI scans and others using diffusion-weighted MRI scans. The scans were assessed using fractional anisotropy (FA), which allows assessment of white matter structure and cortical thickness mapping (Bathelt et al. 2018).

Bathelt et al. (2018) found greater involvement of the corpus callosum and posterior temporal white matter bilaterally in younger children for the executive tasks only, while there was no evidence for any differences when performing verbal or visual tasks (Bathelt et al. 2018). In older children, executive tasks were more linked to the thickness of the left occipitotemporal cortex, with greater thickness in this region being linked to poorer performance in the older age group but not the younger children (Bathelt et al. 2018). The authors conclude, overall, that the executive components of working memory are more likely to be supported by a diffuse white matter structure in younger children and that more localised activation supports executive components in older children (Bathelt et al. 2018).

Cornoldi et al. (2015) explored the impact of training in working memory and metacognition on children's ability to solve mathematical problems. Metacognition describes the beliefs children hold about doing mathematics and also beliefs about monitoring their performance (Cornoldi et al. 2015). Children aged between 8 and 10 years were divided into two groups. Group one undertook training for three months, while group two acted as a control group; then group two trained for three months while group one became the control (Cornoldi et al. 2015).

Each session consisted of a metacognitive task, such as listening to a story and learning to distinguish relevant and non-relevant information, a working memory task and maths problem solving. The researchers found statistically significant improved results for the trained groups in metacognition, working memory and maths problem solving (Cornoldi et al. 2015). They also retested group one after three months and found that these improvements were maintained (Cornoldi et al. 2015). The authors concluded that an intervention combining metacognition and working memory can support improved mathematical problem solving (Cornoldi et al. 2015).

The evidence cited suggests a link between working memory impairments and maths performance. Alloway and Alloway (2015, p. 47) state that such impairments make it harder for children to build a mental 'library of math facts' that can be readily accessed and applied to ongoing maths problem solving. This mental library could include, for example, number bonds that demonstrate which two numbers can be added or subtracted to give another number, knowledge of place value, and multiplication tables. These items are all mandatory within the national curriculum for England (Department for Education 2013).

In line with the findings of Metcalfe et al. (2013), Alloway and Alloway (2015) posit a strong role for the visuospatial sketchpad element of the multicomponent working memory model in solving mathematical problems (Alloway and Alloway 2015). The sketchpad is thought to function as a 'mental blackboard' on which children can work with the crystallised items in their long-term store of maths facts in order to support problem solving (Alloway and Alloway 2015, p. 47). However, a child with working memory impairments does not have a well-developed store of maths facts and therefore has to use working memory capacity when trying to solve basic problems. For instance, when multiplying three and six, the child may need to mentally add three sixes together, rather than rapidly accessing stored knowledge from multiplication tables or number bonds. This requires attentional resources from the central executive and any distraction may cause the child to lose their place while counting, resulting in failure (Alloway and Alloway 2015).

As noted earlier, Metcalfe et al. (2013) found a correlation with visuospatial working memory and performance on language-based maths problems. Alloway and Alloway (2015) concur with this finding. They suggest that the language component of such 'mathematical reasoning' problems adds an extra level of processing with which children with working memory impairments may struggle (Metcalfe et al. 2013, p. 164; Alloway and Alloway 2015).

The view of the visuospatial sketchpad as a 'mental blackboard' fits with one slant on the multicomponent model that divides the visual spatial sketchpad into two components. First, the 'visual cache' is a non-active storage site for visual items (Baddeley 2007, p. 91, 2012). Second, the 'inner scribe' helps maintain this store, but also rehearses and manipulates visual information (Baddeley 2007, p. 91, 2012), This concept also draws on the notion of a 'visual buffer' that is based in the occipital lobes and directs attention to different aspects of a mental image (Kosslyn et al. 2006, p. 136).

The occupational therapist should apply these theoretical insights into task analysis when supporting the child struggling with mathematics as a result of visuospatial working memory impairments. For example, the child may not have number bonds readily available in the visual cache component of the visuospatial sketchpad. In this case, pictures of items illustrating the number bonds could act as a substitute (Alloway and Alloway 2015). This would be an example of bridging between crystallised visual semantic items in the long-term store and new information being dealt with by visuospatial working memory. Similarly, the use of blocks that the child can manipulate could support mathematical operations that another child might accomplish via their inner scribe. In both these cases, working memory could be freed up for problem solving.

In many ways, the therapist's approach will be similar to that for the child with working memory impairments affecting the phonological loop. For example, when assessing the social environment, the therapist should analyse the teacher's presentation manner. It may be the case, for instance, that the working memory demands of the task could be reduced by simplifying any instructions given (Andersson 2008). Also, the presentation format should correspond to the student's working memory abilities (Andersson 2008). For example, Alloway and Alloway (2015) show that vertical rather than horizontal presentation of problems that involve remembering and carrying numbers simultaneously reduces the working memory demands of the task. In addition, simply allowing children more time by reducing the number of problems they have to work on in a given time may help (Alloway and Alloway 2015).

As shown earlier, assessment and use of assistive technology are considered core skills of occupational therapists (College of Occupational Therapists 2016). The therapist may recommend the use of an electronic calculator to support the child with visual working memory impairments. The national curriculum for England (Department for Education 2013) does not permit their use prior to the last part of Key Stage 2, although teachers are asked to judge themselves about when to introduce them. Where the occupational therapist has assessed that a source of the child's problem with maths is a working memory impairment, they should therefore discuss carefully with the teacher their rationale for using this equipment.

Attention Deficit/Hyperactivity Disorder and Working Memory Impairments

ADHD consists of impulsive and hyperactive actions, such as interrupting, not remaining seated in class, restless behaviour and reduced self-restraint, and also poor attention, leading to distraction and errors in school work (Baddeley 2007; Alloway and Alloway 2015). In particular, the child with ADHD may have difficulties with sustained attention (Alloway and Alloway 2015). ADHD is associated with lower educational outcomes, personal relationship difficulties and, in teenage years, high-risk activities (Whitfield 2012). It is estimated that one-third of adolescents with ADHD also have conduct disorder (Whitfield 2012).

Friedman et al. (2018) evaluated the role of working memory and maths calculation skills in children with ADHD. They tested a group of 36 boys diagnosed with ADHD and 33 normally developing boys; all were aged from 8 to 12 years. Tests of central executive and phonological and visuospatial short-term and working memory, applied maths problem solving and maths calculation were administered (Friedman et al. 2018). Maths calculation is the capacity to use mathematical skills and knowledge from the long-term memory store. The researchers found that maths scores were significantly lower for the ADHD group and that the combined effect of central executive and maths calculation explained 79% of the score variance (Friedman et al. 2018). The authors suggest that these children should be supported in improving maths calculation alongside targeting their central executive impairments (Friedman et al. 2018).

Alloway et al. (2009a) used the AWMA battery to test 308 children between 5 and 6 and 8 and 9 years old, all of whom had been identified as having verbal working memory impairments. The children were also assessed on general academic ability and their behaviour was assessed using a teacher-rated scale, as well as the teacher rating executive functions in relation to behaviour (Alloway et al. 2009a). In addition, self-esteem was evaluated using a teacher-rated scale (Alloway et al. 2009a).

Alloway et al. (2009a) found that, while the children had been selected only on the basis of their verbal working memory performance, they also performed poorly on tests of visuospatial working memory (Alloway et al. 2009a).

The authors defined mild impairment in working memory as scoring one standard deviation (SD) below the mean score and found that 95% of the children scored less than this on verbal working memory and 71% scored less than this on visuospatial working memory (Alloway et al. 2009a).

Analysis of the teacher-rated scales showed that the 5–6-year-old group scored 1 SD higher than the normative scores for oppositional and hyperactive segments and 2.5 SDs higher on the attentional segments of the behavioural questionnaire (Alloway et al. 2009a). The mean inattention scores for the older group were 2 SDs higher than the normative scores (Alloway et al. 2009a). It was also found that 39% of the sample had 'vulnerable' levels of self-esteem; the lowest scores for both groups were for 'personal power', which is indicative of the child's knowledge that they can affect change in the world (Alloway et al. 2009a, p. 616).

The authors state that their findings provide strong evidence that children with impaired working memory underachieve in primary school and that the inattention element of ADHD may be related to working memory deficits (Alloway et al. 2009a). Overall, they argue that their findings suggest that about 10% of children in these age bands in mainstream education may experience these difficulties (Alloway et al. 2009a).

Oppositional Defiant Disorder and Working Memory

Schoorl et al. (2018) and Schoemaker et al. (2012) include working memory as a component of executive functions. Schoorl et al. (2018) also invoke the concept of 'cool' and 'hot' executive functions: cool executive functions operate during normal conditions, while hot executive functions are present in emotionally arousing situations (Schoorl et al. 2018). Situations of 'high affective involvement', such as tests, examinations or competitions, may call for more hot executive function (Zelazo and Muller 2002, p. 455). For Schoorl et al. (2018) this is part of 'flexibly adapting to changing environments'; it also underlines the importance, for occupational therapists, of analysing the 'person-in-context' (Pentland et al. 2018, p. 3). For example, during task analysis with a child with working memory impairments, it is important to consider the specific emotional content of the task. A range of research has examined the relationship between working memory and behavioural disorders.

Schoorl et al. (2018) examined boys with oppositional defiant disorder and conduct disorder (ODD/CD). They were interested to know whether this population had concomitant executive function impairments, including working memory and sustained attention, and whether such impairments were affected by stress (Schoorl et al. 2018). Working memory was tested using spatial temporal span, whereby a sequence of squares was presented and the participants had to remember the sequence backwards. Sustained attention was tested by displaying a range of dot patterns and requiring the participants to respond with their left or right hand depending on the number of dots shown (Schoorl et al. 2018).

Two groups of boys were tested: one had ODD/CD and the other had normal development; all were aged from 8 to 12 years. Testing was done in two conditions: stressful and normal. In the stressful condition, the boys watched a faked video of another child performing computer game tasks and were told that this child was competing against them; the child in the video 'won' each game. Following this, the participant performed a series of reaction time tasks in which random delays occurred, while also receiving negative feedback from the child in the video, both intended to increase the participant's level of frustration (Schoorl et al. 2018). After exposure to these stressors, the executive function measures were taken. The participants were also assessed on executive function following performance of the tasks in normal conditions.

Schoorl et al. (2018) found that boys with ODD/CD performed worse than the controls on working memory in *both* the normal and stressful conditions. The authors suggest, therefore, that working memory is important when considering alternative courses of action in changing situations. Further, boys with ODD/CD may have difficulty with this due to working memory impairments, meaning that they could have problems adapting their behaviour in situations provoking emotional arousal (Schoorl et al. 2018).

Schoorl et al.'s (2018) findings suggest that the occupational therapist supporting a child with ODD/CD should include working memory demands as a variable during task analysis. In addition, the occupational therapist should consider the affective aspects of the task. For example, if the task is conceived of as evaluative or involving an element of judgement, the child's performance and behaviour may deteriorate.

Lin and Gau (2017) tested boys with ADHD-related disorders with an average age of 12–13. There were four groups: ADHD with CD; ADHD with ODD; ADHD alone; and a control group with typical development. They were tested using the Cambridge Neuropsychological Testing Automated Battery (CANTAB; Lin and Gau 2017). The researchers found that the ADHD group and the groups who had CD and ODD in addition to ADHD all had impaired spatial working memory and sustained attention. The children with ADHD and ADHD with ODD also had impaired verbal working memory, which was measured via backwards digit span (Lin and Gau 2017). These results point to a link between working memory and attention deficits, ADHD, CD and ODD. Again, occupational therapists working with children with these attentional and behavioural conditions should take into account the possibility that there may be concomitant working memory impairments.

Barnett et al. (2009) explored the relationship between the severity of ADHD and impaired cognition, including spatial working memory. They tested children with ADHD on its own; ADHD with ODD; ADHD with CD; and typically developing controls. All were aged between 6 and 12 (Barnett et al. 2009). They were also tested using CANTAB, which includes a test of spatial working memory (Barnett et al. 2009). In addition, parent-rated measures of children's anxiety symptoms and teacher- and parent-rated measures of behaviour were taken (Barnett et al. 2009).

Barnett et al. (2009) found that all of the children with ADHD performed significantly worse on spatial working memory than the control group. In addition, a large positive correlation was revealed for the teacher-rated measure of ADHD-type behaviours and error scores for spatial working memory for the ADHD and the ADHD with CD groups (Barnett et al. 2009). Overall, the authors suggest that in children with ADHD and ADHD with CD, impaired executive function, in which they include spatial working memory, is linked to the extent of their ADHD symptoms (Barnett et al. 2009).

Jarrett et al. (2016) evaluated working memory performance in three groups of children: a group with ADHD only; a group with ADHD and anxiety; and a group with anxiety only. The two groups with anxiety disorders included children with post-traumatic stress disorder, obsessive-compulsive disorder and generalised anxiety (Jarrett et al. 2016). Working memory was tested via a backwards digit span task. The authors found that the ADHD with anxiety group performed significantly worse than the ADHD only group. They also found that the ADHD with anxiety group did not perform differently from the anxiety group, suggesting that anxiety on its own may have an impact on working memory performance (Jarrett et al. 2016). In addition, the authors comment that working memory scores were lower than average for all three groups, indicating that this may be impaired in children with both ADHD and anxiety (Jarrett et al. 2016).

Schoemaker et al. (2012) explored the relationship between executive function and ADHD and disruptive behaviour disorder (DBD), which encompasses ODD and CD. They examined pre-school children between 3.5 and 5.5 years old with ADHD only; DBD only; ADHD with DBD; and a control group of typically developing children (Schoemaker et al. 2012). Working memory was measured using a delayed alternation task in which the children had to remember the alternating location of a treat, following a distraction task, and also via a task in which they had to remember the location of characters in a sequence of nine boxes (Schoemaker et al. 2012).

Schoemaker et al. (2012) found that, while the ADHD only, DBD only and ADHD with DBD groups all had impaired inhibition, there was no evidence of working memory deficits in any group (Schoemaker et al. 2012). The authors comment that this could be because the working memory evaluation focused more on spatial working memory, while children with DBD may be more likely to experience difficulties with verbal working memory (Schoemaker et al. 2012). They also posit that children with ADHD may not display working memory impairments until later in childhood and adolescence (Schoemaker et al. 2012).

Oosterlaan et al. (2005) tested three research hypotheses. First, is ADHD linked to executive function impairment when ODD/CD is controlled for? Second, is ODD/CD linked to executive function impairment when ADHD is controlled for? Third, is a *combination* of ADHD and ODD/CD linked to executive function impairment? Children were divided into an ADHD group; an ODD/CD group; an ADHD and ODD/CD group; and a group with typical development. The average age was 10.3 years. Working memory was tested using a series of abstract designs in which children had to point to different designs but could not indicate any more than once; the number of errors was measured as the number of times a design was pointed to more than one time (Oosterlaan et al. 2005). The authors found that only the children with ADHD alone made significantly more errors on the working memory test and made more errors as the test got progressively harder. They found no evidence that ODD/CD were linked to working memory performance (Oosterlaan et al. 2005).

The evidence presented suggests a link between working memory impairment and ADHD and also CD. As for language and mathematics, the occupational therapist should apply their knowledge of working memory theory during task analysis. When considering the social environment, the therapist could analyse the way instructions are given by the teacher. Reduced complexity may remove strain from the child's working memory system.

Alloway and Alloway (2015) suggest that a child under 8 years old with ADHD may tolerate only one- or two-step instructions, children with ADHD between 8 and 10 years old may tolerate two or three steps, while those between 11 and 13 years can handle three- or four-step instructions. The task itself may be broken down into shorter timed portions, again putting less pressure on working memory (Alloway and Alloway 2015). As for the other conditions described, the physical environment should be assessed and the student may benefit by working away from distracting noise or clutter. As previously discussed for dementia, the child with ADHD may benefit from reducing the amount of information needed to complete a task, for example by limiting the number of options available to them (Alloway and Alloway 2015).

Alloway et al. (2009b, p. 245) point out the difficulty of assessing for working memory impairments in children via 'casual observation alone'. It may be the case that occupational therapists can use everyday tasks in assessment, drawing on their knowledge of the multicomponent model. For example, a simple food preparation task could test visual–spatial working memory by requiring the child to remember the location of kitchen items needed for a task such as making a cake. The phonological loop aspect might be tested by the child needing to remember spoken or written instructions with several steps, given to them at the start of the session. The child's distractibility and ability to stay on task could be used as an evaluation of central executive function. There are also standardised assessments available for assessing working memory in children and two of these are discussed next.

AWMA is based on the different segments of the multicomponent working memory model (Alloway et al. 2008). Working memory is evaluated in each area with tasks that involve simultaneous processing and caching of memory items (Alloway et al. 2008). For example, in one subtest the examiner reads a number of sentences and the child needs to state whether they are true or false and, at the end, recall the last word of each sentence in the correct order (Alloway et al. 2008). For visual–spatial working memory, a series of pairs of shapes is displayed, the right one of which contains a red dot. The child needs to indicate whether the right shape is the same as the left shape and at the end of the test state the location of the red dots, again in the correct sequence (Alloway et al. 2008). AWMA has been found to have 'good diagnostic validity', suggesting that it can detect working memory impairments in the classroom (Alloway et al. 2008, p. 732). It has also been found to be reliable (Alloway et al. 2008).

The Working Memory Rating Scale (WMRS) contains a list of behaviours considered representative of children with working memory impairments (Alloway et al. 2009b) and is designed to allow teachers to recognise such children (Alloway et al. 2009b). It has been found to have good construct validity and internal reliability (Alloway et al. 2009b). In addition, testing shows that teachers can successfully use WMRS to identify children with working memory difficulties (Alloway et al. 2009b).

Memory and Stressful Life Events in Children and Adolescents

Occupational therapists working within a cognitive behavioural frame of reference are interested in the ways in which cognition affects behaviour. The foci include the person's 'automatic thoughts', which they have little control over, 'beliefs' the person has about themselves and 'core schemas', which are deep, relatively unchanging, convictions developed in early life about themselves (Duncan 2011, pp. 156–157). While Duncan (2011) cautions against the casual use of cognitive behavioural approaches in occupational therapy, an understanding of the ways in which memory and mental health interact is useful.

The psychodynamic frame of reference in occupational therapy has its roots in Freud's psychoanalytic approach (Daniel and Blair 2011). Freud was concerned with the dynamic relationship between the 'ego', the mental structure that mediates between sensory and perceptual input and motor outputs, and the 'id', a realm of primordial sexual desires and memories that are repressed in early childhood (Freud 1991, p. 17). Although many of Freud's positions have been modified or rejected, the psychodynamic approach continues to stress the ways in which memories of childhood trauma can shape current behaviour (Daniel and Blair 2011). Daniel and Blair (2011) suggest that the occupational therapy profession may have its origins in an early twentieth-century attempt to integrate psychoanalysis with contemporary neuroscientific thinking. Psychodynamic occupational therapy may use activities in groups, or with individuals, exploring the ways in which unacknowledged motivations may lead to 'occupational imbalance' (Daniel and Blair 2011, p. 172; Hagedorn 1992).

Both the cognitive behavioural and psychodynamic frames of reference touch on the ways in which unacknowledged or repressed memories might influence current behaviour. It is therefore useful for the occupational therapist working with children and young people within these frames of reference to understand the ways in which trauma, anxiety and depression may affect memory. This section examines this in relation to OAM, which occurs when individuals have problems remembering specific detailed events from their own past (Warne et al. 2019). OAM is linked to MDD, as people with this condition have difficulty recalling detailed personal memories (Warne et al. 2019).

Warne et al. (2019) examined whether exposure to stressful live events in the recent past or over a lifetime led to the development of OAM in children and adolescents. They tested youngsters between 9 and 17 years of age from families with a high risk of depression (Warne et al. 2019). Stressful live events and autobiographical memories were measured in the group. Autobiographical memory was evaluated using the Autobiographical Memory Test, in which participants were asked to recall a memory after hearing six positive emotion cue words and six negative ones (Warne et al. 2019).

Memories were categorised in four ways: specific memories related to particular events; extended memories related to events that happened over more than a day; categoric memories referred to events that took place repeatedly; and 'semantic associates', which referred to responses that were related to a cue word but were not memories (Warne et al. 2019, p. 317). Working memory was assessed using the Wechsler Intelligence Scale for Children (WISC). In addition, 'economic disadvantage' was defined as a family having a median annual income at or below £20 000 (Warne et al. 2019, p. 317).

Warne et al. (2019) found that lifetime exposure to stressful life events was linked to higher numbers of particular autobiographical memories. In addition, it was found that for girls, recent experience of stressful life events was linked to higher numbers of OAMs, while in boys the opposite pattern was found: recent experience of stressful life events was associated with more particular autobiographical memories (Warne et al. 2019). The researchers also found that long-term exposure to stressful life events was linked to lower working memory scores and higher levels of economic disadvantage (Warne et al. 2019). The authors point out that their findings complicate the assumption that OAM is linked to MDD, stating that in their study this effect was related to sex and also how recent the stressful life events were (Warne et al. 2019).

CaR-FA-X

The CaR-FA-X model is an attempt to explain the mechanisms that may result in a predominance of OAM (Gutenbrunner et al. 2019). CaR stands for 'capture and rumination', FA for 'functional avoidance' and X for 'executive control' (Gutenbrunner et al. 2019, p. 759). The model predicts that rumination on negative thoughts, avoidance of negative memories and impaired executive functioning affect memory retrieval in conditions such as anxiety and depression (Gutenbrunner et al. 2019).

The CaR-FA-X model is predicated on the self-memory system model. This was developed by Conway and Pleydell-Pearce (2000, p. 265), who suggested that the 'working self' was constructed from schemas that delineated the possible selves one might become and that the self-memory system involved ensuring that goals generated in this way are compatible with one's autobiographical knowledge. If they were incompatible, this might indicate the presence of a pathological state (Conway and Pleydell-Pearce 2000). The 'working self' was viewed as a control process within the multicomponent working memory model that imposed limits on cognition and action, thereby facilitating efficient function in the world (Conway and Pleydell-Pearce 2000).

Conway and Pleydell-Pearce (2000, p. 264) further proposed that the base of autobiographical knowledge is composed of a hierarchical organisation of 'lifetime period', 'specific events' and 'event-specific' knowledge. Information held at higher levels of the hierarchy can be used as cues that facilitate finding items further down the hierarchy (Conway and Pleydell-Pearce 2000). Overall, this means that when seeking for memories we start at a general level and then work down the hierarchy until we identify specific items (Gutenbrunner et al. 2019, p. 760).

The CaR-FA-X model predicts that 'capture and rumination' will have an impact on the search for memories, as a person may start to ruminate on distracting negative thoughts and terminate the search while still at the more general level (Williams et al. 2007 p. 134). 'Functional avoidance' may also involve terminating the search at the general level in order to avoid negative memories (Williams et al. 2007, p. 134). Meanwhile, 'impaired executive control' indicates that there may be limited inhibition of irrelevant thoughts when searching, resulting in the search being concluded prematurely at the general level (Gutenbrunner et al. 2019; Williams et al. 2007, p. 134). Overall, the effect will be to increase the prevalence of OAM, which may initially be adaptive as a protection against negative feelings, but can eventually prevent retrieval of the specific memories needed to support efficient cognitive function (Gutenbrunner et al. 2019).

Gutenbrunner et al. (2019) tested 323 adolescents annually over four years. They were assessed at each point for depression and on each of the three CaR-FA-X components. Depression was measured with a self-reported scale, and autobiographical memory and memory valence were measured by providing a list of words linked to positive or negative emotions, such as 'happy' or 'angry', and asking the participant to write down a personal memory for each (Gutenbrunner et al. 2019). The authors identified two main subgroups in the sample: a group with lower but rising levels of depression; and a group with 'medium–higher' levels (Gutenbrunner et al. 2019, p. 766).

Gutenbrunner et al. (2019) found that raised avoidance at the third assessment point predicted higher levels of OAM at the fourth point for the medium–higher group, but not for the lower group (Gutenbrunner et al. 2019). They also found that raised avoidance in the medium–higher group predicted more OAMs generated in response to negative emotion words, but that this pattern did not hold in the lower group (Gutenbrunner et al. 2019). Across the whole sample, they found that increased raised avoidance at the third test point predicted increased OAMs at the fourth test, but this was only the case for memories generated in response to the positive words (Gutenbrunner et al. 2019). Overall, the authors argue that their results provide qualified support for the CaR-FA-X model in that the model's predictions were only confirmed for adolescents with medium to high levels of depression (Gutenbrunner et al. 2019).

Fisk et al. (2019) tested the CaR-FA-X model in two groups of adolescents aged 12–17, divided into a depressed and a non-depressed group. They examined the number of autobiographical memories retrieved in response to 10 cue words with positive and negative emotional valence. Functional avoidance was measured by asking participants to recall specific negative aspects of autobiographical memories, with failure taken as an index of avoidance (Fisk et al. 2019). Executive function was measured via a word association task that assessed verbal fluency and a sentence completion task (Fisk et al. 2019). Working memory, which the authors included within executive function, was assessed via a test in which participants had to view a series of words related to six categories and then recall the final word from each category (Fisk et al. 2019).

Fisk et al. (2019) found that participants with depression retrieved a significantly higher number of OAMs and underwent significantly more rumination (Fisk et al. 2019). They also revealed that verbal fluency and working memory were significantly poorer in the depressed group (Fisk et al. 2019). They did not find evidence of raised functional avoidance in the depressed group, which again suggests qualified corroboration for the CaR-FA-X model (Fisk et al. 2019).

Rawal and Rice (2012) conducted a longitudinal study investigating the connection between rumination and executive function and the specificity of autobiographical memory in adolescents at heightened risk from depression. A sample of 10–18-year-olds with depressed parents completed the Autobiographical Memory Test as a baseline and the test was repeated after one year. In addition, rumination and executive function were measured at baseline (Rawal and Rice 2012).

First, the researchers found that age predicted the specificity of autobiographical memory in girls but not boys. Second, they found that, whereas rumination and low executive function predicted low specificity, rumination and high executive function predicted high specificity (Rawal and Rice 2012). The authors suggest that rumination may impair access to autobiographical memory only in the context of low executive function and that, therefore, training focused on improving executive function might help overcome the negative impact of rumination on autobiographical memory (Rawal and Rice 2012).

Hitchcock et al. (2014) conducted a review of literature on OAM in children. They were interested to find out if children experience OAM, how OAM relates to trauma and associated psychopathology, and also to test the assumptions of the CaR-FA-X model (Hitchcock et al. 2014). They found that there was a relationship between OAM and depression and exposure to trauma, although the effect size for both was moderate (Hitchcock et al. 2014). Also, they noted that OAM may be linked to the maintenance of and relapse into depression during adolescence (Hitchcock et al. 2014). They state that their findings give some support to the CaR-FA-X model.

Crane et al. (2016) tested a hypothesis that OAM is a causative factor in depression. They screened over 50 13-year-olds for OAM and then screened them at 16 for a number of life events and mental health outcomes, including thinking about and planning suicide, self-harm and depression. At 13, the participants completed a questionnaire focused on autobiographical memory and at 16, they responded to questions about life events and the identified mental health outcomes (Crane et al. 2016). These authors found no link between levels of OAM at 13 and levels of suicidal thoughts, depression or self-harm at 16 (Crane et al. 2016). They actually identified that OAM may provide some protection, in that there was a 20% increase in planning of suicide for each SD increase in memory specificity (Crane et al. 2016). They suggest that this latter finding may provide evidence that OAM is linked to an impaired ability to formulate goals and plans and that this may have some protective effect (Crane et al. 2016). The authors concluded that OAM is not a predictive factor for later depression in a non-clinical sample from the community (Crane et al. 2016).

One small-scale brain imaging study suggests that MDD can affect cerebral areas linked to memory. Caetano et al. (2007) took MRI scans of the hippocampus and amygdala in 19 children and adolescents with MDD and compared these with 24 individuals without MDD matched for age. All participants were between 8 and 17 years old. The researchers found that the grey matter volume of the left hippocampus was significantly smaller by 5% in the MDD group (Caetano et al. 2007). They did not find any significant differences for the other brain regions compared. The authors suggest that this difference may be connected to increased blood cortisol levels in people with MDD, which may have a neurotoxic effect and lead to destruction of grey matter (Caetano et al. 2007).

Conclusion

Researchers have provided evidence that the multicomponent working memory model predicts performance on English and mathematics in the classroom. In addition, impairments in these areas may underpin conditions that affect reading and writing, such as dyslexia, and those affecting mathematics, such as dyscalculia.

Regarding reading and writing, these findings make sense when one considers that the main approach used to teach these skills in the United Kingdom is underpinned by synthetic phonics. This is based on the sound of the letters and letter combinations. Children with specific impairments affecting the phonological loop may be disadvantaged here.

Evidence also shows that mathematical skills may be underpinned by working memory, particularly the visuospatial sketchpad of the multicomponent model. This may occur because an understanding of place value, for example, depends on grasping the significance of the spatial location of digits in an array of numbers.

As in other chapters, it was argued that occupational therapists should draw on their core skills when approaching these problems. Task analysis of the child in the classroom should take into account the environment. This may be social, for example the style of presentation of the teacher. It may also be the physical environment, for instance the number of distractions in the child's working area. In addition, the nature of the task should be analysed. Techniques such as bridging or chunking items into meaningful units might help.

Conditions affecting behaviour and attention may also involve working memory impairments. Again, this may be incorporated into task analysis. For example, the occupational therapist may consider the emotional content of some classroom tasks and suggest adjusting this, where possible.

The chapter closed with discussion of theories that may be useful for occupational therapists working with children and adolescents with mental health problems. The CaR-FA-X model, for example, offers an explanatory framework that accounts for the ways in which traumatic life experience may affect autobiographical memory retrieval in this population.

Activities

Case Study Vignette 1

Paul is an 8-year-old boy who is in year three of primary school. He struggles to get things down in writing and is frequently 'off task' in class. He sits at the back of the class, next to some brightly coloured wall displays. In addition, the drawers that contain individual students' work and other items are near his table, meaning that children are coming and going to that area throughout the day.

Paul's class is doing a history project on the Tudor period. His teacher has instructed the class to write three paragraphs about Elizabeth I. The teacher is concerned that Paul has so far not written anything.

Katie, Paul's occupational therapist, conducts task analysis of one class teaching session. Katie notices that the teacher presents some words associated with the project on the carpet in the class, holding up handwritten flashcards with the words on. The previous day, however, the teacher had presented these words on the white board, standing at the front of the class.

1. How could Katie apply the multicomponent model of working memory in this case?
2. What changes could be made to Paul's physical environment?
3. How could Katie advise the teacher to adjust his presentation style?

Case Study Vignette 2

Amara is 10 years old. Her teacher reports that she is very distractible and has moved her to the front of the class where she can 'keep an eye on her'. Amara's occupational therapist, Carlos, observes a class teaching session. The teacher instructs the class to 'go to your drawers and get out your pencils. Then, get your maths workbooks. Take your book back to your table and start working from where you finished last week.'

Amara goes to her drawer. There are a lot of other children moving in the same direction. The occupational therapist notices that Amara opens her drawer and looks in it. Then she comes back to her table having left her pencils and workbook in the drawer. When the teacher asks her if she knows what she is supposed to be doing, she answers that she does not. The teacher becomes annoyed with her and Amara appears upset.

1. What changes could Carlos make regarding the teacher's approach to presenting instructions?
2. How could Carlos apply the multicomponent model of working memory in this case?

References

Allen, K., Giofrè, D., Higgins, S., and Adams, J. (2020). Working memory predictors of mathematics across the middle primary school years. *British Journal of Educational Psychology* 90 (3): 848–869.

Alloway, T.P. and Alloway, R.G. (2015). *Understanding Working Memory*, 2e. London: Sage.

Alloway, T.P., Gathercole, S.E., Kirkwood, H., and Elliott, J. (2008). Evaluating the validity of the Automated Working Memory Assessment. *Educational Psychology* 28 (7): 725–734.

Alloway, T.P., Gathercole, S.E., Kirkwood, H., and Elliott, J. (2009a). The cognitive and behavioral characteristics of children with low working memory. *Child Development* 80 (2): 606–621.

Alloway, T.P., Gathercole, S.E., Kirkwood, H., and Elliott, J. (2009b). The working memory rating scale: a classroom-based behavioral assessment of working memory. *Learning and Individual Differences* 19 (2): 242–245.

Andersson, U. (2008). Working memory as a predictor of written arithmetical skills in children: the importance of central executive functions. *British Journal of Educational Psychology* 78 (2): 181–203.

Archibald, L.M.D. and Gathercole, S.E. (2006). Visuospatial immediate memory in specific language impairment. *Journal of Speech, Language, and Hearing Research* 49 (2): 265–277.

Attout, L. and Majerus, S. (2015). Working memory deficits in developmental dyscalculia: the importance of serial order. *Child Neuropsychology* 21 (4): 432–450.

Baddeley, A. (2000). The episodic buffer: a new component of working memory? *Trends in Cognitive Sciences* 4 (11): 417–423.

Baddeley, A. (2003). Working memory: looking back and looking forward. *Nature Reviews Neuroscience* 4 (10): 829–839.

Baddeley, A.D. (2007). *Working Memory, Thought, and Action*. Oxford: Oxford University Press.

Baddeley, A. (2012). Working memory: theories, models, and controversies. *Annual Review of Psychology* 63 (1): 1–29.

Baddeley, A. (2015). Working memory. In: *Memory* (ed. A. Baddeley, M.W. Eysenck, and M.C. Anderson), 67–105. London: Psychology Press.

Baddeley, A.D., Hitch, G.J., and Allen, R.J. (2009). Working memory and binding in sentence recall. *Journal of Memory and Language* 61 (3): 438–456.

Barnett, R., Maruff, P., and Vance, A. (2009). Neurocognitive function in attention-deficit-hyperactivity disorder with and without comorbid disruptive behaviour disorders. *Australasian Psychiatry: Bulletin of the Royal Australian and New Zealand College of Psychiatrists* 43 (8): 722–730.

Bartlett, F.C. (1995). *Remembering: A Study in Experimental and Social Psychology*. Cambridge: Cambridge University Press.

Bathelt, J., Gathercole, S.E., Johnson, A., and Astle, D.E. (2018). Differences in brain morphology and working memory capacity across childhood. *Developmental Science* 21 (3): e12579.

Caetano, S.C., Fonseca, M., Hatch, J.P. et al. (2007). Medial temporal lobe abnormalities in pediatric unipolar depression. *Neuroscience Letters* 427 (3): 142–147.

College of Occupational Therapists (2016). *Entry Level Occupational Therapy Core Knowledge and Practice Skills*. London: College of Occupational Therapists.

Conway, M.A. and Pleydell-Pearce, C.W. (2000). The construction of autobiographical memories in the self-memory system. *Psychological Review* 107 (2): 261–288.

Cornoldi, C., Carretti, B., Drusi, S., and Tencati, C. (2015). Improving problem solving in primary school students: the effect of a training programme focusing on metacognition and working memory. *British Journal of Educational Psychology* 85 (3): 424–439.

Craik, F.I. and Lockhart, R.S. (1972). Levels of processing: a framework for memory research. *Journal of Verbal Learning and Verbal Behavior* 11 (6): 671–684.

Craik, F.I. and Tulving, E. (1975). Depth of processing and the retention of words in episodic memory. *Journal of Experimental Psychology. General* 104 (3): 268–294.

Crane, C., Heron, J., Gunnell, D. et al. (2016). Adolescent over-general memory, life events and mental health outcomes: findings from a UK cohort study. *Memory* 24 (3): 348–363.

Daniel, M.A. and Blair, S.E.E. (2011). An introduction to the psychodynamic frame of reference. In: *Foundations for Practice in Occupational Therapy* (ed. E.A.S. Duncan), 165–178. London: Churchill Livingstone.

Department for Education (2013). *Mathematics Programmes of Study: Key Stages 1 and 2 National Curriculum in England*. London: Department for Education.

Donaldson, J. and Scheffler, A. (2014). *The Gruffalo*. London: Macmillan Children's Books.

Duncan, E.A.S. (2011). The cognitive-behavioural frame of reference. In: *Foundations for Practice in Occupational Therapy* (ed. E.A.S. Duncan), 153–163. London: Churchill Livingstone.

Fisk, J., Ellis, J.A., and Reynolds, S.A. (2019). A test of the CaR-FA-X mechanisms and depression in adolescents. *Memory* 27 (4): 455–464.

Freud, S. (1991). *The Essentials of Psycho-Analysis: The Definitive Collection of Sigmund Freud's Writing*. Harmondsworth: Penguin.

Friedman, L.M., Rapport, M.D., Orban, S.A. et al. (2018). Applied problem solving in children with ADHD: the mediating roles of working memory and mathematical calculation. *Journal of Abnormal Child Psychology* 46 (3): 491–504.

Gathercole, S.E. and Baddeley, A.D. (1989). Evaluation of the role of phonological STM in the development of vocabulary in children: a longitudinal study. *Journal of Memory and Language* 28 (2): 200–213.

Gathercole, S.E. and Baddeley, A.D. (1990). Phonological memory deficits in language disordered children: is there a causal connection? *Journal of Memory and Language* 29 (3): 336–360.

Gathercole, S.E. and Hitch, G.J. (1993). Developmental changes in short-term memory: a revised working memory perspective. In: *Theories of Memory* (ed. A. Collins, S.E. Gathercole, M.A. Conway, and P.E. Morris), 189–210. Hove: Erlbaum.

Gathercole, S.E. and Pickering, S.J. (2000). Working memory deficits in children with low achievements in the national curriculum at 7 years of age. *British Journal of Educational Psychology* 70: 177.

Gathercole, S. and Pickering, S. (2001). Working memory deficits in children with special educational needs. *British Journal of Special Education* 28 (2): 89–97.

Gathercole, S.E., Pickering, S.J., Ambridge, B., and Wearing, H. (2004). The structure of working memory from 4 to 15 years of age. *Developmental Psychology* 40 (2): 177.

Gutenbrunner, C., Salmon, K., and Jose, P.E. (2019). What predicts overgeneral memory in youth? Testing the CaR-FA-X model longitudinally in community adolescents. *Development and Psychopathology* 31 (2): 759–770.

Hagedorn, R. (1992). *Occupational Therapy: Foundations for Practice: Models, Frames of Reference and Core Skills*. Edinburgh: Churchill Livingstone.

Hitchcock, C., Nixon, R.D.V., and Weber, N. (2014). A review of overgeneral memory in child psychopathology. *British Journal of Clinical Psychology* 53 (2): 170–193.

Hogben, L.T., Horrabin, J.F., and Palmer, R. (1938). *Science for the Citizen: A Self-Educator Based on the Social Background of Scientific Discovery*. London: Allen & Unwin.

Howe, M.C. and Briggs, A.K. (1982). Ecological systems model for occupational therapy. *American Journal of Occupational Therapy* 36 (5): 322–327.

Jarrett, M.A., Wolff, J.C., Davis, T.E. 3rd et al. (2016). Characteristics of children with ADHD and comorbid anxiety. *Journal of Attention Disorders* 20 (7): 636–644.

Kielhofner, G. (1995). *A Model of Human Occupation: Theory and Application*, 2e. Baltimore, MD: Williams & Wilkins.

Kosslyn, S.M., Thompson, W.L., and Ganis, G. (2006). *The Case for Mental Imagery*. New York: Oxford University Press.

Law, M., Cooper, B., Strong, S. et al. (1996). The person-environment-occupation model: a transactive approach to occupational performance. *Canadian Journal of Occupational Therapy* 63 (1): 9–23.

Lin, Y.-J. and Gau, S.S.-F. (2017). Differential neuropsychological functioning between adolescents with attention-deficit/hyperactivity disorder with and without conduct disorder. *Journal of the Formosan Medical Association* 116 (12): 946–955.

Luria, A.R. (1973). *The Working Brain: An Introduction to Neuropsychology*. New York: Basic Books.

Metcalfe, A.W., Ashkenazi, S., Rosenberg-Lee, M., and Menon, V. (2013). Fractionating the neural correlates of individual working memory components underlying arithmetic problem solving skills in young children. *Developments in Cognitive Neuroscience* 6: 162–175.

Miller, G.A. (1956). The magical number seven, plus or minus two: some limits on our capacity for processing information. *Psychological Review* 63 (2): 81.

Oosterlaan, J., Scheres, A., and Sergeant, J.A. (2005). Which executive functioning deficits are associated with AD/HD, ODD/CD and comorbid AD/HD+ODD/CD? *Journal of Abnormal Child Psychology* 33 (1): 69–85.

Pentland, D., Kantartzis, S., Clausen, M.G., and Witemyre, K. (2018). *Occupational Therapy and Complexity: Defining and Describing Practice*. London: Royal College of Occupational Therapists.

Rawal, A. and Rice, F. (2012). A longitudinal study of processes predicting the specificity of autobiographical memory in the adolescent offspring of depressed parents. *Memory* 20 (5): 518–526.

Schoemaker, K., Bunte, T., Wiebe, S.A. et al. (2012). Executive function deficits in preschool children with ADHD and DBD. *Journal of Child Psychology and Psychiatry* 53 (2): 111–119.

Schoorl, J., van Rijn, S., de Wied, M. et al. (2018). Boys with oppositional defiant disorder/conduct disorder show impaired adaptation during stress: an executive functioning study. *Child Psychiatry and Human Development* 49 (2): 298–307.

Wallace, S. (2015). *A Dictionary of Education*, 2e. Oxford: Oxford University Press.

Warne, N., Collishaw, S., and Rice, F. (2019). Examining the relationship between stressful life events and overgeneral autobiographical memory in adolescents at high familial risk of depression. *Memory* 27 (3): 314–327.

Whitfield, S. (2012). Treatment and rehabilitation of paediatric/developmental neuropsychological disorders. In: *The Handbook of Clinical Psychology* (ed. J.M. Gurd, U. Kischka, and J.C. Marshall), 471–487. Oxford: Oxford University Press.

Williams, J.M.G., Barnhofer, T., Crane, C. et al. (2007). Autobiographical memory specificity and emotional disorder. *Psychological Bulletin* 133 (1): 122–148.

Zelazo, P.D. and Muller, U. (2002). Executive function in typical and atypical development. In: *Blackwell Handbook of Childhood Cognitive Development* (ed. U. Goswami), 445–469. Oxford: Blackwell Publishing.

6 Occupational Therapy Action Planning and Treatment Implementation for Adults with Memory Impairment Following Acquired Brain Injury

Traumatic brain injury (TBI) often affects the frontal and temporal regions of the brain. This chapter presents evidence that people with TBI may experience executive function problems and working memory difficulties. It is shown that these can lead to problems with long-term memory.

Working memory impairments, and impaired central executive functioning in particular, may have impacts on social functioning for people with TBI. In addition, research is cited showing the impact of environmental factors on executive function in people with TBI.

Acquired brain injury (ABI) encompasses TBI as well as stroke and other conditions. A number of conditions affecting quality of life (QOL) in ABI are outlined, including social inclusion and relationships with others.

Working and prospective memory impairments in brain injury can affect activities of daily living, such as financial management and communication. Working memory difficulties have also been linked to problems with driving abilities and independent living.

The length of time in post-traumatic amnesia (PTA) is a predictor of subsequent levels of occupational performance. For example, people who have been longer in PTA are less likely to transition to independent living after leaving hospital.

The close relationship between working memory impairments, especially in the central executive, and goal attainment is discussed. Approaches for incorporating goal attainment into rehabilitation and therapy include Goal Management Training™ (GMT). The Perceive, Recall, Plan, Perform (PRPP) approach has been developed by occupational therapists as a structured way to analyse task performance and facilitate rehabilitation of people with TBI.

The concept of errorless learning is discussed. This is described in a historical context; however, the approach is shown to have limited applicability to real-world situations. In addition, evidence is presented from situated learning theory and communities of practice concepts showing that techniques such as errorless learning do not pay sufficient attention to the affective aspects of learning.

Evidence is shown that, while declarative memory may be impaired in closed head injury, procedural memory might still be intact. In addition, for adolescents with closed head injury, it is shown that verbal working memory and executive functions are related.

There are two approaches to cognitive rehabilitation: restorative and remedial or compensatory. It is noted that some evidence regarding cognitive rehabilitation in TBI is inconclusive. Indeed, one study shows slightly better results for the control group who did not receive cognitive rehabilitation.

The compensatory approach to cognitive rehabilitation may include the use of assistive technology and three examples of the use of such technology are discussed. It is shown that, if such technology is to be used, it should be tailored carefully to the person's needs.

The method of loci is explained. It is shown that this standard memory training approach has an ancient history. Interestingly, both poets and brain-injured individuals have used imagery linking memory and spatial location when describing memory enrichment and impairments. It shown in this chapter that, if the method of loci is to be used in the rehabilitation of memory in the person with brain injury, extensive training may be required.

There is a lack of evidence regarding the impact of cognitive rehabilitation approaches on return to work, QOL, community integration and performance of activities of daily living in adults with cognitive impairments following TBI.

Traumatic Brain Injury and Acquired Brain Injury

TBI is typically marked by damage to the frontal and temporal regions as well as diffuse axonal injury (Fish et al. 2008). Traumatic axonal injury involves damage at a microscopic level to blood vessels and axons and most frequently affects fronto-temporal and subcortical regions (Finnanger et al. 2015). TBI can cause impairments in memory, attention and executive function. There are a number of differences with stroke, which has a more varied presentation and where the cognitive impairments are dependent on the lesion site (Fish et al. 2008). Furthermore, the age profiles vary: the typical age range for TBI is 15–24, while stroke normally affects those over 65 years of age (Fish et al. 2008).

Finnanger et al. (2015) investigated the self-reported problems experienced by people in the late and chronic periods of moderate and severe TBI. They analysed the impact of variables such as age and educational levels, and also the scope of injury, for example duration of PTA and Glasgow Coma Scale (GCS) levels, or presence of traumatic axonal injury.

The 65 participants in Finnanger et al.'s (2015) study had moderate to severe TBI, were aged between 15 and 65 at the point of their injury and were between two and five years post injury. In addition, there were 75 aged-matched controls who did not have TBI (Finnanger et al. 2015). The participants had to complete a self-report questionnaire on executive function, the Behavior Rating Inventory of Executive Function®–Adult Version (BRIEF®-A). BRIEF-A uses responses on inhibition, shifting, emotional control and self-monitoring to produce a 'behaviour regulation index'. Meanwhile, responses to questions on initiation, working memory, planning and organising, task monitoring and organising materials generate a 'metacognitive index' (Finnanger et al. 2015, p. 4). In this study 49 participants also formed a subgroup who were assessed using neuro-psychological tests three months after injury (Finnanger et al. 2015).

Finnanger et al. (2015) found that the TBI group had significantly more problems with attention, emotional control, anxiety and depression, thought problems and aggressive behaviour (Finnanger et al. 2015). In addition, it was noted that fewer years in education and the presence of depression predicted higher executive dysfunction, while younger age when injured predicted higher levels of aggression and rule-breaking behaviour, which could include substance misuse, lack of empathy and breaking the law (Finnanger et al. 2015).

The subgroup that was tested at three months after injury showed significantly higher levels of memory impairment, reduced speed of processing and impaired executive function (Finnanger et al. 2015). In addition, participants self-reported significantly higher problems with working memory and the authors report that 37% of these problems were within clinical scope (Finnanger et al. 2015). They also found that the presence of traumatic axonal injury was linked to anxiety, depression and difficulties regulating behaviour (Finnanger et al. 2015). These findings highlight the impact on occupational performance in TBI of working memory impairments, and altered executive function generally; environmental influences, such as level of education; and person factors such as age.

The close interaction of working memory and executive function is demonstrated by the fact that working memory deficits may manifest as impairments in planning and attention, and can lead to difficulty following instructions and leaving tasks incomplete (Björkdahl et al. 2013). In addition, Björkdahl et al. (2013) comment that items first need to enter working memory prior to long-term storage, and so working memory impairments may have impacts on long-term memory (Björkdahl et al. 2013). As a result, people with TBI may show difficulties in these areas.

Kersey et al. (2019) wished to identify factors predicting community integration following TBI. They point out that community integration encompasses instrumental activities of daily living (IADL), such as shopping and participation in leisure and social activities. They conducted a scoping review that included 53 research articles (Kersey et al. 2019) and found four categories of predictive factors: demographic; characteristics of the injury; impairments and disability; and environment. Among the characteristics of injury, length of PTA was the factor supported by the strongest evidence as having a relationship with community integration. Among demographic characteristics, race was found to have the strongest relationship with community integration, with white people having better community integration that non-white people (Kersey et al. 2019).

Verdugo et al. (2019) explain that ABI may result from stroke, TBI, anoxia, tumours or infection. ABI is the main cause of death and disability internationally (Verdugo et al. 2019). The authors analysed variables affecting QOL in 421 adults with ABI in Spain (Verdugo et al. 2019). They used an assessment tool based on several domains of QOL: physical, material and emotional well-being; relationships with others; inclusion in society; self-determination; and self-development (Verdugo et al. 2019). The authors found that statistically significant factors for predicting QOL were losing legal capacity; the amount of time since injury, so that a longer time was associated with worse QOL; prior employment; site of injury, meaning that bilateral injuries were linked to lower QOL; and the person's level of dependence (Verdugo et al. 2019).

Clark et al. (2020) evaluated the relationship between cognitive impairments and limitations in everyday function in military veterans with mild to moderate head injuries. In this study, 50 veterans completed the University of California San Diego Performance-Based Skills Assessment–Brief (UPSA-B), which focuses on financial and communication skills, such as writing cheques or changing appointments via telephone (Clark et al. 2020). Participants were also tested on components of neuropsychological function, including working memory and attention, prospective memory and executive function (Clark et al. 2020). Statistically significant negative correlations were discovered between global neuropsychological status and overall functional capability and communication skills. The authors comment that interventions that target cognitive functions, and executive functions in particular including attention and working memory, may help improve the ability of those with mild to moderate head injuries to manage life skills independently (Clark et al. 2020).

Anderson and Knight (2010) conducted research on the impact of dysfunction in the central executive component of the multicomponent working memory model in people with TBI. They were especially interested in the role of the central executive in coordinating memory and attention processes (Anderson and Knight 2010). In their study, 45 people with TBI were compared with 21 non-impaired controls performing a dual task consisting of digit span recollection and tracing a spiral shape. This task was taken as a measure of the 'coordinative function' of the central executive (Anderson and Knight 2010, p. 1075). Participants performed these tasks separately at first and then in combination, and the difference in performance provided a 'change index' (Anderson and Knight 2010, p. 1074).

Significantly worse performance on the dual task was noted only for the proportion of the TBI group who had the most severe TBI-related symptoms following the initial injury (Anderson and Knight 2010). A significant correlation was found between self-reported social competence, covering areas such as initiating conversation, dealing with arguments and seeking help, and dual task performance for the TBI group (Anderson and Knight 2010). These findings suggest that impairments in working memory, and the central executive in particular, are detrimental to occupational performance in the social environment for people with TBI.

Donders et al. (2015) provide a useful overview of executive functions as those that organise and coordinate goal-directed behaviour. Executive functions include direction of attention, working memory, inhibition control, mental flexibility and ability to adapt, planning and organising skills, and application and assessment of problem-solving approaches. The authors point out that executive function is based on a network that encompasses the pre-frontal cortex, cerebellum, basal nuclei and thalamus (Donders et al. 2015). They used BRIEF-A to investigate the correlation of self- and informant-reported estimates of executive function following mild traumatic brain injury (mTBI).

Donders et al. (2015) asked people with mTBI and their informants, who included spouses and parents, to complete BRIEF-A. The patients also completed neuropsychological tests of executive function. First, it was found that patients rated themselves significantly worse than the informants on BRIEF-A. Second, the authors found that higher educational levels and the presence of intracranial lesions on imaging were linked to higher self-rated BRIEF-A behavioural scores, while worse self-rated BRIEF-A behavioural scores were associated with longer time since injury and having a previous psychiatric history (Donders et al. 2015). Third, higher levels of education and evidence of intracranial damage were associated with better BRIEF-A self-rated meta-cognition scores, while worse scores in this category were linked to having a previous psychiatric history and longer time since injury (Donders et al. 2015).

The variable most associated with lower BRIEF-A self- and informant-related performance was previous psychiatric history (Donders et al. 2015). There was no association between findings on the executive function tests and BRIEF-A scores (Donders et al. 2015). The authors conclude that the patients' self-assessment of executive performance following mTBI was mainly a function of factors prior to injury, in this case previous psychiatric referral and educational history, and not of the impairments following from brain injury (Donders et al. 2015). These results underline the impact of environmental factors, such as educational levels, on people with mTBI.

Bottari et al. (2017) examined the correlation between functional magnetic resonance imaging (fMRI) findings, event-related potentials and independence in activities of daily living in three people with mTBI and 12 controls without impairment. Participants performed a working memory task alongside fMRI of the right and left dorsolateral pre-frontal cortex (DLPFC), while event-related potentials were recorded at the same time (Bottari et al. 2017). Another test, the IADL Profile, assessed the participants' ability to obtain information and make a budget (Bottari et al. 2017). It was found that people with mTBI had impaired working memory and delayed completion of budgeting tasks, and that problems with budgeting were linked to decreased activation in the right DLPFC (Bottari et al. 2017).

Sandhaug et al. (2015) examined the levels of community integration in people with moderate and severe TBI two years after the event. They used the Community Integration Questionnaire (CIQ), which assesses areas of home life, including shopping, meal preparation and childcare; productivity, including work, education and transport; and social aspects, which includes seeing friends and leisure activities (Sandhaug et al. 2015). They found that, for the moderate and severe groups, there was a significant difference on the productivity score. Also, they found that significant predictors of a higher CIQ score, indicating greater community integration, included living with a spouse, a higher GCS score during the acute phase, longer stay in rehabilitation and more use of rehabilitation services (Sandhaug et al. 2015). These findings also highlight the importance of environmental factors and therapy in the community integration of people with TBI.

Perna et al. (2012) investigated the link between executive function and performance of IADLs in 65 people with ABI, mainly including stroke and TBI. The Mayo-Portland Adaptability Inventory (MPAI-4) was used to assess IADL performance. Also, tests of intelligence quotient (IQ), speed of processing, working memory and trail making were conducted.

It was found that the sample had low to average working memory scores and that working memory level was strongly correlated with driving ability, money management, independent living and employment (Perna et al. 2012). Overall, working memory level was the strongest predictor of the ability to manage money, employment and independent living; it also correlated significantly with the community participation component of MPAI-4 (Perna et al. 2012).

Post-traumatic Amnesia in Traumatic Brain Injury

The concept of PTA was introduced in Chapter 3. In TBI, PTA has been found to have a subsequent impact on areas that occupational therapists define as occupational performance. This provides further evidence of the role of memory impairment in this population. Some examples of these findings are discussed in this section.

Doig et al. (2001) studied retrospective data on 208 people aged over 15 with brain injury, who were between two and five years post discharge from an inpatient rehabilitation setting. They also followed up these individuals with a mailed CIQ and vocational status self-assessment questionnaire. They were able to identify three distinct clusters among their respondents. Cluster one had returned to work or study following discharge. People in cluster two were 'balanced' and appeared to have achieved a good level of integration in home, productivity and social areas. People in cluster three had achieved low levels of integration in all of the areas examined (Doig et al. 2001).

Doig et al. (2001) found that 83% of cluster three had been in PTA for longer than 30 days, which was significantly longer than for clusters one and two. Also, cluster three had had significantly longer acute hospital stays following the injury than the other two groups (Doig et al. 2001). The return to work level was significantly lower for cluster three than clusters one and two. In addition, this third group required higher levels of support in daily living activities and, for those with children, 35% of childcare was done by someone else, higher than for the other groups (Doig et al. 2001). These results demonstrate the impact of brain injuries even several years after the event and suggest that length of PTA has a relationship with subsequent occupational performance.

Kosch et al. (2010) investigated the relationship between PTA duration, time in hospital and functional status on discharge. In their study, they reviewed data on PTA and Functional Independence Measure (FIM) scores for 611 patients with brain injury admitted to a unit over a 10-year period. They found that PTA duration had strong correlations with total length of hospital stay and length of stay on a rehabilitation unit. They also found that PTA duration was significantly linked to FIM status on admission and at discharge, and that it explained 30–40% of the variance in FIM scores when leaving hospital (Kosch et al. 2010). They conclude that PTA duration is a key predictor of functional outcomes and could be used as a prognostic tool with this population (Kosch et al. 2010).

Brown et al. (2010) also investigated the utility of duration of PTA, often used as a predictor of the severity of TBI, in predicting levels of function one year following TBI. They used data on patients from the Traumatic Brain Injury Model Systems database in the United States (Brown et al. 2010). They found that PTA duration predicted a number of outcomes. PTA into the fourth week post TBI predicted employment status after one year; PTA into the seventh week predicted scores on the FIM; and PTA into the eighth week predicted whether the person was living independently (Brown et al. 2010). Again, this shows that length of time in PTA and occupational performance levels are related.

Trevena-Peters et al. (2018) explain that a higher level of agitation in PTA, which may be characterised by restlessness, disinhibited and impulsive behaviour, and perseveration in verbal and motor domains, is linked to greater levels of impairment in memory, attention and orientation. The authors estimate that 35–70% of patients in PTA become agitated (Trevena-Peters et al. 2018). They evaluated data on agitation levels in PTA using the Agitated Behavior Scale and found that there was no significant relation between agitated behaviour and time spent in treatment, nor was there any significant difference between levels of agitation for the treatment and control groups (Trevena-Peters et al. 2018). The authors conclude that there may be a case for starting active retraining in activities of daily living during the PTA period (Trevena-Peters et al. 2018).

Eastvold et al. (2013) examined the influence of pre- and post-injury factors and severity on work and independent living status one year after brain injury. The sample was 280 military with non-penetrating moderate head injuries, defined as seven or fewer days PTA duration, or severe head injuries, defined as more than seven days PTA (Eastvold et al. 2013).

Eastvold et al. (2013) found that PTA duration was the single greatest predictor of independent living one year post injury. Length of PTA explained 8.8% of the variance in independent living status. In addition, those with fewer than 60 days in PTA were nine times more likely to be living independently at one year and those with fewer than 30 days in PTA were 3.4 times more likely to be living independently at one year, compared with those with longer PTA duration (Eastvold et al. 2013).

Eastvold et al. (2013) also found a strong correlation between PTA duration and length of time taken to enter rehabilitation from the acute hospital setting (Eastvold et al. 2013). According to the authors, the time to enter the rehabilitation setting may therefore also predict future levels of work and independence status. The importance of rehabilitation as a predictive factor is discussed further next.

Sveen et al. (2016) define three stages of rehabilitation in severe TBI. The first is the acute stage, in which the person is in a coma or in an arousal state, and in which the focus is on regulation of sensory experience, mobility and minimisation of complications. The second is subacute, which is often as an inpatient and focuses on activities of daily living, IADL, cognition and coping with new life demands. The third is the post-acute stage, centred on re-entry to the community and social participation (Sveen et al. 2016).

Sveen et al. (2016) examined the treatment pathways of people with severe TBI in Norway, and related these to functional independence levels 12 months after the injury. At 12 months, 71% were independent and 90% were living at home. Factors associated with reduced dependence levels for the whole cohort included younger age, fewer days on ventilation and shorter time in PTA (Sveen et al. 2016). For patients transferred directly to a specialist unit, factors affecting independence included older age, longer time on ventilation and increased stay on a rehabilitation unit (Sveen et al. 2016). Direct transfer from intensive care to a specialist rehabilitation unit was positively correlated with increased levels of functional independence. The key finding is that direct transfer to a specialist rehabilitation setting has a beneficial effect on functional independence levels (Sveen et al. 2016).

Overall, the results described demonstrate the detrimental effects of working memory and prospective memory impairments on occupational performance in people with TBI. In addition, length of time in PTA may be a prognostic factor for later occupational performance. These results underline the importance for this group of environmental factors such as levels of education, relationship status, transfer to a rehabilitation setting and use of rehabilitation services.

The importance of clear goal formulation in memory assessment was discussed in Chapter 4. In relation to people with brain injury, strategies have been developed that encourage the person to set their own goals to guide their behaviour. One of these is GMT.

GMT is a five-step metacognitive approach to task performance aimed at people with executive dysfunction (Emmanouel et al. 2020). The person is taught to formulate goals that fit their present situation, choose from these, and pause during task performance to monitor their behaviour. They are trained to break their goals down into subgoals, then maintain both the goals and the subgoals and assess results in relation to these (Anderson et al. 2012; Emmanouel et al. 2020).

The GMT approach is predicated on the close relationship of working memory and executive function. It was shown in Chapter 4, for example, that some writers assume that executive functions encompass working memory (Schoemaker et al. 2012; Schoorl et al. 2018). In addition, of course, as described in Chapter 1, the multicomponent working memory model includes a 'central executive' component (Baddeley 2003).

Emmanouel et al. (2020) list three key processes as part of executive function: shifting, inhibiting and updating. They argued that impairments in these areas can impede goal attainment. For example, if a person has problems updating items stored and processed in working memory it may be difficult to attain goals and subgoals (Emmanouel et al. 2020). In addition, sustained attention, which may also be impaired in people with brain injuries, may be needed to maintain goals and subgoals in working memory, allowing successful goal accomplishment (Emmanouel et al. 2020). Overall, the behaviour of people with executive impairments may become disorganised, impulsive and subject to distraction (Emmanouel et al. 2020). Executive function, working memory and goal attainment are therefore intertwined.

Emmanouel et al. (2020) evaluated the effect of combined GMT and working memory training in comparison with working memory training alone. Working memory training consisted of visualising a ladder structure that listed the sub-goals of the task (Emmanouel et al. 2020). In this study 18 people with brain injury, including TBI, stroke or post-tumour surgical lesions, were assigned to an experimental group, using GMT with working memory training, or a control group, using working memory training alone. Both groups had 11 training sessions.

Those in the experimental group were trained on the five-step GMT approach, but in the fourth step they were also provided with the visual image of a ladder containing a keyword on each rung to remind them of the subgoals (Emmanouel et al. 2020). The experimental group were tested performing two tasks: purchasing plane tickets online, which had 19 steps; and sending a text message, which had 15 steps. The control group used a bespoke nine-stage working memory strategy to learn two tasks, one concerned with handling money and the other with distributing boxes to different cities; they were also tested on their performance of the tasks. The primary outcome measure was the number of correct steps performed for each task, with one point for each (Emmanouel et al. 2020). It was found that the experimental group performed significantly better than the control group, and the authors suggest that this demonstrates the possibility of combining GMT and working memory training (Emmanouel et al. 2020).

Task Analysis in Traumatic Brain Injury

Nott et al. (2008), working from an occupational therapy perspective, have developed a structured approach to task analysis and training for people with TBI. PRPP involves analysing the cognitive components of a task and linking the analysis with strategies for therapeutic intervention (Nott et al. 2008, p. 670). Analysis is based on quadrants of a circle labelled 'perceive, recall, plan, perform' (Nott et al. 2008). The quadrants are encircled by arrows showing the direction of information-processing flow, as described in theoretical models (Nott et al. 2008).

The PRPP tool measures performance according to 34 descriptors of information processing, which are in turn related to one of the four PRPP components (Nott et al. 2008). For example, processing descriptors related to recall memory include recall of facts, with descriptors 'recognises, labels, categorises'; recall of schemes, with descriptors 'contextualises time, place and duration'; and procedures, with descriptors 'uses objects, uses body, recalls steps' (Nott et al. 2008, p. 671).

In PRPP, the occupational therapist observes the person performing a task and then evaluates the extent to which they display the requisite information-processing skills needed for the task (Nott et al. 2008). The person is taught the strategy of stopping, in order to reach an appropriate arousal level; sensing, so as to be aware of sensory inputs; thinking, so that they can plan a strategy; and doing, when they implement the strategy (Nott et al. 2008). This process is initially modelled by the occupational therapist acting as 'cognitive mediator' between the person and the task (Nott et al. 2008, p. 670). Verbal, visual and physical prompts are used during training, but the role of the therapists 'fades' as the person internalises the strategy (Nott et al. 2008, p. 670).

PRRP is linked to the Occupational Performance Model (Australia) and, according to the authors, offers a synthesis of information theory and occupational performance analysis (Nott et al. 2008). PRPP is a criterion-referenced assessment, meaning that it is not based on norms linked to membership of a group, but is based on task performance (Nott et al. 2008). In this approach, the task requirements, the person's capacities and the context of performance are central to assessment; the authors point out that this is comparable to the stress on person factors, occupation and performance context in occupational therapy assessment approaches (Nott et al. 2008). PRPP has also been found to have moderate inter-rater reliability and a high level of test reliability (Nott et al. 2008).

PRPP presupposes that personal information-processing capacity and ability to deal with the cognitive demands of everyday tasks are observable and identifiable by the occupational therapist (Nott et al. 2009). It aims to pinpoint information-processing problems during performance and develop strategies for treatment (Nott et al. 2009). The outcome measured is the quality of task performance, while the aim is a description of the information-processing skills involved in the performance (Nott et al. 2009). The authors argue that an advantage of PRPP is that it is therefore more ecologically valid than norm-based measurements that, while they may be highly reliable, fail to capture the reality of task performance. They point out that 'Competence for everyday function is not stable. In real world contexts, it depends on how well people can adapt to changes in the performance context, their capacities, and the complexity of task demands' (Nott et al. 2009, p. 310).

While it is rooted in occupational therapy theory, Nott et al. (2009) argue that PRPP is distinct from assessments such as the Assessment of Motor and Process Skills (AMPS), as it provides an account of the cognitive skills underpinning task performance, which, they state, AMPS does not (Nott et al. 2009). In addition, they suggest that the approach diverts from the 'functional versus remedial' divide typical of therapy as it focuses on training the task, training strategy and applying the strategy all at the same time and in the context of occupational performance (Nott et al. 2008).

Nott et al. (2008) conducted a trial of PRPP with eight patients with brain injury who were still in PTA and exhibiting agitated behaviour. The participants had their normal occupational therapy treatment, alternating with PRPP, for six days each week over a four-week period. They were trained, using the techniques described earlier, to stop, sense, think so as to plan a strategy, and then implement the strategy during task performance (Nott et al. 2008). PRPP was used to evaluate their performance.

Nott et al. (2008) found that seven of the participants showed significant improvement when applying information-processing strategies following PRPP training, and that this was significantly better than their performance in the normal occupational therapy condition (Nott et al. 2008). The researchers therefore conclude that PRPP can be used successfully with agitated patients who are still in PTA (Nott et al. 2008).

Table 6.1 shows a worked example of PRPP analysis. 'Recall' is the only 'cognitive processing strategy' shown, as it is germane to the topic of memory

Table 6.1 Example of the application of Perceive, Recall, Plan, Perform (PRPP) task analysis to the task of upper body dressing (Recall quadrant only).

Cognitive processing strategy	Underlying information-processing strategy	Recall	
		Rating[a]	Example from task analysis
Recalling facts	Recognises	2	Recognised shirt with visual prompt only
			Required physical prompt to recognise vest
	Labels	2	Required verbal prompt to label garment as a vest
	Categorises	3	Required physical prompt to realise that vest was an item of clothing
Recalling schemes	Contextualises		
	Time	2	Required verbal prompt to realise that morning time following washing was the appropriate time to dress the upper body
	Place	2	Required gestural prompt to realise that dressing the upper body was best done in the privacy of his bedroom
	Duration	3	Was unable to state an approximate duration for the task, even with a visual prompt (looking at the clock)
Recalling procedures	Uses objects	2	Required physical prompt to put vest on correctly
			Required gestural prompt to put shirt on correctly
	Uses body	2	Required physical prompt to pull vest down over his head
			Gestural prompt needed to place arms in shirt sleeves
	Recalls steps	1	Recalled that vest should be put on before shirt without prompt

[a] 1, Effective for task performance; 2, questionable; 3, not effective.

(Nott et al. 2009, p. 308). The patient is in PTA following TBI and the task analysed is upper body dressing and grooming during morning routine practice on a neurological rehabilitation unit. Here, a shirt and vest have been laid out on the bed for the person to choose from. In addition, other items such as a hairbrush, toothbrush and toothpaste are present on the bed.

Errorless Learning

The concept of errorless learning, as applied to human learning, can be traced back to the ideas of Skinner (1958). This author developed 'thinking machines' that were designed to complement classroom teaching (Skinner 1958, p. 969). The machines required students to respond to questions and only allowed them to progress once a correct response was given. They gave immediate feedback to the students and 'shaped' the students' behaviour via 'contingencies of reinforcement'. The aim was to minimise the errors made (Skinner 1958, p. 970).

In Skinner's plan, teaching would involve reducing information to smaller units, requiring only a single response to each stimulus, giving feedback to the learner straight away, and stipulating that progress to the next stage was only permitted once correct performance had been achieved at the previous one (Clare and Jones 2008). Skinner (1958) argued that the machines could present stimuli that would eventually elicit specific, correct responses. In addition, the machines could present prompts and suggestions that would support the students in learning the appropriate response. Initially, text was presented that supported the students; however this later 'vanished' as the student became capable of providing the correct response independently (Skinner 1958, p. 972). Based on Skinner's work, Glisky contributed the technique of 'vanishing cues', described as 'backward chaining', whereby the person is given progressively fewer cues as performance improves (Clare and Jones 2008, p. 3).

Errorless learning has been used as a technique to teach individuals with impaired memory (Clare and Jones 2008). It involves the removal of mistakes as the person learns. Errorless learning may have five key steps. First, the activity is broken down into smaller, discrete tasks or 'units' (Clare and Jones 2008, p. 1). Second, these tasks are modelled so that the person is able to perform them themselves. Third, the person is required to avoid guesswork when attempting the tasks. Fourth, errors are corrected immediately by the therapist. Fifth, prompts are faded as the person repeats the task (Clare and Jones 2008).

Various techniques have been proposed that may facilitate errorless learning (Clare and Jones 2008). The 'study only' approach means that only the correct responses to stimuli are presented for learning, while the 'vanishing cues' approach requires the clinician to give increasingly weak cues to the person as their performance improves; alternatively, cues may be added and then reduced as errors decrease (Clare and Jones 2008, p. 3). 'Spaced retrieval' requires gradual increases in the time between testing; in one variation, when errors are detected on testing, they are corrected and followed by a reduced time to the next test, with the time only being increased again once the response is correct (Clare and Jones 2008, p. 13).

Glisky (1995, p. 300) describes an experiment involving an errorless learning approach with 'vanishing cues' in order to teach word processing to a person with amnesia following ABI. In the experiment, word processing was broken down into separate components and each component was trained. The participant was required to finish incomplete sentences stating the different steps needed, using the correct word (Glisky 1995). The vanishing cues method meant that if an incorrect response was given, then the participant was provided with a letter from the correct word, with one being added until the response was correct; if the required response was given, then one less letter was given on the next turn.

The participant was eventually able to achieve error-free performance and was also able to use the word programming package at home independently. The author reports that the person was unable to explain the procedures and that performance was only possible when the appropriate cues were present. In addition, he was unable to reflect on his learning. These last two points suggest that learning was implicit (Glisky 1995). Glisky (1995) comments that despite the success of the experiment, it had taken 473 trials over 62 weeks, and such intensive input might be considered uneconomical in clinical practice.

The results described suggest that there are limitations to the application of errorless learning. Skinner (1958) himself argued that his learning machines were designed to shape and maintain *verbal* behaviour only. Clare and Jones (2008), meanwhile, argue that errorless learning is only effective in tasks involving a single domain of cognition. These latter authors do suggest, however, that errorless learning may be beneficial when learning simple information that requires stereotyped responses and no awareness of context (Clare and Jones 2008).

This characterisation of learning in errorless learning echoes the views of Moscovitch on the conditions allowing people with amnesia to learn (Eichenbaum 2012). These are that the task should be formulated so that the goal and the means of accomplishment are clear, the means are part of the person's repertoire, and accomplishment can occur irrespective of the context. However, most activities of daily living require different behaviours in different contexts, for example when deciding which clothes to wear according to the weather. This suggests that a trial-and-error approach can be better than errorless learning, which may only allow 'hyperspecific' learning to occur (Clare and Jones 2008, p. 15). Despite these reservations, some researchers report successful trials of errorless and implicit learning with people with TBI, two of which are outlined next.

Trevena-Peters et al. (2018) conducted a trial of procedural learning using an errorless learning approach in patients with PTA following TBI. The authors suggest that people in this state may still be able to learn via the implicit memory system. They randomly allocated participants to a treatment group or a normal therapy group. The treating occupational therapists first conducted task analysis of areas including self-feeding, personal care and simple meal preparation and the level of support needed to complete the tasks was identified. Types of support were organised in a hierarchical manner, progressing from physical support, verbal prompts, visual cueing, and supervision to complete independence (Trevena-Peters et al. 2018). Personalised goals were set for the treatment group using goal attainment scaling (GAS) and the participants were then trained on the chosen tasks using an errorless learning approach. The primary outcome measure was FIM, taken at admission, following emergence from PTA, discharge and two months after discharge.

The treatment group showed significantly greater improvements on their FIM scores between admission and emergence from PTA and at discharge, although these differences were not maintained at the two month follow-up (Trevena-Peters et al. 2018). The treatment group was 27.76% more likely to show improvement in FIM, leading the authors to argue that the results found were attributable to treatment and not spontaneous recovery, and that errorless learning is feasible and effective for people in PTA.

In subsequent research Trevena-Peters et al. (2019) analysed interviews with the occupational therapists involved in the research just described. The therapists reported that despite the novelty and challenges of the approach, they had found GAS and procedural and implicit memory training useful, and also that the patients had not shown increased agitation during treatment. This was taken as further confirmation of the possibility of treating patients in PTA using the approach outlined (Trevena-Peters et al. 2019).

Evidence that people with TBI can learn fine motor skills via procedural learning comes from Korman et al. (2018). These authors assessed the ability of people with TBI to learn a finger and thumb opposition sequence using procedural learning. In their study, 10 people with TBI were trained on the sequence as well as 10 participants without memory impairment. There was one training session in the first week and four in the second week. The two groups had their performance on the task measured 11 times, including a test at baseline and at one month following training (Korman et al. 2018). Another control group of 10 people with TBI was asked to perform the task without training and was measured at baseline and after six weeks. The outcome measure was the speed and accuracy of task execution (Korman et al. 2018).

Korman et al. (2018) found that during the first week, the TBI trained group and the group without memory impairment showed similar levels of improvement; however, the group without impairment then improved more markedly than the TBI trained group during the second week. Overall, however, the TBI trained group *did* show improvements in speed of performance that were retained four weeks following training, suggesting that procedural learning is possible in this population. The authors also show that that the main improvements took place *between* training sessions and that 9 out of 10 patients evidenced overnight gains, which suggests that learning took place during the consolidation period and was reinforced by sleep (Korman et al. 2018). The authors also maintain that their results support the proposition that the three phases of learning a skill – acquisition, inter-session consolidation and retaining the skills in the long term – that are seen in healthy people are also present in those with TBI (Korman et al. 2018).

Situated Learning in Traumatic Brain Injury

Aadal and Kirkevold (2011) comment that, despite intensive multidisciplinary input, people with severe TBI often make a limited recovery. These authors are critical of the style of rehabilitation outlined earlier, which focuses on isolated cognitive skills. They conducted qualitative research into the rehabilitation experience of two people with TBI, gathering evidence via focus groups with professionals and observing interactions between them and the two patients (Aadal and Kirkevold 2011). The data was analysed from a situated learning perspective, which stresses that learning occurs via participation in 'communities of practice', such as a rehabilitation setting, and as relationships transform as a result of this participation (Aadal and Kirkevold 2011, p. 718). The participants in these communities develop repertoires of skills and experiences that enable them to address frequently occurring problems (Aadal and Kirkevold 2011).

Aadal and Kirkevold (2011) also applied neuropsychological concepts when analysing their findings. They noted, for example, that staff may not take into account the role of procedural memory in routine tasks such as transferring from a wheelchair. In this case, the patient was instructed consistently to wait until a command was given from a staff member, which meant that his active participation in the task was limited. The authors noted that the transfer took place according to identical instructions given each time, meaning that the patient was unable to apply their memories of performing this task to their post-TBI condition (Aadal and Kirkevold 2011). They also found that this patient's social interaction was affected by memory impairment, as he needed to start afresh each time he encountered someone he knew because the storage and retrieval of earlier memories of interacting with the person were compromised (Aadal and Kirkevold 2011).

Aadal and Kirkevold (2011) comment that affective reactions are shaped by long- and short-term memory and may therefore be affected by impaired functioning. In addition, they explain that language use involves memory for syntax and verbal memory (Aadal and Kirkevold 2011), echoing Baddeley's (2003, p. 835) description of language as a crystallised memory system. Aadal and Kirkevold (2011) maintain that while techniques such as errorless learning and vanishing cues might support practice of discrete cognitive functions, they would not be adequate for intensive rehabilitation, meaning that the 'ideology of providing holistic and contextualized rehabilitation' may not, in fact, be realised (Aadal and Kirkevold 2011, p. 720). They argue that a situated learning approach informed by neuropsychological and neurophysiological concepts may offer a way forward (Aadal and Kirkevold 2011).

Adaptations in Acquired Brain Injury

The use of adaptations to encourage occupational engagement is important in occupational therapy (Pentland et al. 2018). Donaghy and Williams (1998) describe a protocol for using a memory journal for people with ABI that builds on the capacities that may be intact: immediate attention, procedural learning and previous knowledge. Their protocol involved baseline testing, a five-level training programme and follow-up on discharge. The baseline tests included testing the patient's awareness of their impairment, their prospective memory capacity and also their higher mental functions (Donaghy and Williams 1998). The person then went through a five-stage training programme that built on semantic and procedural memory capacity.

The first stage involved learning to cross off planned and completed tasks, making notes on the task and then writing down the next tasks to be executed (Donaghy and Williams 1998). Here, training involved role play. At level two, the person used cards to role play cancelling and making new appointments. Only when levels one and two were accomplished was the person given the diary. Level three concerned preparing the diary for use for the coming week, level four was about adding any extra segments that may be needed and level five required the addition of leisure activities to the journal.

Donaghy and Williams (1998) noted that participants in their training programme were sometimes able to use the journal correctly, while being unable to explain formally what they were doing. They suggested that this demonstrates that procedural learning had occurred despite the absence of semantic knowledge (Donaghy and Williams 1998). The key message is that if journal use is to be successful, the clinician needs to build on knowledge of memory theory. In addition, the patient must be able to spontaneously use the journal without the support of the clinician; in the absence of this, the treatment can be judged a failure (Donaghy and Williams 1998).

The Nature of Memory Impairment in Traumatic Brain Injury

Goverover et al. (2010) write that the key impairment in learning and memory for people with TBI is in the acquisition of new information, rather than in the storage and retrieval of items from long-term memory. These authors tested the technique of 'self-generation' with people with TBI. This is based on evidence showing that items that are generated by the person themselves are better remembered (Goverover et al. 2010).

There were 10 people with TBI and accompanying memory impairments and 15 controls without memory impairment participating in the study. They were asked to recall instructions for, and perform, two cooking and two money tasks in 'provided' and 'generated' conditions (Goverover et al. 2010, p. 541). In the provided condition the participants were given all the information needed for the tasks, while in the generated condition some words were missing from the instructions and the person needed to work out the absent items themselves. Verbal recall was tested immediately after the task was learnt, and task performance was evaluated 30 minutes after the presentation (Goverover et al. 2010).

One week later, the participants were tested on their verbal recall of the tasks. The tasks were scored on the recall and performance of each of the 12 steps needed for completion and also on participants' ability to recall the steps in the correct sequence (Goverover et al. 2010). The results showed that both the TBI and the control groups performed significantly better in the generated condition than the provided. The authors suggest that self-generation could be a useful strategy in improving retention of information for those with TBI (Goverover et al. 2010).

Timmerman and Brouwer (1999) conducted an experiment to test the hypothesis that people with closed head injury (CHI) were impaired when accessing declarative memory items, but would still be able to acquire and apply procedural memory. These authors contend that almost any task requires some access to declarative memory, while any information processing necessitates some aspect of procedural memory (Timmerman and Brouwer 1999).

Timmerman and Brouwer (1999) based their hypotheses on Anderson's (1996) adaptive character of thought (ACT) theory, which posits that high-level cognition occurs via the interplay of procedural and declarative processes. Timmerman and Brouwer (1999) propose that declarative knowledge is founded on a nodal network; if a threshold for activation is reached, then the nodes become accessible for use. The more nodes are activated, the stronger they become. However, they suggest that the reduction in processing speed following CHI may be a consequence of decreased strength of nodes resulting from diffuse axonal injury (Timmerman and Brouwer 1999). The experiment is described next.

Four cognitive reaction time tasks were undertaken by 12 people with severe CHI, with an average PTA duration of 33 days, and 12 controls without impairment. The first task, word categorisation, involved the participant deciding whether a presented word belonged to a category, a task considered by the authors to require declarative knowledge. The second was a memory search task, in which the person had to remember a sequence of numbers and then state whether the answer to an addition problem appeared in the sequence or not, which was also considered a declarative activity. Third was a mirror reading task, where the participant learnt to read reversed words; this was considered to have both procedural (mirror reading) and declarative (word recognition) aspects. Fourth was a rotation task, in which participants had to read letters rotated at greater or lesser angles, with some letters also reversed; this was considered to add to the procedural complexity of performance (Timmerman and Brouwer 1999).

The results showed that for the declarative word category and memory search tasks, the CHI group took significantly longer to complete them and made significantly more errors. In the mirror reading task, there were no significant differences between the CHI and control groups for the procedural aspect for speed and number of errors. Similarly, in the procedural rotation task there were no significant differences between the performance of the CHI and control groups (Timmerman and Brouwer 1999). The authors argue that the results supported their hypothesis that declarative memory would be impaired, while procedural memory would still be operational, in CHI (Timmerman and Brouwer 1999).

Proctor et al. (2000) investigated the relationship between executive function and verbal working memory impairments in adolescents with CHI following traffic accidents. They comment that accidents of this sort typically result in acceleration/deceleration injuries in which the person's head is thrown forward and then back; this can result in pre-frontal cortical damage and also ischaemia, oedema, intracerebral haematoma and anoxia or hypoxia (Proctor et al. 2000). These authors based their definition of executive function on Lezak's taxonomy, which covers goal formation, planning, capacity to effect the plan and ability to successfully carry out the activity (Proctor et al. 2000, p. 633). In addition, they describe the multicomponent model of working memory, while also acknowledging that other theorists have posited a unitary model of working memory (Proctor et al. 2000).

In this experiment, Proctor et al. (2000) compared eight adolescents with head injuries to eight matched controls without head injuries. Working memory was assessed using a recognition memory task (RMT), in which the person has to state if a presented word has been previously presented by the examiner (Proctor et al. 2000). Executive function was evaluated using the Pro-Ex, an assessment of everyday task performance that encompasses selecting goals, planning and sequencing, initiating activity, executing action, sense of time, self-monitoring and awareness (Proctor et al. 2000). The emphasis in Pro-Ex, which is scored by someone close to the patient, is on how these executive skills are integrated with daily task performance (Proctor et al. 2000).

Proctor et al. (2000) found a strong positive and statistically significant correlation between Pro-Ex and RMT scores. They then examined the correlations between component scores on Pro-Ex and RMT. They found a strong positive correlation between selecting goals, planning and sequencing, self-monitoring and awareness and RMT scores, and a moderate correlation for initiating, executing and sense of time. The authors conclude that verbal working memory and executive function are related in this population, and also argue that their findings indicate support for the multicomponent model of working memory (Proctor et al. 2000).

Cognitive Rehabilitation

Anderson et al. (2012) comment that the need for rehabilitation arises where the person's cognitive capacities do not fit the requirements of the environment, a view in keeping with the occupational therapy conceptual practice models described in Chapter 4. Cognitive rehabilitation is based on collaboration between the person with brain injury, their family and clinicians. The focus is on restoring cognitive function or compensating for cognitive impairments and the aim is to enhance occupational performance (Anderson et al. 2012; Chung et al. 2013).

The debate on whether restoration of cognitive function or compensation for impairment underpins rehabilitation has a long history. Luria, for example, maintained that cortical damage led to 'functional adaptation' via compensatory activity in intact regions, as opposed to recovery in the impaired region (Luria 1966, p. 73). More recently, Nudo (2007) argued that, while multilevel plasticity is known to occur in the brain following injury, the precise relationship of this to recovery of behaviour is unclear. In addition, Robertson and Murre (1999) argue that, while most research has focused on reorganisation of sensory and motor brain regions following injury, there is also evidence that improvements in sustained attention may be underpinned by renewal in the frontal–parietal pathways serving this function. Chung et al. (2013) suggested meanwhile that cognitive rehabilitation could work by promoting neural plasticity, by increasing awareness of functional impairment and thus supporting the use of compensation, by adapting to the loss of function, or via a combination of these three mechanisms.

The debate about remediation versus compensation in cognitive rehabilitation is not merely scholastic. The occupational therapist, for example, may be faced with a choice of spending valuable time attempting to retrain working memory function in the person with brain injury or adapting their tasks and environment in order to compensate for impairments (Robertson and Murre 1999).

Whichever approach is taken, cognitive rehabilitation is underpinned by an understanding of the relationship between brain impairment and performance (Chung et al. 2013). Also, despite the uncertainties, it is clear that a key modifier of plasticity is the post-injury 'behavioural experience' of the organism, and this is the terrain in which occupational therapists must operate (Nudo 2007,

p. 840; Robertson and Murre 1999). More detailed consideration is given next to restorative and compensatory tactics.

A restorative approach to cognitive rehabilitation could include, for example, the retraining of specific memory skills, GMT and training on behavioural self-control (Chung et al. 2013). Robertson and Murre (1999) point out that restorative treatments for episodic memory impairments have not been successful, and that compensation has been preferred. These authors also maintain, however, that semantic memory impairments may be more receptive to retraining (Robertson and Murre 1999). Fish et al. (2008) comment that overall there is only limited evidence to support restorative treatments and that therefore researchers have tended to focus on compensatory strategies.

A compensatory approach might encompass the use of adaptive technology, modification of the environment or 'self-instruction' strategies in which the person learns to think through the steps required for task completion, in order to offset impaired memory or attention (Chung et al. 2013. p. 3; Fish et al. 2008). Strategies could be internal, such as using mnemonic devices or mental imagery, or external, such as using diaries, pagers and notebooks (Fish et al. 2008). The use of strategies would, however, depend on other cognitive functions being intact. For example, Robertson and Murre (1999) argue that retrograde amnesia does not respond well to a compensatory approach, as the person will often have additional anterograde amnesia.

Taking a compensatory tack, the occupational therapist might analyse the task so as to identify ways to make it simpler. For example, in Chapter 1 it was shown that a task could be adapted by reducing the amount of information needed to make a decision. Therefore, when working with a person with post–brain injury memory impairments in the kitchen, the occupational therapist could lay out the items needed to complete the task, in order of use, within the person's field of vision, so that they do not need to make decisions about the location and sequence of use of the equipment. The therapist could also adapt the environment, for example by reducing clutter in the kitchen, so that the person can focus their attention on the task, or by posting signs that explain the use and safety features of items.

Chung et al. (2013) conducted a systematic literature review on the effectiveness of cognitive rehabilitation as a strategy for treating executive dysfunction in adults with non-progressive acquired brain impairment. These authors argue that while there is no globally accepted definition of what constitutes executive functions, they include planning, initiation, organising skills, inhibition, problem solving, self-monitoring and self-correction of errors (Chung et al. 2013). These authors state that executive functions are activated via working memory mechanisms (Chung et al. 2013). This relates cognitive rehabilitation to the multicomponent working memory model.

Chung et al. (2013) included 13 studies in their meta-analysis, encompassing data from 660 participants. The authors found no statistically significant differences for restorative or compensatory approaches to cognitive rehabilitation when compared to other treatments. Also, there were no statistically significant differences for working memory outcomes for cognitive rehabilitation compared to no treatment and no differences for working memory when using a restorative approach. In addition, there were no statistically significant differences for performance of extended activities of daily living when using cognitive rehabilitation (Chung et al. 2013). Furthermore, there were no differences for working memory outcomes when experimental cognitive rehabilitation techniques were employed, such as intensive neurorehabilitation and group cognitive rehabilitation, when compared with standard approaches to cognitive rehabilitation, such as computer-based approaches (Chung et al. 2013). Overall, the authors state that there is not enough high-quality evidence to support or reject the use of cognitive rehabilitation to treat executive dysfunction in adult with acquired brain impairments (Chung et al. 2013).

Björkdahl et al. (2013) address the issue of rehabilitation of working memory in brain injury. They suggest that transfer of learning from the training context could take place via two mechanisms. First, 'low road' or 'reflexive' transfer involves repetition of the task in a similar context to the one where learning took place (Björkdahl et al. 2013, p. 1658). Second, 'high road' or 'mindful' processes imply 'conscious abstraction' and the search for links to other contexts (Björkdahl et al. 2013, p. 1658).

Björkdahl et al. (2013) point out that an adaptive approach, equivalent to the compensatory approach, implies that transfer is a function of the similarity of task and context as well as the learner's capacity, which remains unchanging. A remedial approach, on the other hand, is based on the idea that training works by *improving* underlying cognitive capacity and is independent of context or baseline capacity (Björkdahl et al. 2013). Overall, these authors argue that the most effective transfer is likely to involve a 'multi-context' approach (Björkdahl et al. 2013, p. 1658).

Salazar et al. (2000) conducted a trial of cognitive rehabilitation with a sample of 120 active members of the military with moderate to severe head injuries. The rehabilitation programme was based on 'neuropsychologically orientated milieu rehabilitation' (Prigatano et al. 1994). This involves the person receiving individualised therapy, including occupational therapy, within a rehabilitation community in which there are expectations of cooperation and responsibility, along with work placement in a supportive setting (Prigatano et al. 1994).

The experimental group experienced eight weeks of inpatient cognitive rehabilitation, including an occupational therapy-facilitated work placement that matched, as closely as feasible, their area of military specialism (Salazar et al. 2000). The control group had a home rehabilitation programme, consisting of written exercises and a weekly 30-minute telephone call from a psychiatric nurse. The principal outcome measures were return to remunerative work or fitness for military service one year following treatment (Salazar et al. 2000). Secondary outcome measures also included verbal, visual and general memory function and QOL measures focused on areas such as antisocial behaviour, social responsibility, apathy and withdrawal (Salazar et al. 2000).

At the end of the year, no significant differences between the experimental and control groups were identified. Indeed, a slightly higher percentage of the control group had returned to work or service (Salazar et al. 2000). The authors do note that some characteristics of the population might make them unrepresentative of the broader TBI population, including high levels of pre-injury education and military standard fitness; the supportive rehabilitation environment offered by the military; and support for return to work (Salazar et al. 2000). One issue with this research is the lack of description of the occupational therapy and other professional approaches taken in the programme, making it difficult to judge the effectiveness of the treatment.

Use of Assistive Technology

As stated earlier, a compensatory approach to cognitive rehabilitation might involve the use of assistive technology. This section offers some examples of research on this area.

Björkdahl et al. (2013) evaluated the use of a computer training program – Cogmed-QM, which focuses on training working memory – in improving everyday function in people with brain injuries. In their experiment, 20 people with working memory impairments following brain injury had standard therapy for five days a week for five weeks, in addition to receiving an equivalent amount of training sessions using Cogmed-QM, while a control group of 18 people with working memory impairments following brain injury received standard therapy only (Björkdahl et al. 2013). Outcome measures included AMPS, the Rivermead Behavioural Memory Test-II (RBMT-II) and an ad hoc working memory questionnaire (Björkdahl et al. 2013). Measurements were taken pre-treatment, immediately post-treatment and three months after treatment (Björkdahl et al. 2013).

The experimental group improved significantly on the working memory questionnaire when comparing pre-treatment measurements with those at the three-month follow-up (Björkdahl et al. 2013). Both groups improved on the motor component of AMPS, while the experimental group showed improvement on the process skills segment of AMPS in comparison with the control group, although this was not statistically significant (Björkdahl et al. 2013). Eight people from the control group were also trained in a second phase using Cogmed-QM and showed significant improvements on RBMT-II (Björkdahl et al. 2013). Overall, the authors state that their results give qualified support to the idea that computer-based training can lead to improvements that can be transferred beyond the training context (Björkdahl et al. 2013).

Fish et al. (2008) conducted a trial of the NeuroPage system, a pager that reminds individuals with brain injuries about tasks they need to perform. The sample consisted of 143 people with ABI, encompassing those with TBI, stroke and other conditions including Alzheimer's disease, learning disability and encephalitis (Fish et al. 2008). The patients and their carers identified goals that the person needed to achieve; these were checked each day and the percentage of goals achieved was the main outcome measure for the study. Baseline neuropsychological function was assessed using RBMT, a map task from the Test of Everyday Attention and the Six Elements Test from the Behavioural Assessment of the Dysexecutive Syndrome (Fish et al. 2008).

Fish et al. (2008) found that both the participants with TBI and those with stroke benefited from using the pager, with around 30% improvement in goal attainment. However, only the TBI group maintained improvement once the pager was removed, while the stroke group regressed to baseline levels (Fish et al. 2008). It was also found that the stroke group performed significantly worse than the TBI group on the Six Elements Test, suggesting a higher level of executive dysfunction. Further analysis revealed that this was the key predictor of the ability to maintain the benefits of using NeuroPage (Fish et al. 2008). So, while both people with TBI and those with stroke may benefit from the use of a paging system, the maintenance of these benefits in the absence of the pager may depend on the level of executive function.

Kim et al. (2000) comment that impairment in prospective memory is one of the most frequent issues experienced by people with brain injuries. They investigated the usefulness of a palm-top computer that gave auditory and visual reminders of tasks. There were 12 people involved in the trial, of whom 9 found the computer useful. When followed up, the authors found that 7 of participants had continued to find the item helpful (Kim et al. 2000). The authors cite researchers who stated that conditions for using electronic items to assist memory may include having average or close to average intelligence, relatively unimpaired reasoning ability, insight into impairments, and ability to initiate behaviours (Kim et al. 2000).

On the basis of this research, it seems that assistive technology may be useful for some people. However, the occupational therapist would need to tailor it to the individual. Issues such as executive capacity, insight and memory status may all have impacts on the person's ability to use such equipment.

Method of Loci

The method of loci, or 'memory palace', is a technique for improving memory using visual imagery (Legge et al. 2012, p. 380). The person is trained to mentally link items they need to remember to different places in a familiar location (Eysenck 2015), by using visual mental imagery to picture a familiar route, linking the items they need to remember to different points on the route, and then mentally moving along the route, observing the items (Massen et al. 2009; Legge et al. 2012).

The method of loci has a very long history. The Roman scholar and orator Cicero wrote in his work *De Oratore* in 55 BCE that it had first been used by the poet Simonides of Ceos 500 years earlier (Cicero et al. 1942). It was also reported that, using the technique, the Roman general Publius Scipio could recognise and name all the 35 000 men in his army (Rose 1992). Later, in early modern Europe, the Dominican friar Giordano Bruno developed the method to such an extent that locations could encompass entire cities or the signs of the zodiac, which could in turn be occupied by thousands of people or different shops, all of which could have items associated with them (Yates 1966).

In the twentieth century, Luria (1975) described the case of a mnemonist called 'S', who used the method of loci to remember vast amounts of information. He converted words from passages to be learnt into images that he would distribute along the visual image of a familiar street, for example Gorky Street in Moscow, placing them at locations such as houses, gates and shops. He could return to these images, which remained intact for years, whenever he wanted and could also view them in reverse order (Luria 1975). In 1934, he was asked to remember a very long but nonsensical mathematical formula. He was able to reproduce it exactly 15 years later and explained that he had converted all of the items in the formula into visual images, for example the square root sign became a tree, d^2 became two houses and so on (Luria 1975). When his memory did fail, this was because the visual image did not work, for example if he had placed an item in an area of his image that was poorly lit; as Luria pointed out, these were not 'defects of memory but defects of perception' (Luria 1975, p. 33).

Poets have also reached for spatial imagery to describe memory. William Wordsworth, who may have known of Giordano Bruno from his collaborator Samuel Taylor Coleridge, who admired Bruno greatly (Coleridge 1812), wrote:

> *...when thy mind*
> *Shall be a mansion for all lovely forms,*
> *Thy memory be as a dwelling-place*
> *For all sweet sounds and harmonies.*
> *(Wordsworth 1904, p. 207)*

Others have used these images to describe the dissolution of memory in dementia. Philip Larkin (2012, p. 81) wrote:

> *Perhaps being old is having lighted rooms*
> *Inside your head, and people in them, acting.*
> *People you know, yet cannot quite name;*
> *... or sometimes only*
> *The rooms themselves.*

T.S. Eliot (1963, p. 26), meanwhile, described how, in mental illness,

> *Whispering lunar incantations*
> *Dissolve the floors of memory*
> *And all its clear relations,*
> *Its divisions and precisions.*

Perhaps most interesting of all, N.N., the patient with brain injury discussed in Chapter 1 who had severely impaired episodic memory, resorted to comparable images when describing his experience of trying to think about the future: 'It's like being in a room with nothing there and having a guy tell you to go find a chair, and there's nothing there' (Tulving 1985, p. 4).

Could the method of loci help in memory rehabilitation for people with brain injuries? Wilson (1987) reported on an experiment with 20 people with brain injury, 10 of whom had TBI, and 20 controls without memory impairment. Each was given five lists of words to learn using different techniques, including the method of loci, but also visual imagery, cueing using the initial letter of each item, and embedding the items in a story narrated by the researcher (Wilson 1987). For the method of loci, the person was asked to associate each list item with a location in their abode and then imagine walking around it recalling the items (Wilson 1987). Following this, they were asked to recall the lists after a 24-hour delay. It was found that for the group with brain injury recall was significantly better for all the techniques when compared with using no strategy at all. However, the method of loci was no more effective than the other approaches, and the most effective was the use of a story to embed the items (Wilson 1987).

It may be the case that further research is needed on effective ways to use the method of loci in the treatment of people with memory impairment following TBI. First, it is important to note that successful use of the method requires several training sessions (Legge et al. 2012). Second, the locations used seem to make a difference, as Massen et al. (2009) noted that participants recalled more items when deploying imagery of a walk to work as opposed to imagery centred on their house. Third, mental imagery can be visual, where the person imagines the appearance of the environment, or kinaesthetic, where they imagine the feel of moving (Malouin et al. 2004). It may be important to include these variables in future work.

Conclusion

TBI most frequently affects people in adolescence or early adulthood. The brain region involved is generally the frontal and/or temporal regions and there may also be diffuse axonal injury. In keeping with the brain regions affected, executive and working memory impairments are key issues for this population.

Working memory impairments have been linked to a range of problems in activities of daily living in these patients. In addition, executive impairments are associated with reduced social participation.

In keeping with themes explored elsewhere in this book, it has been shown that environmental factors, including those linked to social class, may affect the lived experience of brain injury. For example, educational levels and access to rehabilitation services may have an impact on outcomes.

PTA is a key issue in TBI. Several sources have supported the view that the length of time in PTA is a predictive factor for subsequent recovery of occupational performance. There is, however, evidence that rehabilitation can be carried out effectively with people while still within PTA.

Goal setting was discussed in detail in Chapter 5. This chapter has shown that for people with TBI, working memory impairments, particularly those involving the central executive, can hamper their pursuit of goals. As a response, occupational therapists have developed approaches to rehabilitation such as PRPP that encourage the person to monitor their ongoing task performance.

Errorless learning was discussed. It was shown that it has its origins in the behaviourist school of psychology. For behaviourists such as Skinner, the learning process was reduced to discrete units, devoid of analysis of the impact of the environment or affective factors that influence learning and memory. Researchers have pointed out that errorless learning has allowed people with brain injury to learn some information. However, it seems to be a relatively inflexible approach that requires a great deal of effort in order to learn a limited number of items.

It was shown that people with brain injury may benefit when they themselves generate the information to be learnt. Meanwhile, other researchers have stressed the environmental aspects of learning and have recommended a 'communities of practice' approach.

The chapter also covered the topic of cognitive rehabilitation. The two main approaches here are remedial/restorative and compensatory. The first is based on the assumption that some improvement in the underlying cognitive impairment is possible. The second stresses that such improvement is unlikely, but that the person can be taught to adapt to impairments. Overall, however, there is limited evidence to support the cognitive rehabilitation approach.

Finally, the method of loci was examined. The ancient history of this technique was explained. It may be useful for people with brain injury, but could require careful training and attention to the nature of the imagery used.

Activities

Case Study Vignette 1

Niamh is a 24-year-old solicitor. She fell and struck her head on a stone step while out with friends. She has TBI affecting the frontal and temporal regions and has difficulty with working memory and episodic memory.

Niamh is planning to return to work. A key skill she will need is the ability to use a computer to process information contained in spreadsheets.

Simulation Task 1

You have taken Niamh to the occupational therapy treatment area to see if she can open a spreadsheet. You have also put some mock data on a sheet that she will need to input into the spreadsheet cells.

Using Table 6.1 to guide you, complete this simulation task by analysing the recall components of the spreadsheet task. Imagine that you are working with Niamh and you are observing her perform the task. Complete the blank PRPP analysis form shown in Table 6.2.

Table 6.2 Blank form for Perceive, Recall, Plan, Perform (PRPP) task analysis of using a computer spreadsheet (Recall quadrant only).

Recall			
Cognitive processing strategy	**Underlying information-processing strategy**	**Rating**[a]	**Example from task analysis**
Recalling facts	Recognises		
	Labels		
	Categorises		
Recalling schemes	Contextualises		
	Time		
	Place		
	Duration		
Recalling procedures	Uses objects		
	Uses body		
	Recalls steps		

[a] 1, Effective for task performance; 2, questionable; 3, not effective.

Using the method for errorless learning described by Clare and Jones (2008) and discussed in this chapter, write down a strategy for retraining this task.

1. Break the task down into separate smaller steps.
2. Explain how you would model these steps so that Niamh could follow them.
3. Ask Niamh to perform the steps. State what prompts you could use so that Niamh does not have to guess what she should be doing at each step. Prompts could be verbal, visual or physical.
4. Explain how you would immediately correct any errors in performance.
5. State how you would fade prompts as Niamh's performance improves. Explain what order the prompts could be faded in. For example, would you fade visual prompts before verbal prompts?

Simulation Task 2

Complete two intervention plans for Niamh based on the spreadsheet training task. The first should use a compensatory approach; the second should use a restorative approach.

Case Study Vignette 2

Charles is a 33-year-old classroom assistant and has TBI following a road traffic accident. His episodic memory has been affected and he has antero- grade amnesia. In particular, he has difficulty remembering people's names and faces. He is hoping to return to work in a school.

1. Explain how the method of loci could be used to help him remember the names and faces of his colleagues.
2. Explain how Charles could be taught to embed the names and faces of his colleagues in a story to support his memory.

References

Aadal, L. and Kirkevold, M. (2011). Integrating situated learning theory and neuro- psychological research to facilitate patient participation and learning in traumatic brain injury rehabilitation patients. *Brain Injury* 25 (7–8): 717–728.

Anderson, J.R. (1996). ACT: a simple theory of complex cognition. *American Psychol- ogist* 51 (4): 355–365.

Anderson, T.M. and Knight, R.G. (2010). The long-term effects of traumatic brain injury on the coordinative function of the central executive. *Journal of Clinical and Experimental Neuropsychology* 32 (10): 1074–1082.

Anderson, N.D., Winocur, G., and Palmer, H. (2012). Principles of cognitive rehabili- tation. In: *The Handbook of Clinical Psychology* (ed. J.M. Gurd, U. Kischka, and J.C. Marshall), 50–77. Oxford: Oxford University Press.

Baddeley, A. (2003). Working memory: looking back and looking forward. *Nature Reviews. Neuroscience* 4 (10): 829–839.

Björkdahl, A., Akerlund, E., Svensson, S., and Esbjörnsson, E. (2013). A randomized study of computerized working memory training and effects on functioning in everyday life for patients with brain injury. *Brain Injury* 27 (13–14): 1658–1665.

Bottari, C., Gosselin, N., Chen, J.-K., and Ptito, A. (2017). The impact of symptomatic mild traumatic brain injury on complex everyday activities and the link with alterations in cerebral functioning: exploratory case studies. *Neuropsychological Rehabilitation* 27 (5): 871–890.

Brown, A.W., Malec, J.F., Mandrekar, J. et al. (2010). Predictive utility of weekly post-traumatic amnesia assessments after brain injury: a multicentre analysis. *Brain Injury* 24 (3): 472–478.

Chung, C.S.Y., Pollock, A., Campbell, T. et al. (2013). Cognitive rehabilitation for executive dysfunction in adults with stroke or other adult non-progressive acquired brain damage. *Cochrane Database of Systematic Reviews* 2013 (4): CD008391. https://doi.org/10.1002/14651858.CD008391.pub2.

Cicero, M.T., Sutton, E.W., and Rackham, H. (1942). *De Oratore*. Cambridge, MA: Harvard University Press.

Clare, L. and Jones, R.S.P. (2008). Errorless learning in the rehabilitation of memory impairment: a critical review. *Neuropsychology Review* 18 (1): 1–23.

Clark, J.M.R., Jak, A.J., and Twamley, E.W. (2020). Cognition and functional capacity following traumatic brain injury in veterans. *Rehabilitation Psychology* 65 (1): 72–79.

Coleridge, S.T. (1812). *The Friend: A Series of Essays*. London: Gale and Curtis.

Doig, E., Fleming, J., and Tooth, L. (2001). Patterns of community integration 2–5 years post-discharge from brain injury rehabilitation. *Brain Injury* 15 (9): 747–762.

Donaghy, S. and Williams, W. (1998). A new protocol for training severely impaired patients in the usage of memory journals. *Brain Injury* 12 (12): 1061–1076.

Donders, J., Oh, Y.I., and Gable, J. (2015). Self- and informant ratings of executive functioning after mild traumatic brain injury. *Journal of Head Trauma Rehabilitation* 30 (6): E30–E39.

Eastvold, A.D., Walker, W.C., Curtiss, G. et al. (2013). The differential contributions of posttraumatic amnesia duration and time since injury in prediction of functional outcomes following moderate-to-severe traumatic brain injury. *Journal of Head Trauma Rehabilitation* 28 (1): 48–58.

Eichenbaum, H. (2012). *The Cognitive Neuroscience of Memory: An Introduction*, 2e. Oxford: Oxford University Press.

Eliot, T.S. (1963). *Collected Poems, 1909–62*. London: Faber and Faber.

Emmanouel, A., Kontrafouri, E., Nikolaos, P. et al. (2020). Incorporation of a working memory strategy in GMT to facilitate serial-order behaviour in brain-injured patients. *Neuropsychological Rehabilitation* 30 (5): 888–914.

Eysenck, M.C. (2015). Improving your memory. In: *Memory* (ed. A. Baddeley, M.W. Eysenck, and M.C. Anderson), 469–493. London: Psychology Press.

Finnanger, T.G., Olsen, A., Skandsen, T. et al. (2015). Life after adolescent and adult moderate and severe traumatic brain injury: self-reported executive emotional and behavioural function 2–5 years after injury. *Behavioural Neurology* 2015: 329241.

Fish, J., Manly, T., Emslie, H. et al. (2008). Compensatory strategies for acquired disorders of memory and planning: differential effects of a paging system for patients with brain injury of traumatic versus cerebrovascular aetiology. *Journal of Neurology, Neurosurgery, and Psychiatry* 79 (8): 930–935.

Glisky, E.L. (1995). Acquisition and transfer of word processing skill by an amnesic patient. *Neuropsychological Rehabilitation* 5 (4): 299–318.

Goverover, Y., Chiaravalloti, N., and DeLuca, J. (2010). Pilot study to examine the use of self-generation to improve learning and memory in people with traumatic brain injury. *American Journal of Occupational Therapy* 64 (4): 540–546.

Kersey, J., Terhorst, L., Wu, C.-Y., and Skidmore, E. (2019). A scoping review of predictors of community integration following traumatic brain injury: a search for meaningful associations. *Journal of Head Trauma Rehabilitation* 34 (4): E32–E41.

Kim, H.J., Burke, D.T., Dowds, M.M. Jr. et al. (2000). Electronic memory aids for outpatient brain injury: follow-up findings. *Brain Injury* 14 (2): 187–196.

Korman, M., Shaklai, S., Cisamariu, K. et al. (2018). Atypical within-session motor procedural learning after traumatic brain injury but well-preserved between-session procedural memory consolidation. *Frontiers in Human Neuroscience* 12: 10.

Kosch, Y., Browne, S., King, C. et al. (2010). Post-traumatic amnesia and its relationship to the functional outcome of people with severe traumatic brain injury. *Brain Injury* 24 (3): 479–485.

Larkin, P. (2012). *The Complete Poems*. London: Faber and Faber.

Legge, E.L.G., Madan, C.R., Ng, E.T., and Caplan, J.B. (2012). Building a memory palace in minutes: equivalent memory performance using virtual versus conventional environments with the Method of Loci. *Acta Psychologica* 141 (3): 380–390.

Luria, A.R. (1966). *Higher Cortical Functions in Man*. New York: Basic Books.

Luria, A.R. (1975). *The Mind of a Mnemonist: A Little Book About a Vast Memory*. Harmondsworth: Penguin.

Malouin, F., Belleville, S., Richards, C.L. et al. (2004). Working memory and mental practice outcomes after stroke. *Archives of Physical Medicine and Rehabilitation* 85 (2): 177–183.

Massen, C., Vaterrodt-Plünnecke, B., Krings, L., and Hilbig, B.E. (2009). Effects of instruction on learners' ability to generate an effective pathway in the method of loci. *Memory* 17 (7): 724–731.

Nott, M.T., Chapparo, C., and Heard, R. (2008). Effective occupational therapy intervention with adults demonstrating agitation during post-traumatic amnesia. *Brain Injury* 22 (9): 669–683.

Nott, M.T., Chapparo, C., and Heard, R. (2009). Reliability of the perceive, recall, plan and perform system of task analysis: a criterion-referenced assessment. *Australian Occupational Therapy Journal* 56 (5): 307–314.

Nudo, R.J. (2007). Postinfarct cortical plasticity and behavioral recovery. *Stroke* 38 (2): 840–845.

Pentland, D., Kantartzis, S., Clausen, M.G., and Witemyre, K. (2018). *Occupational Therapy and Complexity: Defining and Describing Practice*. London: Royal College of Occupational Therapists.

Perna, R., Loughan, A.R., and Talka, K. (2012). Executive functioning and adaptive living skills after acquired brain injury. *Applied Neuropsychology, Adult* 19 (4): 263–271.

Prigatano, G.P., Klonoff, P.S., O'Brien, K.P. et al. (1994). Productivity after neuropsychologically oriented milieu rehabilitation. *Journal of Head Trauma Rehabilitation* 9 (1): 91–102.

Proctor, A., Wilson, B., Sanchez, C., and Wesley, E. (2000). Executive function and verbal working memory in adolescents with closed head injury (CHI). *Brain Injury* 14 (7): 633–647.

Robertson, I.H. and Murre, J.M.J. (1999). Rehabilitation of brain damage: brain plasticity and principles of guided recovery. *Psychological Bulletin* 125 (5): 544–575.

Rose, S.P.R. (1992). *The Making of Memory*. London: Bantam.

Salazar, A.M., Warden, D.L., Schwab, K. et al. (2000). Cognitive rehabilitation for traumatic brain injury: a randomized trial. *JAMA* 283 (23): 3075–3081.

Sandhaug, M., Andelic, N., Langhammer, B., and Mygland, A. (2015). Community integration 2 years after moderate and severe traumatic brain injury. *Brain Injury* 29 (7–8): 915–920.

Schoemaker, K., Bunte, T., Wiebe, S.A. et al. (2012). Executive function deficits in preschool children with ADHD and DBD. *Journal of Child Psychology and Psychiatry* 53 (2): 111–119.

Schoorl, J., van Rijn, S., de Wied, M. et al. (2018). Boys with oppositional defiant disorder/conduct disorder show impaired adaptation during stress: an executive functioning study. *Child Psychiatry and Human Development* 49 (2): 298–307.

Skinner, B.F. (1958). Teaching machines: from the experimental study of learning come devices which arrange optimal conditions for self-instruction. *Science* 128 (3330): 969–977.

Sveen, U., Røe, C., Sigurdardottir, S. et al. (2016). Rehabilitation pathways and functional independence one year after severe traumatic brain injury. *European Journal of Physical and Rehabilitation Medicine* 52 (5): 650–661.

Timmerman, M.E. and Brouwer, W.H. (1999). Slow information processing after very severe closed head injury: impaired access to declarative knowledge and intact application and acquisition of procedural knowledge. *Neuropsychologia* 37 (4): 467–478.

Trevena-Peters, J., McKay, A., Spitz, G. et al. (2018). Efficacy of activities of daily living retraining during posttraumatic amnesia: a randomized controlled trial. *Archives of Physical Medicine and Rehabilitation* 99 (2): 329–337.

Trevena-Peters, J., Ponsford, J., and McKay, A. (2018). Agitated behavior and activities of daily living retraining during posttraumatic amnesia. *Journal of Head Trauma Rehabilitation* 33 (5): 317–325.

Trevena-Peters, J., McKay, A., and Ponsford, J. (2019). Activities of daily living retraining and goal attainment during posttraumatic amnesia. *Neuropsychological Rehabilitation* 29 (10): 1655–1670.

Tulving, E. (1985). Memory and consciousness. *Canadian Psychology/Psychologie Canadienne* 26 (1): 1.

Verdugo, M.A., Fernández, M., Gómez, L.E. et al. (2019). Predictive factors of quality of life in acquired brain injury. *International Journal of Clinical and Health Psychology* 19 (3): 189–197.

Wilson, B.A. (1987). *Rehabilitation of Memory*. New York: Guilford Press.

Wordsworth, W. (1904). *The Poetical Works of William Wordsworth*. London: Henry Frowde.

Yates, F.A. (1966). *The Art of Memory*. London: Routledge & Kegan Paul.

7 Occupational Therapy Action Planning and Treatment Implementation for Older Adults with Memory Impairment

The concept of occupational therapy as a 'non-pharmacological treatment' in dementia is explored in this chapter. It is shown that occupational therapy approaches may be even more effective than the currently available pharmacological approaches to treatment. Examples are also given of researchers who have used qualitative approaches in order to capture the effects of occupation-based approaches for treatment of people with dementia.

The client-centred approach in dementia treatment is explained. Its key principles include a focus on the person, as well as on those close to them, and also a collaborative approach to treatment planning.

Researchers have contrasted the 'old culture' of dementia care, which had a narrow medical focus and a rather pessimistic view of the person's future, with a 'new culture' that has a more occupational focus. This new culture is supported by a number of theoretical resources, including Kitwood's concept of 'positive person work' and Allen's 'cognitive disabilities' model. The latter was developed from within occupational therapy.

A strong theme is that interventions aimed at dementia in general, and memory impairments in particular, should be tailored to the individual. Approaches such as the home Environmental Skill-building Program (ESP) and Care of Persons with Dementia in Their Environments (COPE) are described. The extensive Tailored Activity Program (TAP) for people with dementia at different stages is discussed. Evidence from large-scale trials of TAP are reported, showing positive results for the intervention. In addition, this

Memory Impairment and Occupation: A Guide to Evaluation and Treatment, First Edition.
Jonathon O'Brien.
© 2024 John Wiley & Sons Ltd. Published 2024 by John Wiley & Sons Ltd.

non-pharmacological approach has been researched using race as a variable, revealing differing results for Black and white person–carer dyads.

Problems related to lack of awareness of disease in dementia, particularly in Alzheimer's type dementia (ATD), are discussed. It is shown that such problems may be related to memory impairments. In addition, lack of awareness is compared with lack of insight and impaired social cognition. It is suggested that impaired social cognition, resulting from a diminished 'theory of mind', may originate in hippocampal damage and compromised episodic memory in ATD.

Researchers have argued that rehabilitation is a useful organising concept when working with people with dementia, and one that also fits well with the social model of disability. Evidence regarding the effectiveness of cognitive rehabilitation for this population is reviewed; it is shown that the picture remains unclear and that results are mixed.

Cognitive stimulation therapy (CST) is discussed in some detail. The history of its development is described and it is shown that the underlying principles fit well with occupational therapy. However, CST does not seem to have any effect on memory per se.

The behavioural and psychological symptoms of dementia (BPSD) are discussed, and it is shown that these may be linked to memory impairments. In addition, the impact of the environment on such symptoms is explored. Some occupational therapy approaches to analysing the impact of the environment on behaviour in dementia are outlined.

Memory Impairments and Occupational Performance

Cordier et al. (2019) identified a link between subjective reports of memory impairment in older people and problems in performing activities of daily living (ADL) and instrumental activities of daily living (IADL). IADL involve maintenance of independence and community activities, for example shopping; they are considered to be more complex than ADL and require higher cognitive capacity (Cordier et al. 2019). Cordier et al. (2019) used data on 3721 women born between 1921 and 1926, which had been gathered as part of the Australian Longitudinal Study on Women's Health (ALSWH). ALSWH takes repeated measurements of subjective memory complaints and changes in ADL/IADL performance (Cordier et al. 2019).

Cordier et al. (2019) found that women who began the survey with more subjective memory complaints had a significantly higher number of ADL problems. Also, they found that there was a significant positive correlation between change in memory complaints over time and increase in reported ADL problems (Cordier et al. 2019).

Similar findings were made for IADL. Women with a higher starting level of memory complaints had significantly higher levels of IADL difficulties, and tended to have a higher rate of increase in IADL problems (Cordier et al. 2019). In the case of ADL performance, the authors point out that decline is more likely to be linked to physical impairments, while IADL are more affected by cognitive impairment (Cordier et al. 2019).

Occupational Therapy as a Non-pharmacological Treatment in Dementia

Chapter 3 described current pharmacological treatments for dementia and showed that these have limited success and, generally, do not treat the underlying disease process (Yuill and Hollis, 2011). As a result, non-pharmacological treatments, which include occupational therapy, are preferred in the first instance (Gitlin et al. 2017; Yuill and Hollis, 2011).

Evidence for the effectiveness of occupational therapy approaches comes from a randomised controlled trial of occupational therapy with people with mild to moderate dementia and their carers (Graff et al. 2006); 68 of the patients received occupational therapy, while 67 were allocated to a control condition (Graff et al. 2006). The content of the occupational therapy treatment was decided by consensus of a panel of experienced occupational therapists. It focused on cognitive and behavioural approaches to using aids that helped the person adapt to cognitive impairment. In addition, carers were educated on ways to adjust to dementia-related behaviour and on supervising the person (Graff et al. 2006). Outcome measures included the process component of the Assessment of Motor and Process Skills (AMPS). The occupational therapy treatment groups showed significant improvements on all outcome measures at six weeks and three months. The authors also show that the effect sizes were greater than those for pharmacological treatments and recommend that occupational therapy should be used as a treatment in this area (Graff et al. 2006).

Some support for occupation-orientated approaches in dementia treatment was provided by Pöllänen and Hirsimäki (2014). These researchers used a phenomenological approach to examine the responses of three women with dementia in a residential care facility while engaging in craft activities. The authors argued that craft skills may survive where other procedural capabilities are impaired in dementia (Pöllänen and Hirsimäki 2014). Also, craft can invoke reminiscence, which can orientate the individual in relation to their earlier life roles and interests (Pöllänen and Hirsimäki 2014).

Pöllänen and Hirsimäki (2014) found that engaging in craft facilitated attention over extended periods. It also supported non-verbal communication. In addition, they noted body movement, looking, haptic responses and smelling of craft items, as well as verbal responses (Pöllänen and Hirsimäki 2014). The authors stated that the crafts allowed their participants to 'position themselves in time and space' (Pöllänen and Hirsimäki 2014, p. 424). They recommend the use of bespoke craft activities that connect to the person's earlier life, as well as training carers to incorporate proprioception and touch when interacting with people with dementia (Pöllänen and Hirsimäki 2014).

There is a range of dementia treatment approaches that focus on ADL and are closely aligned with occupational therapy. One feature of these treatments, however, is that they do not generally focus on memory impairments per se. This may be because, as shown in Chapter 3, memory is only one of the areas affected in dementia. Indeed, it is only ATD that has memory deficit as the initial impairment. It will be recalled from Chapter 1, though, that occupational therapy theorists have defined memory as one of the cognitive skills that underpin occupational performance (Kielhofner, 2008). In this sense, these packages are implicitly concerned with memory alongside other cognitive domains.

Another aspect of the occupational therapy treatment approaches discussed in this chapter is a concern with what might be described as client-centred practice. This is a long-established principle in occupational therapy (Creek 2003) and Parker (2011) has gone so far as to describe client-centred practice as an occupational therapy frame of reference. It involves making the person the focus of the planning and intervention, as opposed to being led by a medical diagnosis of dementia.

In this approach, the concept of 'client' may be expanded to include carers as well as the person themselves (Parker 2011). This is affirmed by Cordier et al. (2019, p. 236), who highlight the importance of 'dyadic interventions', focusing on the person with dementia and their carer, in cases of severe cognitive impairment.

Client centredness also entails a collaborative approach to treatment planning, whereby the person is engaged as a partner by the occupational therapist (Parker 2011). This means that goals should be negotiated between the therapist and the person (Parker 2011). A further notion is 'contextual congruence', referring to the importance of understanding the specific 'roles, interests, culture and environments' of the client (Parker 2011, p. 141). These principles infuse some of the non-pharmacological approaches to treating memory impairments.

Du Toit et al. (2019) reviewed literature on client-centred practice and meaningful engagement in dementia care in residential facilities, using a critical interpretive synthesis approach. They identified two main conceptual constructs in their review: the promotion of a collaborative care culture; and the concept of the person with dementia as someone with a past, a present and a future. The first of these, collaborative care, involves a shift from a 'biomedical' approach to the person with dementia as a 'patient' to a condition where residents are engaged in decision making about their situation (Du Toit et al. 2019, p. 349). The second construct involves exploring the person's life narrative and experiences and drawing on their interests in designing challenging and engaging therapy (Du et al. 2019). The authors point out that past skills may be part of the person's procedural memory and can be tapped by the therapist. Du Toit et al. (2019) also highlight the role of the Assessment Tool for Occupation and Social Engagement (ATOSE), an open-access outcome measure based on principles of occupational justice (Du Toit et al. 2019), which is discussed further on in this chapter.

Du Toit et al. (2019) conclude that, while occupational therapists support principles of client-centred practice and seek to develop relationships between carers and residents, they should also consider building relationships between the residents themselves based on co-occupation. They comment that there is often a focus on 'doing' in occupational therapy practice in this area, while the roles of belonging, and connection and contribution to the 'microcommunity' of the residential setting, may be neglected (Du Toit et al. 2019, p. 352).

Old and New Cultures of Dementia Care

Warchol (2006, p. 215) describes an 'old culture' of dementia care, which is about making sure the person is safe, delivering basic care and meeting physical requirements; it is dominated by medicine and regards dementia as a progressive condition that eventually eliminates personhood. Opposed to this is the 'new culture', which focuses on the maintenance of personhood and regards the quality of care as important in the person's experience of their condition; it regards care as the responsibility of the entire multidisciplinary team and emphasises the importance of carers understanding the person's interests, capacities, values and spirituality (Warchol 2006, p. 215).

Warchol (2006) outlines a number of theoretical resources that can support this new culture. The first is Kitwood's 'positive person work', which focuses on the maintenance of personhood in dementia and the promotion of well-being, and is discussed later (Kitwood and Brooker 2019, p. 151). Second, Reisberg's concept of 'retrogenesis' suggests that the death of neurons and the accompanying functional losses occur in the reverse order to normal development, so that the developmental stages of childhood correlate with different stages of dementia (Warchol 2006, p. 218). In this view, the carer needs to recognise the capacities of the person at each stage and match tasks and communication to these, just as the carer of a child does (Warchol 2006). Third is Allen's 'cognitive disabilities' model, which outlines the capacities of people at different stages of dementia and gives ways to adapt tasks to match their level of function (Warchol 2006, p. 219). Both Allen's and Reisberg's approaches have associated assessment tools and outcome measures, and in Allen's model the person is engaged in both working and procedural memory tasks (Warchol 2006).

Warchol (2006, p. 221) describes her own 'forget-me-not' approach, which builds on these resources. In this approach, the cognitive level of the person is assessed so as to utilise their extant capacities. Activities are then adapted to their level. Furthermore, the life story, interests and tastes of the individual are taken into account, allowing the therapist to draw on the person's long-term and procedural memory when planning treatment.

Home Environmental Skill-Building Program, Care of Persons with Dementia in Their Environments and Tailored Activity Program

A systematic review of 13 randomised controlled trials examined the most effective non-pharmacological treatments aimed at reducing functional decline in people with dementia living at home (Scott et al. 2019). The authors found that occupational therapy focused on teaching carers from the family to set task-based goals that were tailored to the individual was associated with lower levels of dependence in ADL. In addition, they found that individually tailored cognitive rehabilitation was associated with reduced functional decline, but that group-based cognitive rehabilitation showed no benefits (Scott et al. 2019).

Overall, the authors argue that effective therapy should be bespoke to the individual and needs to be home based (Scott et al. 2019). They also note that focus on the dyad of the person with dementia and their carer appears to be effective (Scott et al. 2019).

Gitlin et al. (2003, p. 532) investigated the effects on such dyads when taking part in the home ESP. The authors state that ESP is built on the notion of 'competence-environmental press' and 'personal control theory' (Gitlin et al. 2003, p. 533). The aim is to reduce the press of the environment on the dyad by focusing on stressors that can be modified (Gitlin et al. 2003).

In ESP, the environment is analysed as having physical, task and social components; the aim is to increase the congruence of 'environmental press' and caregiver competence by improving the carers' skills to adjust aspects of the environment (Gitlin et al. 2003, p. 536). It will be recalled from Chapter 4 that this emphasis on environmental influences on behaviour is a feature of occupational therapy conceptual practice models.

In Gitlin et al.'s (2003) evaluation of ESP, their sample consisted of carers of people with moderate to severe dementia. There were 89 carers who were randomly allocated to a treatment group and 101 to a control group, and all 190 were interviewed six months after commencing (Gitlin et al. 2003). There were four components of ESP. First, the carer was educated about dementia and the influence of environment on behaviour. Second, they were trained to problem solve and adjust the physical and social environment. Third, bespoke strategies for adapting the environment were applied; and fourth, the strategies were generalised to new problems as they emerged (Gitlin et al. 2003).

The strategies taught to carers in ESP align well with the approaches to treating memory impairment discussed elsewhere in this book. They included modification of the physical environment, for example with equipment, placement of items for personal care and dressing, and labelling items or using contrasting colours (Gitlin et al. 2003). There was also emphasis on simplifying tasks by giving the person with dementia verbal or tactile cues and improving communication techniques, or using a planned routine and graded activities. In addition, the programme included modification of the social environment via communication with support networks and providers of care (Gitlin et al. 2003).

ESP had an 'active phase' for the first six months, followed by six months of 'maintenance' (Gitlin et al. 2003, p. 533). After six months, the ESP group carers reported significantly less disruptive behaviour, fewer problems with memory-linked problematic behaviour, and less need for help from friends or family (Gitlin et al. 2003). Women carers reported reduced numbers of days needing help with ADL and better affect and sense of mastery. They also reported improved management capability and well-being (Gitlin et al. 2003). ESP builds on occupational therapy skills of task analysis, education and environmental adjustment.

Gitlin et al. (2005) subsequently evaluated the long-term effects of ESP. Carers of people with dementia were randomised to ESP or a control intervention and measured at baseline, following 6 months of active treatment and at 12 months, following a 6-month maintenance period. At 6 months it was found that carers reported improved skills, requiring less help to give assistance and fewer occurrences of problem behaviours (Gitlin et al. 2005). However, at 12 months it was found that only caregivers' affect had improved (Gitlin et al. 2005). The authors suggest that the active phase of ESP treatment may need to be extended if the results found at 6 months were to be maintained (Gitlin et al. 2005).

Another approach is COPE (Gitlin et al. 2010, p. 984), which involves occupational therapists interviewing carers about the person's roles, habits and interests. The therapists then train them to adjust the environment, their communication with the person and ADL, so that they are matched with the person's capacity (Gitlin et al. 2010).

Gitlin et al. (2010) conducted a randomised controlled trial of COPE. Occupational therapists produced a plan of action for person–carer dyads (Gitlin et al. 2010). Outcome measures included a rating of functional independence that covered IADL, such as shopping, preparing meals and managing finance, and personal activities of daily living (PADL), for example dressing, using the toilet, eating and transferring to and from bed (Gitlin et al. 2010). In addition, the researchers measured the frequency of agitation, engagement in activities, well-being, the confidence of carers in use of the activities and the carers' perception of the benefits of COPE (Gitlin et al. 2010). Over four months 209 dyads were assessed: 102 were treated with COPE and 107 with a control treatment. After four months, the COPE group showed significantly lower functional dependence and dependence in IADL, greater levels of engagement and higher well-being for the carers, although no changes were found for agitated behaviour (Gitlin et al. 2010).

The TAP approach entails the therapist producing bespoke 'activity prescriptions' for people with dementia (Regier et al. 2017, p. 988). TAP trains the therapist to prescribe activities that are matched to the capacities and motivations of the person with dementia, as well as delivering training to caregivers (Regier et al. 2017).

Gitlin et al. (2008, p. 231) explain that TAP is based on the linked ideas of increased vulnerability to the environment and a reduced stress threshold. These concepts suggest that those with dementia are less able to tolerate stressful stimuli and are therefore more vulnerable to environmental stressors. Problematic behaviours in dementia are thus a result of interaction between neurological, environmental and psychosocial factors (Gitlin et al. 2008). It will be recalled that a focus on the impact of environment on occupational performance is also a key feature of occupational therapy conceptual practice models, discussed in Chapter 4.

Gitlin et al. (2008) conducted a trial of TAP with 60 patient–carer dyads. The focus was on reducing neuropsychiatric behavioural disturbance, increasing engagement and improving the well-being of carers. Of the dyads, 30 were assigned to TAP and 30 to a waiting list control group (Gitlin et al. 2008). Occupational therapists interviewed the TAP group in order to identify the patients' interests and roles and also observed dyadic interactions and the environment (Gitlin et al. 2008). An 'activity prescription' was developed for each patient, based on assessment of their capabilities in memory, language, concept formation, attention and construction (Gitlin et al. 2008, p. 231). The therapists determined the cues required by the person, their ability to follow instructions and problem solve, and also their previous interests and roles. There were three activities in each prescription, which ranged in complexity from those with multiple steps to one or two steps or basic sensory activities (Gitlin et al. 2008).

After four months, Gitlin et al. (2008) found that the TAP treatment group had a significantly lower number of problematic behaviours, specifically repetitive questioning and shadowing, and higher activity engagement, and also that carers reported fewer hours doing things for patients (Gitlin et al. 2008). The treatment group reported five fewer hours 'on duty', while the control group reported two hours more (Gitlin et al. 2008). No difference was found for carer quality of life (QOL) or levels of depression (Gitlin et al. 2008). The authors conclude that TAP may work by ameliorating the 'allostatic load', meaning that it reduces the strain on the patient's information-processing and sensory capabilities (Gitlin et al. 2008, p. 236).

Regier et al. (2017, p. 988) assessed 158 activity prescriptions formulated by occupational therapists as part of TAP. These authors found that differences in the type of activities prescribed and the degree of simplification and support needed varied according to disease severity. People with moderate dementia were more likely to be prescribed musical and entertainment activities than those with mild or severe dementia, and also had an increased likelihood of being prescribed more complex arts and crafts (Regier et al. 2017). Those with severe dementia were more likely to be prescribed basic sorting, sensory or manipulation activities. Also, reminiscence activities were prescribed less for those at the severe stages than those at mild–moderate stages (Regier et al. 2017).

Regier et al. (2017) found that the average time for the prescribed activities varied. For those with mild dementia it was 28 minutes; for those with moderate dementia it was 24 minutes; and for those with severe dementia it was 15 minutes (Regier et al. 2017). Furthermore, the degree of support needed varied: those with mild dementia required reorientation and cues 68% of the time, while people with moderate–severe dementia needed such support 78% of the time. People with mild dementia required assistance to initiate activity less than 50% of the time, while those with moderate–severe disease needed this support more than 50% of the time (Regier et al. 2017).

Regier et al. (2017) conclude that meaningful activity can be used therapeutically at all disease stages. However, they point out that the approach should be varied according to disease stage: people with severe dementia may need activities simplifying to one or two steps and to those that include more tactile and auditory cueing to allow initiation and sequencing of the activities (Regier et al. 2017). The authors also maintain that at the severe stage the person is less able to engage for longer periods, but that as little as 10 minutes engaged in meaningful activity may be beneficial (Regier et al. 2017).

Gitlin et al. (2017, p. 575) tested the feasibility of implementing a variant of TAP, the Tailored Activity Program for Hospitals (TAP-H), with people with disturbed behaviour linked to dementia. TAP-H consists of 11 sessions that include an interview with family members about the person's roles, habits and interests. In addition, occupational therapists meet with the person twice after admission to assess their attention, likelihood of falling, capacity for following instructions and problem solving, ability to learn new information, social behaviour and functional abilities (Gitlin et al. 2017). Bespoke activities are then chosen for the person by the occupational therapists, who also complete structured observation of the person's room and hospital environment and their interactions with staff; this is considered important since, the authors suggest, people with dementia may be more vulnerable to environmental factors (Gitlin et al. 2017). An activity prescription is then designed that includes a targeted activity; a time schedule, for example 10 minutes daily prior to meals or bedtime; and instructions to the staff on implementation, for example cueing or setting up the activity (Gitlin et al. 2017, p. 577).

The authors note that prescribed activities for people with lower-level cognitive impairments included activities such as card games or crochet; for those with moderate impairment levels, repetitive activities with few steps, such as towel folding; and those with severe impairments were more likely to be prescribed passive sensory activities such as music listening (Gitlin et al. 2017).

Following treatment with TAP-H, the occupational therapists completed a questionnaire on the person's level of engagement. In addition, the researchers observed video recordings of the participants performing standardised activities and the activities prescribed via TAP-H (Gitlin et al. 2017). These structured 10-second observations covered verbal, non-verbal and affective behaviours, which were then coded (Gitlin et al. 2017). The person's family also completed a questionnaire on their satisfaction with the programme.

The occupational therapists reported high levels of engagement, which increased as the sessions progressed (Gitlin et al. 2017). The researchers noted an increased percentage of behaviours expressing pleasure, such as laughing and smiling, from 11% at baseline to 17% during the TAP-H activities, and a reduction in behaviour expressing anger or anxiety, from 25% at baseline to 7% during TAP-H (Gitlin et al. 2017). Families also reported high levels of satisfaction with TAP-H (Gitlin et al. 2017). The authors argue that TAP-H is effective as it aims at a 'just right' fit between activity and person and focuses on engagement in that activity, rather than training new skills, and it involves families and care staff (Gitlin et al. 2017).

Gitlin et al. (2022) comment that, despite African American people having higher rates of dementia alongside later diagnosis and generally worse outcomes, there is little research on non-pharmacological treatments for dementia that treat ethnicity as a variable. These authors conducted a randomised controlled trial of TAP comparing results for 90 Black and 145 white carer–person with dementia dyads (Gitlin et al. 2022, p. 3105). TAP consisted of eight occupational therapist–led sessions, where three preferred activities were identified in collaboration with the carer and the person with dementia. There was also carer education on how to use the activities, adapting the environment, communication strategies, stress reduction, BPSD and the disease (Gitlin et al. 2022). The control group was treated with eight educational sessions on disease and home safety. The principal outcome measure was the Neuropsychiatric Inventory–Clinician (NPI–C), a carer-rated scale measuring frequency of agitation and aggression (Gitlin et al. 2022).

Gitlin et al. (2022) found that African American people showed a statistically significant greater reduction in aggression, aggression frequency and aggression severity. In addition, Black dyads reported a 34.5% reduction in such behaviours, compared with 11.9% of white dyads. Furthermore, only 2.6% of Black dyads showed *worse* aggression and agitation scores, compared with 16.7.% of white dyads (Gitlin et al. 2022). This is despite the fact that the TAP sessions tended, by chance, to be slightly shorter for the Black dyads, meaning that over the course of the study they received almost two hours less treatment (Gitlin et al. 2022). Overall, the results suggested that Black families had benefited more from TAP.

Gitlin et al. (2022) cite evidence that Black carers may have a more positive attitude to their role, and may therefore benefit more from training. In addition, they point out that recruiting from the community rather than clinical settings made the aetiology of dementia difficult to control for, and that Black people may be more likely to have 'vascular pathology', which may also explain the differing results (Gitlin et al. 2022, p. 3113). The authors also make the point that race is a 'societal construct' and that disparities between Black and white families may reflect African American people's poorer access to services and the impact of racism on the lives of Black carers (Gitlin et al. 2022). They suggest that understanding the impact of such factors should be a priority for future research (Gitlin et al. 2022).

It will be noted that, like other research on dementia, the focus in ESP, COPE and TAP is not specifically on memory impairment. However, it may be the case that the underlying cause of much agitated and/or aggressive behaviour is the frustration of living with an impaired memory. In this sense the results are germane to the topic of this book.

Training is available for both COPE and TAP. These websites provide details, along with additional resources:

- TAP: `https://duo.online.drexel.edu/new-ways-for-better-days`
- COPE: `https://duo.online.drexel.edu/cope`

Gaps Between Evidence and Practice

Despite the high-quality research that supports the use of person-centred, occupation-focused treatment approaches for people with memory impairments resulting from dementia, researchers have demonstrated that there are challenges to occupational therapists engaging this population in meaningful activity. Cations et al. (2019), for example, asked nine occupational therapists to report on a total of 244 consultations with people with dementia and their carers. They found that 67% of consultations were focused on assessing the person's needs; 47% involved providing equipment or assistive technology; 31% were focused on preventing falls or pressure care; and only 24% of consultations involved areas such as meaningful activities, skill development or strategies to support memory (Cations et al. 2019). This research was carried out in Australia, which, the authors point out, has specific challenges connected to low density of population, and also involved a small sample of occupational therapists (Cations et al. 2019). The authors conclude nonetheless that strategies need to be developed to support translation of evidence into clinical practice (Cations et al. 2019).

Rahja et al. (2018) audited 87 case notes in a study of occupational therapy practice with people with dementia in Australia. They were interested in finding out the extent to which Australian guidelines that occupational therapy intervention with this population should involve 'multiple components', such as training carers and engagement in activity bespoke to the person, were being implemented (Rahja et al. 2018, p. 566). Their key finding was that intervention was mainly limited to assessments of the risk of falling, safety in the home and the person's daily living functions (Rahja et al. 2018). Interventions mainly involved referrals to other services, environment modification advice and prescription of equipment (Rahja et al. 2018). Overall, they concluded that there was a gap between evidence-based recommendations and the reality of occupational therapy practice with the population (Rahja et al. 2018).

Reduced Awareness, Anosognosia, Lack of Insight and Social Cognition in Memory Impairment

Awareness is defined as the ability to internalise perceived external happenings (Leocadi et al. 2023). Leocadi et al. (2023, p. 2) point out that 'awareness' has been used interchangeably with other terms such as 'anosognosia', 'lack of insight' and 'reduced autonoetic awareness'. It is considered important for participation in activity, for example by allowing a person to link their choices to their capabilities and also for adaptation to different situations (Leocadi et al. 2023). It may also affect areas such as memory and social cognition, and can have impacts on management of finances, driving, social relationships and other areas (Leocadi et al. 2023). That awareness can involve memory impairment is clear if we consider that reduced awareness can occur in ATD and fronto-temporal dementia (Leocadi et al. 2023). Overall, it is an important issue for occupational therapists and is dealt with in more detail in this section.

Leocadi et al. (2023) conducted a literature review using several search terms linked to reduced awareness and also searched for brain imaging data concerning the neural substrates of these different conditions. They found evidence of pronounced anosognosia (reduced awareness of impairment) in ATD, focused particularly on the person's general condition and their levels of executive function (Leocadi et al. 2023). Other authors have stated that the prevalence of anosognosia in ATD is anywhere between 20% and 80% (Flores-Vázquez et al. 2021).

Leocadi et al. (2023) also found that people with ATD, and those with mild cognitive impairment (MCI) who exhibited anosognosia, have more impairments in working and episodic memory when compared with patients without agnosia. In particular, they note that people with MCI show anosognosia for activities involving a strong memory component, and that this tendency is more marked in those who later transition to ATD (Leocadi et al. 2023).

It is interesting to note that imaging evidence consistently highlights alterations in the hippocampus and medial temporal lobe in anosognosia, indicating that the condition is likely to be underpinned by impairments in memory, particularly autobiographical episodic memory (Flores-Vázquez et al. 2021). In addition, anosognosia for memory impairments in ATD may be present prior to demonstration of full-blown dementia (Leocadi et al. 2023). It seems that in these conditions memory impairments and anosognosia may be linked.

Insight describes the ability to foresee the consequences of actions that stem from one's diseased state. Impairments in this area are more typically a feature of fronto-temporal dementia than ATD (Leocadi et al. 2023). Reduced insight has been linked to atrophy in pre-frontal and ventro-medial regions (Leocadi et al. 2023). A lack of insight may have an impact on mental capacity to make specific decisions, and should therefore be taken into account when occupational therapists are involved in assessing mental capacity, which was discussed in Chapter 6.

'Social cognition' refers to the faculties that allow us to interact with others and take into account their feelings and thoughts. A key component of social cognition is 'theory of mind' (ToM), which is the capacity to know one's own mental state or that of others (Leocadi et al. 2023). In people with fronto-temporal dementia, impaired ToM is associated with changes in lateral temporal and parietal areas, the striatum and medial frontal regions (Leocadi et al. 2023). People with ATD who have impaired ToM show evidence of impairment in the hippocampal regions and also problems with episodic memory, and these problems appear to underpin their ToM impairments.

Moral reasoning facilitates judgement about the morally correct way to act and is underpinned by the ability to retrieve information about social norms (Leocadi et al. 2023). In one experiment, individuals with ATD and fronto-temporal dementia took part in a game of trust where investments were made with individuals who acted in trustworthy or untrustworthy ways. Patients did worse than people who did not have cognitive impairments, while better memory for interactions in the game was linked to being less financially vulnerable in people with ATD, and this was also associated with having less damage in medial temporal and temporal–parietal regions (Leocadi et al. 2023). These findings should be taken into account when occupational therapists are assessing the hazards that may be faced by people with memory impairments, for example on discharge from hospital.

Flores-Vázquez et al. (2021) state that the occurrence of anosognosia in people with amnesic mild cognitive impairment (aMCI) is predictive of future transition to full ATD. The authors point out that anosognosia may present problems with ADL and inhibition of risk-taking behaviour, and places an increased burden and stress on carers (Flores-Vázquez et al. 2021). They point to evidence for the involvement of the medial temporal lobe, the insula and medial frontal and orbito-frontal regions (Flores-Vázquez et al. 2021). The majority of these areas are part of a 'default mode network' that is implicated in autobiographical memory and 'introspection' and that becomes impaired early in the progress of ATD (Flores-Vázquez et al. 2021, p. 2).

Flores-Vázquez et al. (2021) conducted magnetic resonance imaging (MRI) scans on the brains of 6 people with aMCI combined with anosognosia; 12 people with MCI without agnosia; 6 people with ATD and agnosia; and 9 people with ATD without agnosia (Flores-Vázquez et al. 2021). It was found that people with aMCI and anosognosia had significantly lower grey matter volume in the hippocampus bilaterally when compared with those with aMCI without agnosia. Also, the authors found that the average density of the hippocampi in people with aMCI and anosognosia was similar to that of all the people with ATD, with or without agnosia (Flores-Vázquez et al. 2021). The association of anosognosia in this study with alterations in the hippocampus suggests a role for impaired episodic memory in anosognosia, with a possibility that this leads to dependence on 'remote personal semantics' to assess behaviour and therefore poor self-evaluation (Flores-Vázquez et al. 2021, p. 7).

Cognitive Rehabilitation
in Dementia Treatment

Clare et al. (2013) describe approaches to the treatment of early-stage ATD, vascular dementia and mixed dementia. First, restorative approaches make the most of existing capabilities and use instructions and prompts. Here, techniques such as spaced retrieval and errorless learning may be used (Clare et al. 2013). Second, compensatory approaches make use of adaptations and aids, such as diaries and smartphones. Meanwhile, rehabilitation is concerned with adaptation to impairment in order to attain optimal well-being and function (Clare et al. 2013).

Clare et al. (2013) comment that the concept of rehabilitation fits with the social model of disability, in that the focus is on ameliorating functional disability stemming from environmental or social factors, rather than reducing underlying impairments (Clare et al. 2013). The authors propose that rehabilitation may provide a helpful 'conceptual framework' within which to consider supporting and caring for those with dementia and from which to derive treatment approaches (Clare et al. 2013, p. 4). They describe cognitive rehabilitation as a specific approach to rehabilitation for the person with cognitive impairment (Clare et al. 2013). They suggest that identifying meaningful goals in collaboration with the person is essential to cognitive rehabilitation and also underpins 'person-centred practice' (Clare et al. 2013, p. 2).

Kim (2015) evaluated the effectiveness of cognitive rehabilitation for people with early-stage ATD. An experimental group of 22 people took part in 30 minutes of group and 30 minutes of individual cognitive rehabilitation once per week over 8 weeks. The group sessions consisted of place and time orientation, fitting names to faces, and memory and attention training. The individual sessions involved work on personal goals identified using the Canadian Occupational Performance Measure (COPM), along with practical techniques such as diary use and stress control. The control group consisted of 21 people, who watched videos and engaged in conversation with the researcher. The experimental group showed evidence of significantly improved performance and satisfaction scores on COPM, improved scores on the Quality of Life in Alzheimer Disease (QOL-AD) measure and also on the orientation subsection of the Mini-Mental State Examination (MMSE; Kim 2015).

Chandler et al. (2016) conducted a systematic review of literature on the treatment of people with a diagnosis of MCI using cognitive approaches. People with MCI show evidence of cognitive impairment when tested, but do not meet the threshold for a dementia diagnosis, and may experience few difficulties with ADL (Chandler et al. 2016). The diagnosis helps in those at risk of developing ATD (Hampstead et al. 2014).

Chandler et al. (2016) reviewed 14 articles with treatments delivered by therapists. The treatments included errorless learning and training on using external aids such as calendars. They found that the largest effects were for the outcome of metacognition, which means the person's views or feelings about their cognitive state, for example their confidence in using cognitive strategies in everyday life. Slightly smaller though still positive effects were found for ADL performance (Chandler et al. 2016). The researchers also examined 'multimodal' approaches, which entail combining non-pharmacological techniques, and found that the largest effects on ADL performance came from a combination of cognitive and exercise programmes (Chandler et al. 2016, p. 225).

Hampstead et al. (2014) reviewed 36 studies of people with MCI in order to produce a clearer description of the techniques used in clinical practice. They identified a range of issues, including variation in diagnostic criteria, treatment techniques used, outcome measures and the dosage of treatment (Hampstead et al. 2014). These authors make a useful distinction between cognitive training, which aims to improve particular cognitive capacities, and cognitive rehabilitation, which focuses on enhancing the functioning of the person in the outside world (Hampstead et al. 2014).

Hampstead et al. (2014) describe different approaches to treatment in MCI, including rehearsal-based approaches such as spaced retrieval, where the person remembers specified items with widening delays; repeated exposure; vanishing cues; procedural learning; computer training programmes; and modelling of behaviour (Hampstead et al. 2014). The authors also list compensatory approaches such as the use of external aids, including notebooks, calendars, lists, and smartphones; and guided cueing and internal mnemonic strategies, such as semantic organisation, semantic elaboration, mental imagery and the method of loci (Hampstead et al. 2014).

Hampstead et al. (2014) note the limitations of many techniques that are available. For example, rehearsal-based approaches, such as spaced retrieval, are specific to the items learnt and mean that all new information has to be rehearsed as well. Meanwhile, compensatory techniques, such as keeping lists, become cumbersome as they multiply to match the number of items to be remembered. Internal approaches, such as using mental imagery, semantic organisation and elaboration, can be difficult for people who are cognitively impaired, and their complexity means they may not be practical in everyday situations where more quotidian approaches such as making a list may be warranted (Hampstead et al. 2014).

These authors propose a hierarchical model for assessing the effectiveness of mnemonic strategies. At the first stage, the clinician should ask if the strategy enables the patient to learn particular items or improve specific cognitive abilities; if not, then it should be discarded (Hampstead et al. 2014). At the second stage, the clinician needs to find out if the patient can use the technique independently in order to learn other items in similar conditions. If not, then the clinician should revert to techniques that were effective according to the stage one criteria. At stage three, the technique should be capable of being used in a wider range of ecological, or real-world, situations. Where this is not the case, the clinician should return to an approach that was effective at stage two (Hampstead et al. 2014). The authors point out that this hierarchy progresses from content-based to rule-based approaches (Hampstead et al. 2014). They stress that cognition is imprecise and complex and that no one technique, or combination of techniques, is equipped to meet the challenges of daily living (Hampstead et al. 2014).

Bahar-Fuchs et al. (2013) conducted a systematic review of cognitive training and cognitive rehabilitation for people with mild to moderate ATD and vascular dementia. These authors explain that cognitive training involves specific standard tasks that focus on attention, memory and problem solving. It may also involve training on strategies such as using imagery and the method of loci and may be delivered in groups or to individuals (Bahar-Fuchs et al. 2013). Cognitive rehabilitation involves designing bespoke treatment for the person with dementia and their carers that focuses on everyday activities; there is no assumption that this will generalise to improvements in other areas as well (Bahar-Fuchs et al. 2013). Cognitive training, on the other hand, aims to improve or maintain underlying cognitive function, and may be based on existing memory skills or performance of everyday tasks; it can use approaches such as errorless learning and spaced retrieval, memory aids or adaptations to the environment (Bahar-Fuchs et al. 2013).

Bahar-Fuchs et al. (2013) identified one randomised controlled trial of cognitive rehabilitation that reported improved goal attainment after treatment and greater satisfaction with memory performance six months following treatment. The carers in this study also reported improved relations with the person six months after treatment and there was evidence of changes in relevant brain areas in a subgroup of the sample (Bahar-Fuchs et al. 2013). However, the authors did not identify any positive or negative effects for cognitive training (Bahar-Fuchs et al. 2013).

Ciro et al. (2014, p. 1) describe another rehabilitation programme, Skill-building through Task-Oriented Motor Practice (STOMP). This involves identification of goals for the person with mild–moderate dementia; massed practice delivered in blocks; praise for the person between stages; and an errorless learning approach to training.

STOMP was developed from the concept of 'learned non-use', usually applied to motor rehabilitation in stroke. Here, the authors state that the person with dementia may react negatively to a failure in ADL performance, leading their carer to perform the task for them, when in fact they could execute it themselves with minimal support; this results in 'learned ADL disability' (Ciro et al. 2014, p. 2).

The authors wished to discover if there was any advantage to delivering STOMP in the home compared to the clinical environment (Ciro et al. 2014). The intervention was given five days per week for three hours per day over two weeks, with 10 people in the home and 6 people in a laboratory-delivered group. Outcome measures included COPM, goal attainment scaling (GAS) and the Caregiver Burden Scale. In addition, clinicians recorded the number of task iterations in each session, the time taken to accomplish each task and the number of neuropsychiatric behaviours, including wandering, violent outbursts and inappropriate sexual behaviour (Ciro et al. 2014). Measures were taken pre and post treatment and then at 90 days following treatment.

Ciro et al. (2014) found significantly different improvements for ADL performance post treatment and these effects were maintained at 90 days. However, no differences were noted between the home and clinic groups. Neither were any differences noted for the time needed to accomplish the tasks nor for reductions in neuropsychiatric behaviours (Ciro et al. 2014). The authors suggest that the key contribution of this research is to show that massed practice can be effective with this population, although no advantages were demonstrated for home versus laboratory settings, as they had originally hypothesised (Ciro et al. 2014).

Cognitive Rehabilitation, Cognitive Training and Cognitive Stimulation Therapy

Occupational therapists are engaged in more specific treatment of memory impairments in people with dementia. Robert et al. (2010) aimed to establish which cognitive treatments were being deployed via a survey of 65 occupational therapists working with people with ATD in an urban setting in Australia. They identified three main types of cognitive treatment, which are described in this section.

First, 82% of occupational therapists were using cognitive rehabilitation, which was described in detail in Chapter 6 in relation to brain injury as well as earlier in this chapter. Cognitive rehabilitation was noted to involve individualised treatment focused on everyday activities. This approach was considered appropriate for early-stage ATD and could involve memory aids such as diaries and calendars, spaced retrieval, training using procedural memory and dual cognitive support (Robert et al. 2010; Kim 2015). Cognitive rehabilitation also involves goal setting with the person and their families (Chandler et al. 2016). Goals can aim at restoration of baseline function and may be remedial, focusing on improving function, or compensatory, aimed at adapting to impairments (Chandler et al. 2016).

The second approach that Robert et al. (2010) noted being used by 50% of the occupational therapist respondents in their survey was cognitive training. This entails training on specific cognitive skills via task performance. It is a remedial approach, premised on the idea that practice can improve function. It could involve reduced cueing, errorless learning, repetition and concentration, among other strategies (Robert et al. 2010). Techniques could involve, for example, practising recall of items from a word list with guidance from a therapist (Yuill and Hollis 2011). The approach focuses on promoting particular functions, such as memory and problem solving (Chandler et al. 2016). It has been criticised for neglecting the real-life contexts of those with dementia and for a lack of evidence to support its advantages (Yuill and Hollis 2011).

Third, CST was being used by 62% of the sample. This approach involves group activities aimed at promoting 'global' cognitive activity (Chandler et al. 2016; Robert et al. 2010, p. 11). This could include reminiscence, which entails discussion of events, activities and experiences from the past, and may involve the presentation of items that stimulate such conversation (Yuell and Hollis 2011). It may also use validation therapy, in which the person's individual experience is shown as valuable (Robert et al. 2010), as well as reality orientation, which is supported with memory via aids that orientate the person to themselves and their context (Robert et al. 2010; Yuill and Hollis 2011). Finally, CST may involve goal-directed home activities for carers (Yuill and Hollis 2011).

Spector et al. (2001) described the original protocol for a CST programme, which was divided into four stages. The first was a focus on sensory stimulation, such as taste, with unusual food items, sound, vision and touch. Second, there was reminiscence about the past. Third, there was naming items and individuals from the person's family, members of the group and from the staff team (Spector et al. 2001). The fourth stage was a focus on practical money management and way finding.

Spector et al. (2001. p. 384) also describe five 'guiding principles' that underpinned their protocol: experience-based learning, in order to promote memory and cognitive stimulation in general; a focus on ADL; a focus on the person with dementia's cognitive performance and emotional state; a non-didactic approach to skill instruction, based on the notion of implicit learning; and an emphasis on the person with dementia and their carer learning together about their mutual capacities (Spector et al. 2001).

Spector et al. (2001) comment that these principles were influenced by Kitwood and Brooker's (2019) views on the maintenance of personhood in dementia, which argued that personhood was sustained by recognition of the transcendent nature shared by all humans; ethical commitment to the concept that each person has absolute value; and the notion that self-esteem is sustained by social recognition (Kitwood and Brooker 2019). In addition, Kitwood and Brooker (2019, p. 164) described the concept of 'rementing', whereby people with dementia, when cared for in this way, might display slowed cognitive decline or even improvement in cognitive capacities that were thought to be irreversibly impaired. These values connect to the concept of client-centred practice in occupational therapy described earlier.

CST aims to promote optimal cognitive performance within the context of ADL (Yuill and Hollis 2011). It recognises that cognitive functions such as memory are linked to relationship and life quality and also performance of everyday tasks (Yuill and Hollis 2011). It is also intended to be inclusive and pleasant for the person with dementia (Yuill and Hollis 2011).

Yuill and Hollis (2011) argue that CST fits well with occupational therapists' core skills of task and activity analysis, activity grading and promotion of participation in occupation. In addition, it takes a client-centred approach (Yuill and Hollis 2011). In a systematic review of evidence, Yuill and Hollis (2011) identified evidence of some 'relatively modest' improvement or maintenance of cognitive function for people with mild–moderate dementia.

Spector et al. (2003) describe a randomised controlled trial of CST for people with dementia. This consisted of 14 sessions of 45 minutes spread over 7 weeks (Spector et al. 2003). There were 115 people in the treatment group and 86 in a control group, who either did nothing or recreational activities such as craft and bingo. The key outcome measures were scores on the MMSE and Alzheimer's Disease Assessment Scale–Cognitive Subscale (ADAS-Cog) (Spector et al. 2003). It was found that the treatment group scored significantly higher on both of these measures than the control group (Spector et al. 2003). These results suggest that CST is linked to improvement in general cognitive function. However, is CST linked to improvement in memory performance?

Spector et al. (2003) used data from the randomised controlled trial and analysed data from the subtests of the ADAS-Cog. While there were significant improvements in tests of language function, there were no differences in memory scores between the treatment and control groups. This suggests that CST does not have an impact on memory per se (Spector et al. 2003).

Coe et al. (2019) tested the effectiveness of an occupational therapy 'memory strategy education group' (MSEG). The MSEG provided participants with subjective memory complaints, MCI and early-stage dementia with a range of external memory strategies that could be applied to everyday life situations such as remembering names, appointments and tasks (Coe et al. 2019). The

MSEG focuses on goal achievement and has a compensatory approach (Coe et al. 2019).

In Coe et al.'s (2019) study, MSEG consisted of six one-hour weekly sessions structured around different memory categories, including attention, short-term memory, long-term memory and prospective memory (Coe et al. 2019). Measurements were taken prior to attending the MSEG using the Rivermead Behavioural Memory Test (RBMT), a dementia QOL measure (DEMQOL), a non-standardised measure of the use of external memory strategies and COPM.

After taking part in the MSEG, significant improvements were found on RBMT, the DEMQOL cognitive function subtest, the use of external strategies to support memory, and COPM performance and satisfaction scores (Coe et al. 2019). This is evidence that training can both improve memory performance and lead to increased use of external strategies. However, the study did not include a control group, and it would be interesting to see how use of MSEG compares in other treatment conditions.

Errorless Learning in Dementia

The errorless learning approach, as used in treating people with brain injuries, was introduced in Chapter 6. Clare et al. (2000) conducted an experiment to assess the application of errorless learning in people with early-stage ATD. Three participants used errorless learning to remember lists of names, one to learn personal data and two to learn how to use external memory aids, including calendars, diaries and memory boards (Clare et al. 2000). The participants learning names used different combinations of expanded rehearsal, vanishing cues and repeated presentation. All three also used 'verbal elaboration', based on distinctive facial features of the people to be remembered (Clare et al. 2000). Errorless learning was facilitated by instructing participants to respond that they did not know an answer rather than giving a wrong response. When using the memory aids, the participants were given consistent feedback when the specified behaviour took place (Clare et al. 2000).

Five of the participants showed changes on the measures used. Participants one, two and three demonstrated significant improvement on remembered names, participant four showed significant improvement on the amount of personal information remembered and participant five showed a significant reduction in repeated questioning of the person's partner (Clare et al. 2000). Participants one, two and three were found to benefit from verbal elaboration in particular. Despite these positive results, it will be recalled from Chapter 6 that errorless learning is more suited to learning non-complex information that does not depend on context for memorisation.

Treatment of Behavioural and Psychological Symptoms Linked to Dementia

Gitlin et al. (2012) describe a range of behavioural symptoms that may affect people with dementia, which include restlessness, repetitive questioning, repeated vocalisations, depression, psychosis, delusional beliefs, disturbed sleep, shadowing the carer, being argumentative and resisting care (Gitlin et al. 2012). Specific problems associated with impaired memory include disorientation and difficulties recognising objects (Gitlin et al. 2012).

Bennett et al. (2019) conducted a systematic literature review of the effect of occupational therapy on reducing BPSD, QOL of people with dementia and QOL of their carers, and also carer burden and depression. The authors state that the majority of studies reviewed described a dyadic approach, whereby the person with dementia and their carer were involved in bespoke interventions with specific goals (Bennett et al. 2019, p. 4). Carers and the person with dementia were given assistance in identifying activities they wished to work on for improvement; carers were shown how to make activities simpler, employ compensatory techniques and adapt the environment (Bennett et al. 2019). An educational approach was also often used, with the occupational therapist giving information on areas such as knowledge of dementia and managing stress (Bennett et al. 2019).

Bennett et al. (2019) found that occupational therapy was linked to improvements in overall performance of ADL and also of IADL. They noted a reduced incidence of BPSD when occupational therapy was compared to other treatments (Bennett et al. 2019). In addition, improved QOL was found for both the person with dementia and the carer, with reduced stress reported in relation to the person's behaviour reported by the occupational therapist and less time spent helping the person (Bennett et al. 2019). Bennett et al. (2019, p. 8) conclude that occupational therapy's strength is an integral 'multicomponent' approach, where the therapist works with the individual and their carer to identify bespoke activities and adapts the environment with the aim of raising engagement and participation levels.

Gitlin et al. (2012) argue that, while brain impairment plays a role in behavioural symptoms, people with dementia are more vulnerable to interacting environmental factors. These may be external, such as overstimulation from their surroundings or complicated communication, or internal, such as feelings of pain or fear (Gitlin et al. 2012). There may be a poor fit between the person's environment and their capacity for processing and responding to cues, demands and expectations (Gitlin et al. 2012). The authors show that some behaviours may be expressions of needs that have not been met and are then reinforced by environmental factors, such as learning that screaming draws the carer's attention. The authors stress that some of these factors may be open to modification (Gitlin et al. 2012).

Gitlin et al. (2012) suggest that pharmacological treatments for behavioural symptoms usually consist of prescribing antipsychotic medication outside the terms of its licence. They point out that such treatment may not be effective at treating the most distressing symptoms and also that they have side effects such as increasing the risk of falling and mortality (Gitlin et al. 2012). It is better, according to these authors, to use non-pharmacological approaches as the first step in treatment. Treatments may include repetitive two-stage tasks such as sheet folding or placing money in a jar, tasks that may require carer initiation (Gitlin et al. 2012). Education and support can also be given to the carer. For example, they may be trained to allow more time for communication; to reduce choice, so that the person with dementia has only two options; and to use a soothing tone and light touch (Gitlin et al. 2012).

The environment can be made less complex by reducing clutter and using signs and labels to help the person find their way. On the other hand, the person's surroundings may be *under*-stimulating, and items for touching and feeling can be introduced and lighting improved (Gitlin et al. 2012). Tasks can be broken down and supplemented with tactile and verbal cueing; it may also be important to maintain an organised daily routine (Gitlin et al. 2012). Specific interventions for memory impairment could involve labelling objects to support recognition; removal of unnecessary items; only introducing one item at a time; or including all of the objects needed for a specific task, such as washing, in one labelled container (Gitlin et al. 2012).

Certainly, Gitlin et al.'s (2012) description of non-pharmacological treatments for behavioural issues in dementia fits well with occupational therapy skills and conceptual practice models. Their emphasis on the impact of the environment also jibes with occupational therapy conceptual practice models. The next section describes research that focuses on the interaction of the person with dementia and their environment.

Impact of the Environment on People with Dementia

Lawton and Rich (1968, p. 76) outlined an early programme for the study of ageing in the context of human ecology, stating that the person should be viewed in relation to their 'environment . . . resources and . . . social and cultural patterns' and that these factors should be tracked across the 'entire life span'. These themes were taken up by psychologists such as Proshansky (1976, p. 308), who decried the behaviourist, laboratory-based approach to the study of human behaviour, and called for the development of 'environmental psychology' that would examine the interaction of the person with the built environment and also the 'social, organisational and cultural properties' of the space in which movement, gesture, posture and feeling occurred. Proshansky (1976, p. 310) argued that these events must be studied over time and should encompass the whole person, as opposed to isolated stimuli; in that sense environmental psychology was a 'sociohistorical behavioral science'.

Another writer in this tradition, Rowles (2000, p. 59S), shows how the person becomes part of their environment and that the environment also exists within them, a situation of 'autobiographical insideness'. He suggests that the person is embedded in a matrix of actions, meanings and relationships, which are 'inextricably linked' and are in a state of 'homeostasis', providing that none of the components is disrupted, for example by illness or the death of a community member (Rowles 2000). Rowles (2000, p. 61S) bases his arguments on the theory of complexity, which posits both a 'state', the fundamental structure of a system, and 'dynamic', rules describing how the structure changes in time. He further maintains that occupational therapists must aim at promoting the person's sense of 'being in place' and should be able to detect patterns of habit, routine and ritual (Rowles 2000, p. 64S).

The specific impact of the environment on people with dementia was highlighted in the work of Powell Lawton (2001), who stated that the environment should facilitate a reduction in disturbed behaviour, which he interpreted as an expression of anxiety or inner agitation; an increase in chances for social behaviour, while avoiding overstimulation; opportunities for increased activity, even if this was relatively low level; and an overall increase in positive feelings. He argued that the components of QOL in care settings were autonomy, so that residents were still able to take the initiative; individuality, meaning that preferences and interests were considered by staff; privacy; dignity; enjoyment; meaningful activity; relationships; and security (Powell Lawton 2001, p. S59).

Calkins (2003) stresses the far-reaching impact of Powell Lawton's (2001) ideas in the design of residential facilities for people with dementia in the United States. Calkins (2003) states that Powell Lawton's key contribution is in the legacy of five principles of environmental design for this population: orientation, meaning that facilities should be visible to individuals who are less able to rely on memory; negotiability, indicating that there will be preservation of autonomy for ADL; personalisation of surroundings; social interaction; and safety (Calkins 2003).

These views on the impact of the environment on the person and those with dementia in particular have informed some contemporary research on this topic, including work by occupational therapists. Richards et al. (2015) explored the impact of residential care settings for people with dementia on occupational engagement. These authors describe 'traditional' settings that prioritise physical and care requirements and pharmacological treatment. Such locations may be austere and present restricted opportunity for engagement in occupation (Richards et al. 2015, p. 339). Opposed to this are 'non-traditional' facilities that may have open floor plans, ready access to outdoor areas and features similar to home, and where clinical aspects are not obviously visible (Richards et al. 2015, p. 339).

Richards et al. (2015) compared a traditional and a non-traditional care facility, both located in a rural part of Australia, using the Residential Environment Impact Survey (REIS). REIS is based on Model of Human Occupation (MOHO) concepts and requires a visual survey of the environment, structured observation of three activities and interviews with staff and residents, although the researchers in this case only interviewed staff (Richards et al. 2015).

The authors found that the non-traditional environment provided more chance for engagement with staff and in meaningful activities. For example, staff were visible to residents while completing routine tasks and residents were able to assist in tasks such as setting the tables (Richards et al. 2015). Also, the non-traditional facility gave easier access to communal areas and the kitchen was accessible to residents and their families, while the nurses' station was placed in a communal area and pharmaceuticals were kept in a 'camouflaged' secure area (Richards et al. 2015, p. 444). The less restricted flow of movement within the non-traditional environment encouraged more interaction with objects, staff members and other residents, and, the authors suggest, gave more opportunity for occupational engagement (Richards et al. 2015).

Morgan-Brown and Chard (2014) examined the impact of environment on the occupational engagement of people with dementia via structured observations of two nursing homes in Ireland. The homes were being renovated, moving from a traditional model, with separate sitting and dining rooms, rigid timetabling and food prepared in a kitchen shielded from residents' view, to a 'household model', with open planning of the dining and seating areas, a kitchen located within the communal area and a more flexible and spontaneous approach to meal times (Morgan-Brown and Chard 2014, p. 51). The household model also employed a member of staff in a 'homemaker' role; this person prepared breakfast when residents wished, facilitated hobby-based activities and games and encouraged residents to take part in domestic tasks (Morgan-Brown and Chard 2014, p. 50).

Morgan-Brown and Chard (2014) based their work on theories of environmental impact on people with dementia. They refer to Lawton's 'competence press hypothesis', which suggests that insufficient press from the environment results in boredom and reduced capacity, while excessive press leads to stress and anxiety (Morgan-Brown and Chard 2014, p. 50). In addition, they cite Lawton's 'environmental docility theory', which suggests that the environment presses most on individuals with the lowest levels of competence (Morgan-Brown and Chard 2014, p. 50), a point echoed by Gitlin et al. (2017). They also cite findings by Proshansky that an unaltered environment can lead to a 'continuity of behavior', even when the personnel in the environment has changed (Morgan-Brown and Chard 2014, p. 50).

Morgan-Brown and Chard (2014) evaluated the environment of the two facilities using ATOSE, which is based on 12 five-minute observations over one hour. These observations happen twice a day between certain times (Morgan-Brown and Chard 2014, p. 51). ATOSE uses observation of an entire room and observable occupational interactions and engagement in social interaction between everyone in the space (Morgan-Brown and Chard 2014).

Morgan-Brown and Chard (2014) found that in the traditional facility residents were passive 76% of the time, whereas in the household setting this was reduced to 59%. Also, behaviour that was interactive and engagement increased from 24% of the time in the traditional setting to 41% of the time in the household residency, while engagement between residents and employees increased from 24% in the traditional home to 36% in the household setting (Morgan-Brown and Chard 2014). The authors maintain that it is essential for occupational therapists to remember that 'a whole environment occupational space is composed of physical, operational, and social elements, and all the people within it' and suggest that a tool such as ATOSE gives a practical way of assessing this (Morgan-Brown and Chard 2014, p. 56).

Morgan-Brown and Brangan (2016) went on to analyse the environment of a traditional residential home in Ireland using ATOSE. They noted that residents were passive and unengaged in meaningful interaction or activity 83% of the time and that staff were busy 99% of the time, while 43% of this time was spent in activity that did not involve the residents (Morgan-Brown and Brangan 2016). They noted that social, physical and occupational aspects of the environment did not support occupational engagement. Rooms were bare and did not contain personal objects that might have stimulated interaction or chat; residents were seated around the television, which they paid little attention to, but whose sound was 'omnipresent' and frequently broadcast 'high emotional content' (Morgan-Brown and Brangan 2016, p. 7). It was noted, in addition, that a female resident was discouraged from helping set the table at lunch and that residents sometimes were unable to initiate conversation but were 'outpaced' by staff (Morgan-Brown and Brangan 2016, p. 8). The authors recommend that staff should be trained to start conversations and also that the physical, sensory, social and occupational environment should be reformed to facilitate occupational engagement (Morgan-Brown and Brangan 2016).

Nagayama et al. (2016) reflect on results such as these, commenting that most residents in care facilities spend the majority of their time with nothing to do and with limited communication with care staff. In order to address this the authors developed the Aid for Decision-making in Occupation Choice (ADOC; Nagayama et al. 2016, p. 1). This is based on 95 pictures of occupations, presented on an iPad, that facilitate collaborative choice and occupation-focused goal setting between the older person and the occupational therapist.

The authors evaluated the use of ADOC with service users in a residential home. An experimental group of 23 care home residents set occupation-based goals created using ADOC and their treatment was based on meaningful activity towards achieving these goals (Nagayama et al. 2016). The control group consisted of 23 residents who were treated according to an impairment-based approach, focused on restoration of capacity. Each group received 20 minutes of treatment per week over four months.

At the end of the treatment period, it was found that the experimental group had significantly higher Barthel index scores (Nagayama et al. 2016). The authors do not provide measures of memory impairment. They do, however, report that the mean MMSE score of the treatment group was 23 and that of the control group was 21, so it is possible that the participants did have memory deficits (Nagayama et al. 2016). It is also likely that the 'visual cue' provided by ADOC to support goal setting might benefit people with dementia (Nagayama et al. 2016, p. 8).

It will be recalled from Chapter 3 that occupational therapy conceptual practice models have developed an extended view of the environment that may encompass the person's social interactions. Chard et al. (2009) addressed these aspects in a study that evaluated the impact of teaching carers verbal cueing and reinforcement techniques, alongside modifying the environment, on performance of ADL for people with ATD living in a residential care setting.

Chard et al. (2009) used AMPS to identify two valued ADL for each person and also as a pre- and post-treatment outcome measure (Chard et al. 2009). It will be recalled that AMPS provides a measurement of motor skills, which are defined as observable actions used to move the self or items needed for a task, and process skills, which are defined as observable actions to sequence skills in time and to select and use tools and materials and also respond to problems occurring during task performance (Chard et al. 2009).

Chard et al. (2009) included five people and their carer from the facility. The carer was trained on verbal cueing and reinforcement techniques and environmental modifications included labelling items, arranging the workspace so that needed items could be seen, and taking away items that may have led to distraction (Chard et al. 2009). Following treatment it was found that all participants showed statistically significant improvements in process skills, while two also showed significant improvements in motor skills (Chard et al. 2009).

Although not explicitly addressing the interaction of memory and the environment, these studies provide a picture of the effects of environmental deprivation on the person with dementia. Further research is required to determine the precise effects on memory.

Conclusion

It has been shown in this chapter that memory impairments in older people are linked to a range of everyday problems. In addition, a key message is that occupational therapy, as a non-pharmacological approach to dementia treatment, has advantages over medical approaches.

One theme running through the range of treatment options developed by occupational therapy researchers, or by those working with occupational therapists, is the importance of a client-centred approach. This is apparent in contemporary approaches to residential dementia care.

In addition, researchers have developed quite involved treatment programmes that focus on activities that are meaningful to the person with memory impairments. One major example is TAP. While not specifically linked to occupational therapy, TAP reflects some key principles of the profession, including client centredness and a focus on tasks that have meaning for the person.

Occupational therapists should be proud of the developments described in this chapter. However, evidence also suggests that occupational therapists may be spending a lot of their time with people with dementia and their families on more basic safety and personal care issues.

The challenge of lack of insight and impaired social cognition for people with dementia was discussed. It was shown that, for people with ATD, this could be linked to hippocampal and hence memory impairments.

The concept of cognitive rehabilitation was considered in relation to dementia treatment. It is interesting to note that this has been linked to the social model of disability. Overall, however, there is limited evidence available to support this approach. This also underlines the importance of programmes such as TAP.

CST is used by occupational therapists when working with people with dementia. A brief historical overview of this intervention demonstrated that it is also underpinned by client-centred approaches to treatment. It was shown that it may be an effective treatment, although it does not target memory in isolation.

Finally, it was shown that a number of researchers have explored the impact of the environment on people with dementia. Practical applications of environmental approaches include the open-access ATOSE.

Overall, research tends to confirm the importance of evaluating the impact of the environment on the person with memory impairment during task performance. The interaction of these factors of the person with memory impairment, their occupations and their environment has been a central concern of this book.

Activity

Clive, a resident in a care home, is 87. He has a diagnosis of ATD. It has been reported that he has become more disorientated in recent months. His son, Chris, has stated that Clive has had difficulty remembering whether his family members have visited, although someone from the family visits daily. Chris says that Clive does not seem to know where he is, sometimes stating that he is in prison; at these times he becomes anxious and demands to be set free.

You are a community occupational therapist and have been asked to assess Clive. You attend the residential home and spend some time observing the communal area. You note that while you are there the television is switched on permanently. Clive is seated with other residents around the television and there is no interaction between them. The television is showing a daytime tabloid talk show with the volume turned up quite loud. A member of staff turns the channel over, but Clive and the other residents do not respond to this and carry on watching.

You also note that a game of bingo is being prepared by a staff member in the communal space. Some residents walk over to take part. Clive pays no attention to this and carries on watching the television.

Later, lunch is prepared in the communal area. Two members of staff walk over to the residents who are watching television and ask them to come to eat. Clive remains seated and the two members of staff attempt to encourage him to move from sitting to standing by gently pushing on his shoulders from behind. At this point he becomes agitated, looks around and tells the two staff members to leave him alone. After the staff members make several attempts to move him using the same technique, he gets up and comes to the lunch table independently.

Following lunch, Clive is guided back to the television area. He sits back in the same chair. A member of staff switches on the television again without asking the residents what they would like to watch.

Later, Chris comes to visit Clive, who is still seated with other residents watching television. You notice that after saying hello to his father, Chris sits in a chair next to him and does not speak again. After a few minutes, Chris picks up a magazine and starts to read. He does not attempt to include Clive in this activity.

1. Describe the features of the environment that may be having a negative impact on Clive's dementia symptoms.
2. State what could be changed about Clive's environment in order to improve his symptoms.
3. Select one of the approaches discussed in this chapter in order to define a bespoke occupation-based approach for Clive.
4. Explain how Chris could be included in your planning.

References

Bahar-Fuchs, A., Clare, L., and Woods, B. (2013). Cognitive training and cognitive rehabilitation for persons with mild to moderate dementia of the Alzheimers or vascular type: a review. *Alzheimer's Research & Therapy* 5 (4): 35–35.

Bennett, S., Laver, K., Voigt-Radloff, S. et al. (2019). Occupational therapy for people with dementia and their family carers provided at home: a systematic review and meta-analysis. *British Medical Journal Open* 9 (11): e026308.

Calkins, M.P. (2003). Powell Lawton's contributions to long-term care settings. *Journal of Housing for the Elderly* 17 (1–2): 67–84.

Cations, M., Radisic, G., de la Perrelle, L. et al. (2019). Post-diagnostic allied health interventions for people with dementia in Australia: a spotlight on current practice. *BMC Research Notes* 12 (1): 559–559.

Chandler, M.J., Parks, A.C., Marsiske, M. et al. (2016). Everyday impact of cognitive interventions in mild cognitive impairment: a systematic review and meta-analysis. *Neuropsychology Review* 26 (3): 225–251.

Chard, G., Liu, L., and Mulholland, S. (2009). Verbal cueing and environmental modifications: strategies to improve engagement in occupations in persons with Alzheimer disease. *Physical and Occupational Therapy in Geriatrics* 27 (3): 197–211.

Ciro, C., Poole, J.L., Skipper, B., and Hershey, L.A. (2014). Comparing differences in ADL outcomes for the STOMP intervention for dementia in the natural home environment versus a clinic environment. *Austin Alzheimers and Parkinsons Disease* 1 (1): 1003.

Clare, L., Wilson, B.A., Carter, G. et al. (2000). Intervening with everyday memory problems in dementia of Alzheimer type: an errorless learning approach. *Journal of Clinical and Experimental Neuropsychology* 22 (1): 132–146.

Clare, L., Bayer, A., Burns, A. et al. (2013). Goal-oriented cognitive rehabilitation in early-stage dementia: study protocol for a multi-centre single-blind randomised controlled trial (GREAT). *Trials* 14 (1): 152–152.

Coe, Á., Martin, M., and Stapleton, T. (2019). Effects of an occupational therapy memory strategy education group intervention on Irish older adults' self-management of everyday memory difficulties. *Occupational Therapy in Health Care* 33 (1): 37–63.

Cordier, R., Chen, Y.-W., Clemson, L. et al. (2019). Subjective memory complaints and difficulty performing activities of daily living among older women in Australia. *Australian Occupational Therapy Journal* 66 (2): 227–238.

Creek, J. (2003). *Occupational Therapy Defined as a Complex Intervention*. London: College of Occupational Therapists.

Du Toit, S.H.J., Shen, X., and McGrath, M. (2019). Meaningful engagement and person-centered residential dementia care: a critical interpretive synthesis. *Scandinavian Journal of Occupational Therapy* 26 (5): 343–355.

Flores-Vazquez, J.F., Ramírez-García, G., Marrufo-Meléndez, O.R. et al. (2021). Anosognosia in amnestic mild cognitive impairment is related to diminished hippocampal volume comparable to Alzheimer's disease dementia: preliminary MRI findings. *Frontiers in Aging Neuroscience* 13: 739422.

Gitlin, L.N., Winter, L., Corcoran, M. et al. (2003). Effects of the home environmental skill-building program on the caregiver–care recipient dyad: 6-month outcomes from the Philadelphia REACH initiative. *Gerontologist* 43 (4): 532–546.

Gitlin, L.N., Hauck, W.W., Dennis, M.P., and Winter, L. (2005). Maintenance of effects of the home environmental skill-building program for family caregivers and individuals with Alzheimer's disease and related disorders. *Journals of Gerontology. Series A, Biological Sciences and Medical Sciences* 60 (3): 368–374.

Gitlin, L.N., Winter, L., Burke, J. et al. (2008). Tailored activities to manage neuropsychiatric behaviors in persons with dementia and reduce caregiver burden: a randomized pilot study. *American Journal of Geriatric Psychiatry* 16 (3): 229–239.

Gitlin, L.N., Winter, L., Dennis, M.P. et al. (2010). A biobehavioral home-based intervention and the well-being of patients with dementia and their caregivers: the COPE randomized trial. *Journal of the American Medical Association* 304 (9): 983–991.

Gitlin, L.N., Kales, H.C., and Lyketsos, C.G. (2012). Nonpharmacologic management of behavioral symptoms in dementia. *Journal of the American Medical Association* 308 (19): 2020–2029.

Gitlin, L.N., Marx, K.A., Alonzi, D. et al. (2017). Feasibility of the tailored activity program for hospitalized (TAP-H) patients with behavioral symptoms. *Gerontologist* 57 (3): 575–584.

Gitlin, L.N., Marx, K., Piersol, C.V. et al. (2022). Differential race effects of the tailored activity program (TAP) on dementia-related behaviors: a randomized controlled trial. *Journal of the American Geriatrics Society* 70 (11): 3105–3115.

Graff, M.J.L., Vernooij-Dassen, M.J.M., Thijssen, M. et al. (2006). Community based occupational therapy for patients with dementia and their care givers: randomised controlled trial. *British Medical Journal* 333 (7580): 1196–1199.

Hampstead, B.M., Gillis, M.M., and Stringer, A.Y. (2014). Cognitive rehabilitation of memory for mild cognitive impairment: a methodological review and model for future research. *Journal of the International Neuropsychological Society* 20 (2): 135–151.

Kielhofner, G. (2008). *A Model of Human Occupation: Theory and Application*, 4e. Baltimore, MD: Lippincott, Williams & Wilkins.

Kim, S. (2015). Cognitive rehabilitation for elderly people with early-stage Alzheimer's disease. *Journal of Physical Therapy Science* 27 (2): 543–546.

Kitwood, T.M. and Brooker, D. (2019). *Dementia Reconsidered, Revisited: The Person Still Comes First*, 2e. London: Open University Press.

Lawton, A.H. and Rich, T.A. (1968). Ecology and gerontology: an introduction. *Gerontologist* 8 (2): 76–77.

Leocadi, M., Canu, E., Paldino, A. et al. (2023). Awareness impairment in Alzheimer's disease and frontotemporal dementia: a systematic MRI review. *Journal of Neurology* 270 (4): 1880–1907.

Morgan-Brown, M. and Brangan, J. (2016). Capturing interactive occupation and social engagement in a residential dementia and mental health setting using quantitative and narrative data. *Geriatrics* 1 (3): 15.

Morgan-Brown, M. and Chard, G. (2014). Comparing communal environments using the assessment tool for occupation and social engagement: using interactive occupation and social engagement as outcome measures. *British Journal of Occupational Therapy* 77 (2): 50–58.

Nagayama, H., Tomori, K., Ohno, K. et al. (2016). Effectiveness and cost-effectiveness of occupation-based occupational therapy using the aid for decision making in occupation choice (ADOC) for older residents: pilot cluster randomized controlled trial. *PLoS One* 11 (3): e0150374.

Parker, D.M. (2011). The client-centred frame of reference. In: *Foundations for Practice in Occupational Therapy* (ed. E.A.S. Duncan), 139–152. London: Churchill Livingstone.

Pöllänen, S.H. and Hirsimäki, R.M. (2014). Crafts as memory triggers in reminiscence: a case study of older women with dementia. *Occupational Therapy in Health Care* 28 (4): 410–430.

Powell Lawton, M. (2001). The physical environment of the person with Alzheimer's disease. *Aging & Mental Health* 5 (1): 56–64.

Proshansky, H.M. (1976). Environmental psychology and the real world. *American Psychologist* 31 (4): 303–310.

Rahja, M., Comans, T., Clemson, L. et al. (2018). Are there missed opportunities for occupational therapy for people with dementia? An audit of practice in Australia. *Australian Occupational Therapy Journal* 65 (6): 565–574.

Regier, N.G., Hodgson, N.A., and Gitlin, L.N. (2017). Characteristics of activities for persons with dementia at the mild, moderate, and severe stages. *Gerontologist* 57 (5): 987–997.

Richards, K., D'Cruz, R., Harman, S., and Stagnitti, K. (2015). Comparison of a traditional and non-traditional residential care facility for persons living with dementia and the impact of the environment on occupational engagement. *Australian Occupational Therapy Journal* 62 (6): 438–448.

Robert, A., Gélinas, I., and Mazer, B. (2010). Occupational therapists use of cognitive interventions for clients with Alzheimer's disease. *Occupational Therapy International* 17 (1): 10–19.

Rowles, G.D. (2000). Habituation and being in place. *Occupational Therapy Journal of Research* 20 (1): 52S–67S.

Scott, I., Cooper, C., Leverton, M. et al. (2019). Effects of nonpharmacological interventions on functioning of people living with dementia at home: a systematic review of randomised controlled trials. *International Journal of Geriatric Psychiatry* 34 (10): 1386–1402.

Spector, A., Orrell, M., Davies, S., and Woods, B. (2001). Can reality orientation be rehabilitated? Development and piloting of an evidence-based programme of cognition-based therapies for people with dementia. *Neuropsychological Rehabilitation* 11 (3–4): 377–397.

Spector, A., Thorgrimsen, L., Woods, B. et al. (2003). Efficacy of an evidence-based cognitive stimulation therapy programme for people with dementia: randomised controlled trial. *British Journal of Psychiatry* 183 (3): 248–254.

Warchol, K. (2006). Facilitating functional and quality-of-life potential: strength-based assessment and treatment for all stages of dementia. *Topics in Geriatric Rehabilitation* 22 (3): 213–227.

Yuill, N. and Hollis, V. (2011). A systematic review of cognitive stimulation therapy for older adults with mild to moderate dementia: an occupational therapy perspective. *Occupational Therapy International* 18 (4): 163–186.

Index

Please note that page references to Figures will be followed by the letter 'f', to Tables by the letter 't'